The Complete Pregnancy Guide

For Expectant Mothers

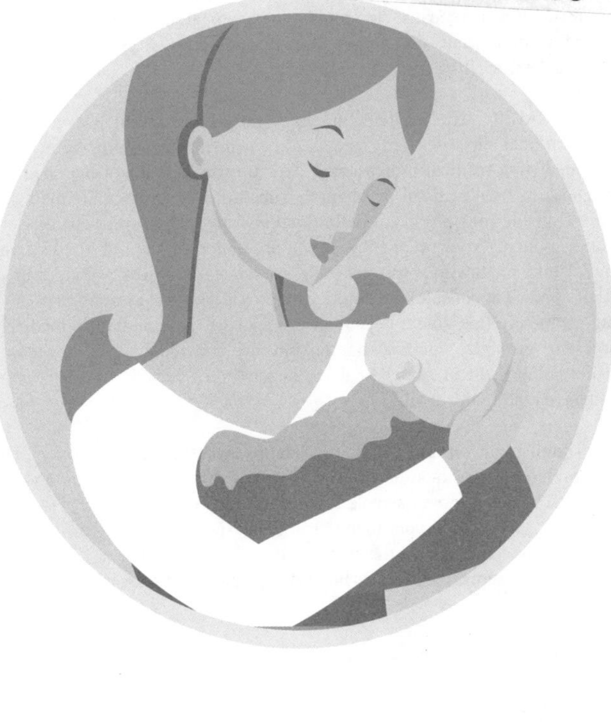

Everything a Mom Needs to Know About Pregnancy and Motherhood

By Alex A. Lluch, Author of Over 4 Million Books Sold
& Dr. Benito Villanueva, M.D., Obstetrics and Gynecology

The Complete Pregnancy Guide for Expectant Mothers

By Alex A. Lluch, Author of Over 4 Million Books Sold
& Dr. Benito Villanueva, M.D., Obstetrics and Gynecology

Published by WS Publishing Group
San Diego, California 92119

For Inquiries:
Log on to www.WSPublishingGroup.com
E-mail info@WSPublishingGroup.com

ISBN: 978-1-936061-29-7

Printed in China

Table of Contents

Table of Contents . . . .

Table of Contents

Introduction

FINDING OUT YOU ARE PREGNANT may very well be the single most exciting moment in your life. Having a baby is amazing, thrilling and somewhat overwhelming, all at once. If you became pregnant soon after making the decision to go for it, you are probably thrilled that it worked out so quickly and easily. On the other hand, if you have been trying for some time to conceive, the positive sign on the pregnancy test wand is the amazing moment of relief and joy you have been waiting for. Finally, if you were not expecting to become pregnant, you will soon appreciate all the potential for happiness that having a baby adds to your life.

There is no doubt that things are about to change. Over the next weeks and months, you and your baby will go through amazing changes. Having a baby will also affect your relationship with your partner, your career, friendships, and possibly even your world outlook and politics. Issues that did not concern you before suddenly matter more than anything else, such as the condition of the schools in your area, affordable daycare, breast-feeding in public, and toy safety standards. Your shifting concerns, interests, and responsibilities can cause your relationships to change but, of course, all these adjustments are worth it, as there is possibly nothing as rewarding as being a parent.be a difficult transition but, ultimately, your friends and family will adjust along with you and love your child almost as much as you do. And of course, all these adjustments are worth it, as there is possibly nothing as grand in this world as being a parent.

Throughout your pregnancy, there will be much to do to make yourself more comfortable and prepare your home and family for the big arrival. There are many decisions that you must make as your pregnancy progresses and your baby's birth draws near.

One such decision that should be made very early on is what kind of health care provider you prefer. Selecting an OB/GYN or a midwife is mostly up to you, but if you have pre-existing medical conditions, a midwife may insist that a doctor follow your pregnancy. When selecting a doctor, visit a few of them to find out if your personalities will gel, and if your philosophies on childbirth match up. By the way, it is perfectly normal at this point to be thinking, "What if I don't have a childbirth philosophy?" You may not have one right now, but as your pregnancy progresses you will discover what is important to you. This is why asking your doctor a ton of questions—such as his rate of Cesarean deliveries, how often he does episiotomies, how many patients he attends, and who delivers you if he is on vacation—will help you to form opinions about what matters most to you. Do not worry if some of these terms are unfamiliar to you—they will all be explained in this book.

Indeed, you can expect to do a lot of learning over the next nine and a half months. You have taken the first step by buying this book! We will talk you through your pregnancy day by day, which will be comforting and educational. You can also take other steps to educate yourself on what your pregnancy will be like. It is a good idea to subscribe to a few parenting magazines, join an online pregnancy chat community, and take childbirth-preparation classes. In addition, seek out friends and acquaintances who have recently had babies and find someone willing to mentor you throughout your pregnancy. Make sure this person had a positive experience and that she will allow you to have your own experience without constantly comparing it to hers. If you can, make a friend who is pregnant at the same time. It will help to go through this experience with another woman. This is where online chat rooms and message boards come in extremely handy. Having support while you are pregnant is the most valuable tool you can ask for—support can come from a variety of sources, but the point is to not go through it alone. The online world that exists makes it possible to participate in a community and receive support even if your loved ones are no longer with you.

In fact, many women are unable to anticipate how becoming pregnant will highlight other absences in their lives, such as the loss of a partner, parent, or previous pregnancies. It is perfectly normal to mourn these losses as if they were fresh when filled with all of this new potential. It is to be expected that you would want to share this news and the life of your subsequent child with those who have passed away and are still dear to you. Becoming pregnant will likely heighten your respect—now more than ever—for the cycle of life and death, and help you to appreciate the wonder and joy that is coming in just 9 months.

If you have already seen your doctor to have your pregnancy confirmed, you are probably wondering why you are two weeks farther along according to his calculations than you are according to this book. This because your doctor estimates your due date based on your last menstrual period (LMP)—about two weeks before you were pregnant—for the sake of easily marking time. However, the lunar calendar will follow your baby's actual development, which starts at conception and is generally two weeks after your last menstrual period. So, when your doctor tells you that you are eight weeks pregnant at your first prenatal visit, you will know that your baby is six weeks into her development. So, you will actually be pregnant for approximately 266 days.

If the fact that you will be pregnant for hundreds of days has you feeling nervous, realize that you are about to embark on a very special and short time in your life. Indeed, the average American woman is fertile for 30 to 40 years, and yet only spends a tiny fraction of that time pregnant—about 18 months in an entire lifetime! The time a woman is pregnant is to be cherished. You will be surprised how quickly the next 266 days go. Be sure to capture this rare time in your life by keeping a journal, taking monthly photos of your changing body, and by making only the healthiest choices for you and your baby. And when it feels like you've been pregnant forever, consider that humans get off easy with such a short gestation period. Some creatures, such as elephants, are pregnant for 23 months in a row! The nine and a half months you spend warming your bun in the oven are a drop in the hat, comparatively.

Each of the 266 days of your pregnancy will be covered in this book. At the beginning of each month, you will read an extension introduction to the lunar month you are about to experience. We will cover what you can expect from that month, how much weight you should gain, potential symptoms you may experience and how you can alleviate them, how you should exercise, what changes your baby will undergo, and ways others can help you as you and your baby grow throughout the month. Each week of your pregnancy is also covered, helping you digest the enormous amount of information there is to know about each step of pregnancy. Finally, each daily entry explains what is happening within your body and also tracks your baby's development. Each day also includes one of the following: Pregnancy Fact, Food for Thought, Tips and Advice, or For Your Health. These facts and ideas will give you useful, insightful, and interesting information that is not specifically covered in the Mom and Baby sections. Inspirational quotes from authors, activists, and other notable people are sprinkled throughout the book to help you reflect on what it means to be pregnant and to become a mother. Overall, the information included in this book will help you to feel more informed and less anxious about the miracle that is happening within your body. Congratulations, and cheers to the beginning of a very special time in your life.

Notes . . . .

Getting Ready for Parenthood

EATING FOR TWO—THE RIGHT WAY

Even before you know you are pregnant, for the health of your child (and you, of course), you should be paying attention to your diet. The nutrients you consume make a difference in some of the most critical moments in a child's life: the first week or two after conception.

What kinds of food should you eat?

Most health professionals say that during the first few weeks after conceiving, the single most important nutrient a woman should have is folic acid. One of the B vitamins, folic acid is necessary for the proper development of a baby's nervous system—the brain and the spinal cord. Because folic acid is so important at such an early stage of development, your health care provider has probably already started you on a prenatal vitamin supplement that includes plenty of folic acid.

Even if you are taking a supplement, you should be eating foods that are high in folic acid. Good sources of folic acid include green, leafy vegetables like broccoli and spinach, red meats, and fruits. You need 400 micrograms of folic acid per day to support a healthy pregnancy. Most breakfast cereals are fortified with folic acid as well. Not only will a bowl of cereal with milk each day supply you with folic acid, but it will provide calcium, which your baby needs. Studies show that most women in the U.S. fail to get enough calcium, so if you are pregnant you almost certainly will need to make some changes in your diet. Currently, government authorities recommend that pregnant women aged 19 to 50 get 1,000 milligrams of calcium per day; younger pregnant women need more—1,300 milligrams per day.

In addition to calcium and folic acid, you need to be certain that you are getting enough other vitamins and minerals. To ensure that you are getting the necessary nutrients, eat seven servings of fruits and/or vegetables per day. That may sound like a lot, but it really isn't. One serving of fruit, for example, is the equivalent of one medium-sized apple or ¾ of a cup of juice. You can get the equivalent of one serving of vegetables by eating just ½ cup of most cooked or raw vegetables. An excellent way to get your daily dose of fruits and vegetables is to drink them in a smoothie. An orange-banana-mango-berry smoothie will be chock full of vitamins and minerals. So will a juice blended from apples, carrots, beets, and celery.

You should also be eating six to nine servings daily of whole-grain foods such as bread and pasta. These foods are a source of folic acid and also supply you with other vitamins, minerals, and fiber. For healthy choices, select whole wheat bread and pasta products. These have more nutrients per serving, and taste just as good as their white-flour counterparts.

How much food should you eat?

Almost as important as what you eat is how much you eat. Although you do need to eat more because you are eating for two, doctors say that for most of your pregnancy, you should only consume an extra 300 calories per day. That's not much when you consider that a plain bagel can have almost 250 calories. If you eat too much extra food, especially if it is high in fat, you will put on too much weight, which is potentially harmful to both you and your baby. Eating steamed green vegetables or lean red meats will help you get the folic acid and other vitamins and minerals you need without taking on too many extra calories.

Be careful, though, not to starve yourself. The federal government's National Women's Health Information Center advises women to avoid low-calorie diets while pregnant. According to federal authorities, if you don't get enough calories you'll start burning stored fat. A by-product of burning fat is ketones, which if produced constantly will cause mental retardation in your child.

How much weight should you gain?

Although you should be careful not to overeat, you should gain weight as your pregnancy progresses. After all, the baby is growing, and the protective amniotic fluid and placental tissue are going to add weight as well. Doctors say that as a rule, women should gain two to four pounds during the first trimester, and then an additional three to four pounds per month during the second and third trimesters. Health authorities say that on average, a woman should gain 25 to 30 pounds over the course of her pregnancy.

Another reason you should avoid gaining too much weight during your pregnancy is that it will be much harder to lose the extra weight after your baby is born. According to the National Women's Health Information Center, studies have shown that women who gain too much weight during their pregnancy and who fail to lose that weight within six months of delivering their baby are at increased risk of being obese 10 years later.

Watch the seafood!

One way to avoid gaining too much weight—and generally maintain your health—is to eat foods that are low in fat. That means eating vegetables, fruits, lean meats, and fish. Doctors agree that fish is a good source of protein and substances called omega-3 fatty acids, which are good for your heart. However, some fish also can contain a harmful substance, mercury. Scientists say that pregnant women should completely avoid eating fish like shark, king mackerel, white snapper, and certain kinds of tuna. In any case, to avoid ingesting harmful amounts of mercury, you should not consume more than 12 ounces of fish per week.

Eating for two the right way really isn't that hard. With just a few minor adjustments to your diet, you and your partner can enjoy your meals and give your baby a healthy start in life.

STAYING IN SHAPE

Health authorities agree that it is important for you to stay in shape. Keeping fit will help you feel better while you are pregnant, especially as your baby grows larger. Women who stay in shape generally have easier deliveries than those who are less fit. And of course, being fit will help you keep up with your little one, once he or she starts walking!

Is it safe to exercise?

Doctors agree that if you are basically healthy when you get pregnant, moderate exercise is completely safe. In fact, the American College of Obstetricians and Gynecologists (ACOG) says that healthy pregnant women should try to get 30 minutes of moderate exercise almost every day of the week. However, according to the federal government's Department of Health and Human Services, you should consult your doctor before beginning an exercise program because some women develop complications during their pregnancy that can be aggravated by exercise.

Indeed, not every pregnant woman should exercise. Women who have conditions such as heart or lung disease, severe diabetes, thyroid conditions, or are subject to seizures should be especially wary of exercising during pregnancy. Also, women who have high blood pressure from their pregnancy, are having premature labor, bleeding that continues during the second or third trimester, or complications with past pregnancies may be told that exercise isn't a good idea.

What kind of exercise is appropriate?

The American College of Obstetricians and Gynecologists recommends low-impact exercise, meaning that the activity you choose shouldn't be something that jars your spine or puts stress on your knees and hips. Good examples of low-impact exercise are cycling, walking, and swimming. Your exercise should be gentle enough so that you can talk, and you should take frequent breaks. The ACOG also says you should avoid exercise that could involve sustaining blows to your abdomen. Contact sports, such as soccer or tae kwon do, should be avoided. You should also avoid exercising at high altitudes—over 6,000 feet (1829 meters), since the lack of oxygen at high altitude could be harmful to your baby.

How late in pregnancy can I exercise?

You can continue exercising throughout your pregnancy, although the type and duration of your exercise will change as time goes on. Particularly in your second and third trimesters, you should avoid exercises that involve lying on your back. Doctors say that as your pregnancy advances, your expanding uterus can put pressure on certain blood vessels, interfering with circulation.

No matter what stage you are at in your pregnancy, doctors say that you should stop and seek medical attention any time you experience symptoms such as pain in your abdomen, headache, dizziness, or chest pain. If you notice fluid leaking from your vagina, vaginal bleeding, or contractions, you should stop and get to a doctor.

The bottom line, when it comes to exercise, is that you should let your body tell you what's appropriate. But moderate exercise should not only benefit you by strengthening the muscles you'll use during your delivery, but by making it easier for you to lose weight following your delivery.

COPING WITH PREGNANCY

No matter how prepared you think you are for pregnancy, there will be times when you feel overwhelmed and unable to cope. When that happens, it may help to remember that pregnancy doesn't last forever (even though it may seem otherwise!). There are also some specific strategies that will help you either avoid or deal with the most unpleasant aspects of pregnancy.

Dealing with morning sickness

Nausea and/or vomiting first thing in the morning are common complaints among pregnant women and often are experienced at other times of the day or night as well. Experts say that for most women, symptoms of morning sickness greatly diminish or disappear after the first trimester.

As with nausea from other causes, morning sickness can be greatly helped by eating smaller amounts of food. Because you and your baby need nutrition, though, you must make an extra effort to get the food you need. This may mean eating more meals each day so that your overall food intake is adequate. Experts also advise avoiding fatty or spicy foods, which tend to make nausea worse.

In many cases, eating foods that are starchy will help ease symptoms of nausea. Drinking carbonated beverages, such as ginger ale or lemon-lime soda can also help. Carbonated water, since it contains no sugar or artificial sweeteners, may be an even better option.

Getting the rest you need

Your body is working overtime to produce a baby. As a result, you will feel very tired most of the time. The good news is that, like morning sickness, fatigue will probably ease after the end of the first trimester.

You may need to adjust your lifestyle and/or your work schedule to accommodate your need for more rest. If you have a full-time job outside the home, be certain that your supervisor knows you are expecting a baby. Pregnancy is, after all, a medical condition and your employer is obligated to make accommodations so that you can do your job. Even if you aren't ready to announce your pregnancy to the world at large, it is in your interests to make certain your boss is aware of your status. There's a good chance that he or she can arrange your work schedule so you can take a short break during the day, or at least make your schedule less demanding.

Emotional ups and downs

Having a baby—especially your first child—is potentially the most life-changing event you will ever experience. It is natural, therefore, to feel a whole range of emotions. No doubt, if this pregnancy is something you and your partner have been hoping for, you are thrilled to know that you are going to be parents. But even if your pregnancy is something you and your partner have long desired, it is likely that you'll have moments in which you question the wisdom of having a child: Can we afford to feed and educate this person? Will we be good parents? Are we ready to give up our carefree lifestyle? Such questions are perfectly normal.

You'll find, too, that any misgivings will gradually fade as the baby's birth approaches.

As your hormone levels change to accommodate and support your pregnancy, you may experience some emotional turmoil as well. You may feel uneasy, sad, or frightened by changes—or a combination of these emotions. You might also feel upset without being able to identify the emotion! If this happens to you, perhaps you'll take comfort in knowing that this is completely normal!

Stress and what to do about it

The emotional upheaval you experience is almost certainly the result of feeling a certain amount of stress. Even if you have confidence in your ability to be a good parent, it is inevitable to experience some worry. For example, if you work outside the home, there's a good chance that you'll find yourself having to make room in your already-busy schedule for doctor's appointments. If your pregnancy has been called "high-risk," meaning that there are serious chances of miscarriage or health problems for you, you'll probably be told to take it easy—causing even more stress as you try to figure out how to meet all your work and family commitments.

Fortunately, there are some steps you can take to reduce stress. For example, yoga has proven to be an excellent stress-reliever. Yoga is an ancient discipline that teaches people how to stretch their muscles in healthy ways and to relax. Sometimes, too, yoga instructors encourage their students to engage in meditation. Especially during the first trimester of your pregnancy, you should be able to engage in yoga without any real discomfort. In fact, most centers that offer yoga classes offer specific classes called prenatal yoga. These focus on poses and movements that are beneficial and/or protective of your pregnant body. Organizations like the YMCA offer yoga classes for people of differing abilities and levels of fitness. Your local school district may offer yoga through its adult education program. You can also ask your doctor about help with stress-reduction. He or she may know of stress-reduction classes that you can attend.

Another excellent way to reduce stress is to look for opportunities to increase your sense of control over your surroundings. For example, being conscientious about keeping your doctor's appointments will help you rest assured that your pregnancy is proceeding normally and that you are doing everything that can be done to produce a healthy baby.

Of course, many studies have shown that regular exercise, in addition to promoting physical health, can relieve stress. As long as your health care provider has given you the green light for moderate exercise, take advantage of this opportunity to decompress.

Finally, keep in mind that unless you are a national political leader (and there's no second-in-command), the world will not come to an end if you leave something undone. You are in the process of becoming a mother, and that entitles you to let someone else sweat the small stuff!

YOU AND YOUR SPOUSE

Becoming a mom is not, as a general rule, something that you can do alone. Somebody, after all, contributed half the genetic material that went into making the baby that's now growing inside you. In order to make pregnancy as stress-free as possible and for you to concentrate on giving your baby the best start in life, you are going to need to keep your relationship with the baby's father strong.

Sex during pregnancy

One of the first questions many couples ask their doctor is whether it is safe to continue to have sex during pregnancy. The answer is an unequivocal yes! The baby is well-protected in your uterus, so there is very little chance that the physical motions involved with intercourse will harm the baby.

Of course, all the rules for preventing sexually transmitted diseases (STDs) still apply during pregnancy. Not only can diseases such as syphilis, gonorrhea, and AIDS be serious or deadly for you, all of these can be passed along to your baby during the birthing process. If you and your partner are not committed to being monogamous, you should encourage your partner to use a condom.

As your pregnancy advances and your body changes shape, you may find that the sexual positions you are accustomed to are no longer comfortable. Especially late in your pregnancy, the so-called "missionary position" may be uncomfortable—and because lying on your back for long periods of time may not be healthy for you or your baby, you'll probably want to avoid this traditional position. This can be an opportunity to experiment with new positions and techniques that you may find rewarding even after the baby is born!

Keeping dad involved

It is natural for you to feel possessive toward the baby that's growing inside you. That said, it is important for you to help your partner feel involved in the pregnancy. By involving your partner now, you'll be helping him develop a habits and attitudes that you'll appreciate months from now, after the baby is born.

One way you can help your partner be involved is by teaching him how to do some of the household chores you won't have the time or energy for once the baby arrives. As capable as you might be, it is unlikely you are going to be able to cook meals, clean the house, and do laundry while caring for a newborn. You don't need to make your spouse into a gourmet cook, but showing him how to make simple breakfasts and how to assemble a nutritious dinner will save you some stress and give him something to do.

Sometime during your second trimester, you'll probably be offered the opportunity to take birthing classes of some sort. The content of these classes can vary, but they usually entail teaching both you and your partner about the birthing process and how you can work together to help labor and delivery go as smoothly as possible. No matter how much or how little coaching your partner is able to offer, attending these birthing classes will help him feel more involved.

Your partner is likely to also appreciate whatever tips these birthing classes offer on what to do once the baby is born and everyone is back home. The dad-to-be may not be confident that diaper-changing or comforting a crying infant is something he can do; birthing classes are excellent venues for voicing his misgivings—and for having those doubts laid to rest!

KEEPING YOUR BABY SAFE

From the moment you learn you are pregnant, nothing you do is quite as important as guarding the welfare of the baby. Because you supply the growing fetus with all its nutrients through the placenta, anything that enters your body has the potential to affect the baby. Fortunately, by being vigilant you can minimize the risk that your baby will be exposed to anything that is potentially harmful.

Medications to avoid

The federal government's Food and Drug Administration (FDA)

rates all prescription medications for their safety for pregnant women. Drugs given an A rating are considered safe; ratings of B, C, and D are assigned to drugs that are either considered less safe for pregnant women or drugs whose effects on pregnant women and their fetuses are unknown. Prescription drugs that the FDA knows can harm a fetus are assigned an X rating. It is always a good idea to query your doctor about the safety of any prescription medicine. The pharmacist who fills a prescription should also be asked about safety; he or she may have more recent information about a drug and its side effects than your doctor has.

Non-prescription, or over-the-counter (OTC), medications can pose just as great a risk to your baby as a prescription drug. Some medicines, such as ibuprofen and aspirin, can be harmful, particularly during the third trimester. The FDA doesn't rate the safety of over-the-counter medications; instead, the agency requires that the makers of non-prescription medicines carry a warning on their labels about what risks they pose to pregnant women and their fetuses. The iron-clad rule for any medications is that you should ask your doctor about the risks before taking them.

Don't make the mistake of assuming that so-called "natural" remedies are risk-free. The herbal concoctions sold in many health food stores and even in many drug stores can have serious effects on your baby. Be wary, too, of medications that are called homeopathic. The ingredients in many natural, herbal, or homeopathic preparations can have the same effects as their synthetic counterparts. In addition, the FDA does not require the manufacturers of herbal preparations to check their safety for pregnant women, so their effects are often unknown.

Dietary supplements are also something to be wary of if you are pregnant. Some supplements, such as folic acid or multivitamins, are considered safe (your doctor may well advise you to take these), but just as is true of herbal or natural preparations, most dietary supplements have not been studied for their effects on you and your baby. You should check with your doctor before taking any dietary supplement.

X-rays and other forms of radiation

The federal government's National Women's Health Information Center says that X-rays are usually safe for your unborn baby and that if your doctor says you absolutely need to be X-rayed for some reason, you should follow his or her advice. On the other hand, because there is a very slight chance that X-rays can cause cancer in your baby, you should avoid unnecessary X-rays. Sometimes, it is possible to use a different diagnostic procedure, such as ultrasound, instead of an X-ray; in other cases, it may be possible to delay having the X-ray until after your baby is born.

Other types of radiation exposure should be avoided as well, particularly in the earliest stages of pregnancy. The federal government's Centers for Disease Control says that large doses of radiation—the equivalent of more than 500 chest X-rays—during the first two weeks of pregnancy can kill the embryo, since at this point it consists of relatively few cells. Exposure to radiation in weeks 3 to 15 of a pregnancy can result in a baby being brain-damaged or mentally retarded, since this is a time when the first brain cells are developing.

Of course, the chances of your being exposed to radiation powerful enough to harm your baby are extremely small. However, if your job involves the handling of radioactive substances, it would be a good idea to ask your employer for a different assignment, at least until after your baby is born.

Alcohol and tobacco

Doctors almost all agree that you should not smoke or consume alcohol during your pregnancy. Alcohol consumption—especially in large amounts—can seriously damage your baby's brain. Pregnant women who drink alcohol risk giving birth to babies with what is known as fetal alcohol syndrome (FAS). As babies with fetal alcohol syndrome grow up, they often have difficulty learning. Children with FAS sometimes have vision or hearing difficulties. They also tend to have behavior problems. Worse still, FAS is incurable; FAS babies face a lifetime of disabilities.

Tobacco products can also cause problems for your baby. If you smoke, chew tobacco, or use a nicotine patch, you are exposing your baby to nicotine, which can cause low birth weight, premature birth, and even stillbirth. You should immediately give up smoking or chewing tobacco and stop using nicotine patches. Secondhand smoke—that is, the smoke from someone else's cigar or cigarette—can also harm your baby. If someone in your household smokes, it would be a good idea to ask him or her to indulge in their habit outside your home.

Caffeine

Another substance you should try to avoid—or at least limit—is caffeine. Studies have linked consumption of more than 150 milligrams of caffeine per day to an increased risk of miscarriage. Since the average cup of drip coffee contains 137 milligrams of caffeine, you are putting your pregnancy at increased risk if you have two cups per day. And since the amount of caffeine in a cup of coffee varies depending on the type of bean and the brewing method, you cannot be certain how even a single cup will affect you and your baby. As an alternative, try drinking decaffeinated coffee. The flavor of good decaf is the same as regular coffee, and there's a good chance that just drinking the hot liquid will make you feel alert and ready to start (or continue) your day.

Remember that coffee is not the only source of caffeine. Tea, whether it is green or black, has significant amounts of caffeine. Many soft drinks contain caffeine as well. Unless you are vigilant, then, by the end of the day you could well be over the limit of what's considered a safe amount of caffeine.

Food-borne illness

It is also important to avoid certain foods that can carry harmful organisms. You should avoid eating foods like sushi and sashimi, since the uncooked fish can be a source of food-borne illness. In fact, you should be extra-cautious to avoid any foods that are undercooked, since these can be sources of serious diseases like salmonella, listeriosis, and toxoplasmosis. You should cook all meats thoroughly and be careful to wash and/or peel fresh fruits and vegetables.

Certain dairy products, such as soft cheeses, should be avoided. Avoid blue-veined cheeses like bleu cheese, stilton, and Roquefort, and fresh cheeses like feta and queso fresco. These products can be sources of organisms that can cause serious birth defects or even death for your baby.

Keeping your baby safe can seem a daunting task. However, the good news is that safety is mostly straightforward. By paying attention to what your surroundings and the things you eat and drink, you can make sure your baby gets the best possible start.

GETTING THE CARE YOU NEED

From the very beginning of your pregnancy, it is important that you get the proper prenatal care. That means finding a health care provider who meets your needs, making certain that you get the information you want in a form that you can use, and selecting a hospital for the delivery.

Finding the right doctor

The first person to tell you that you are definitely pregnant may be your family doctor. This individual may be the one who treats you for minor illnesses, gives you your annual checkup, and gives you the vaccinations you require from time to time. Once your pregnancy is confirmed, your family doctor (often known by health insurers as your primary care physician) may refer you to a specialist in obstetrics and gynecology. Although any doctor knows the basics about delivering a baby, this specialist has extra training and can handle any complications that might arise during your pregnancy.

If you have what is known as a high-risk pregnancy, it is especially important that you get care from a specialist in obstetrics and gynecology, or OB/GYN for short. If you are diabetic or suffer from high blood pressure, your primary care physician will almost certainly refer you to an OB/GYN. You might also be advised to see such a specialist if you have a history of miscarriages or if you've had fertility problems. Even if your pregnancy is not considered high-risk, you should ask for a referral to an OB/GYN if that makes you feel more at ease.

There's also no need for you to accept the first OB/GYN you are referred to. This is a person you'll be seeing often in the coming months (once a month for the first six months, every two weeks in months seven and eight, and once a week in the final month), so it is important for you to feel comfortable with this doctor. Do you like to be given lots of information? Do you have strong feelings about which medical school the doctor attended? Do you prefer a woman doctor? Sometimes, deciding on a doctor comes down to a matter of "chemistry"—your instinct that this is the right person to manage your care throughout your pregnancy.

The nurse/midwife option

If your pregnancy is considered low-risk, you might even consider going to a nurse or a midwife instead of an OB/GYN. Nurses and midwives are not doctors, but they are trained to manage pregnancies and deliver babies. If you expect your pregnancy to require a minimum of medical intervention (e.g., anesthesia), a nurse or midwife might be the right choice. Although some hospitals allow nurses and midwives to care for patients, it is more common for nurses and midwives to see their patients in facilities known as birthing centers. Sometimes, too, nurses and midwives will arrange to deliver a patient's baby at home.

Because they are not doctors, nurse and midwives cannot do surgery. If it turns out that your baby needs to be delivered by Cesarean section, an OB/GYN will handle the operation. However, nurses and midwives can handle many pregnancy-related issues. Especially if this isn't your first pregnancy and your previous deliveries went smoothly, a nurse or midwife might be an option worth considering.

Selecting a pediatrician

No matter how comfortable you are with the OB/GYN or nurse/midwife who cares for you during your pregnancy, that person's responsibility for your baby will end soon after the delivery. At that point your baby will need a pediatrician. This specialist in the care of babies and children will probably see your baby almost immediately after your delivery. Because this doctor may be overseeing your child's medical care for the next 18 years, it makes sense for you to be careful in selecting someone with whom you are comfortable.

As you decide who your child's doctor will be, you can use some of the same criteria you used for choosing your OB/GYN. For example, is the doctor willing to provide you with the amount of information you want? Does it matter to you where the doctor received his or her medical training? Do any of your friends or acquaintances take their children to this doctor?

Another factor that is worth considering is the pediatrician's office hours. Because many of their patients are school children, some pediatricians maintain office hours on Saturdays. This can be a real benefit for you if you have a job outside the home that keeps you busy during weekdays.

Of course, you will want to ask about what insurance plans the doctor accepts. Although you cannot put a price on getting good care for your child, knowing whether a doctor can and will bill your insurance company directly can help you decide between two physicians who are otherwise equal in your mind.

Where to have the baby

Just as you have a number of options regarding who cares for you and your child, you also have several options for where you give birth. Your choice will probably depend to some degree on who you selected to provide your prenatal care. As we have already noted, a nurse/midwife is more likely to deliver your baby at a birthing center or at your home; on the other hand, an OB/GYN may be willing to handle the delivery in one of these settings as well.

The main advantage of a birthing center is a more relaxed atmosphere than you are likely to find in a hospital. Your husband will almost certainly be allowed to be present during the delivery, and other family members may be allowed as well. The staff at a birthing center will try to make the delivery of your baby as natural an experience as possible. For example, you won't be given anesthesia. Overall, the setting will probably remind you more of a room in an upscale hotel than a hospital room.

If your pregnancy is considered to be extraordinarily low-risk, giving birth at home might be an option. A nurse/midwife is more likely than an OB/GYN to offer home-birthing, but you can ask the doctor if he or she would be willing to do the delivery at your home. Of course, home-birthing involves the absolute minimum of medical technology. The person providing your care will probably bring oxygen and some basic supplies, but if you decide that you need anesthesia, or if complications crop up, you'll be taken to a hospital to complete the delivery.

Although birthing centers and home-birthing are gaining in popularity, the majority of births take place in a hospital. Even in hospitals, though, an effort is often made to make the experience of giving birth seem more natural and relaxed. You'll almost certainly be given the option of delivering without anesthesia, for example. The delivery rooms in many hospitals are equipped with amenities like stereos and DVD players. Your partner will almost certainly be allowed to be with you during labor and delivery as well.

The main thing to remember is that having a baby may be the most memorable experience of your life. Your choices should aim to make your memories of this event as pleasant and as safe as possible.

GETTING YOUR HOME READY

From the moment you walk through your front door with your baby in your arms until months (or even years!) later, you are likely to feel that there just aren't enough hours in the day to do even a fraction of the things that need doing. You and your partner will almost certainly be sleep-deprived and will probably feel overwhelmed. The last thing you'll want to be doing after the birth is decorating and equipping the nursery. You'll be able to concentrate on being a good mom if all the preparations have been done well in advance.

As you may already have noticed, the bill for equipping your home to accommodate the new family member mounts up quickly. Unless you are wealthy, it makes sense to prioritize your purchases. Buy the things you know you'll need immediately, such as diapers, changing supplies, a crib, and changing table. If your friends or family members are planning a baby shower, you can tactfully let them know what other items you need. The checklist later in this book will give you some ideas of items that will make life with your new arrival easier.

Furnishing the nursery

When you start shopping for baby furniture, you'll quickly discover that the options (and the amount you can wind up spending) are almost limitless. For example, cribs can be made from a number of materials—metal, wood, or particle board, for example. The most expensive cribs are made from hardwood and may be so fancy that they're more like works of art! The crib's mattress may be a simple pad, or it may resemble a shrunken version of the mattress on your bed, with inner springs. Some cribs are constructed in such a way as to allow them to be converted into what's known as a "youth bed," for use when your baby grows into a toddler. The main thing to look for in a crib is ease of use. Keep in mind that you'll be having to lay your baby down in the crib and pick him or her up from it—probably many times each day. One side of the crib will be designed so that it can be lowered to make that task easier; try the display model in the store and make sure that it can be lowered and raised again with a minimum of effort (and with a minimum of noise).

Another "must" for the nursery is a changing table. Although you might get by using a dresser, bed, or other piece of furniture for this purpose, a changing table has the advantage of compartments for storing supplies such as wipes, lotion, and clean diapers. As is the case with cribs, changing tables come in a wide variety of styles; prices vary widely. Unless you've got your heart set on all of the nursery furniture matching, there's no need for the changing table to be very elaborate. Within a year, your baby will have grown too large for the table, at which time you'll either be putting this piece of furniture in storage or disposing of it in some way.

If you don't already have one, consider buying a rocking chair. Many new mothers find that rocking in a chair soothes a crying infant and helps them get some much-needed rest as well. (You might, however, need to shoo Dad out of the chair first!) You can put the rocker wherever you are most likely to use it. If there's room for it in the nursery, that will give you a place to sit while you give your baby a 2 a.m. feeding.

Nursery supplies

After you've purchased the furnishings for the nursery, don't forget to stock up on basic supplies: You are unlikely to want to stop on the way home from the hospital to buy diapers and wipes! Although the hospital may provide you with a small supply of diapers, you will want to have enough to last you at least a week or two. In addition, you should have a package or two of wipes on hand. Although wipes usually are advertised as having lotion incorporated into them, you should also have some petroleum jelly or some other kind of soothing ointment to apply to your baby's backside before you put a fresh diaper on him or her.

Even if you plan to breast-feed your baby, you will want to be prepared to feed him or her with a bottle as well. Not every new mother finds that breast-feeding comes naturally, for example. Sometimes, too, it can take a day or two before your own milk begins to flow in amounts adequate for feeding your baby. It is a sensible precaution, then, to have a supply of nipples, bottle liners or clean bottles, and formula available. You can always return unopened items to the store if you find you don't need them.

Childproofing your home

Your new baby will be utterly dependent on you for his or her mobility, but that will change quickly. In as little as nine months (possibly even sooner!) your little one will be able to crawl, "furniture-cruise," or walk a few steps. At this point, the possibilities for getting into things that are potentially harmful are virtually boundless. The time to make your home safe for a curious baby is before he or she can move about independently. And since you and your partner will be tired and quite busy after the birth, you will both be happier if childproofing has already been done before you come home with a newborn in your arms.

The first step in keeping your baby safe at home is to make certain that all cupboards and drawers have safety latches. You can find the necessary supplies at your local hardware store, home improvement center, or baby-supply store. Many different styles of latches are available. You may need to experiment to find a style that fits the design of your cabinetry and that you can install easily. You don't absolutely have to install latches on cupboards that are more than four feet off the floor, but such hardware is also a useful precaution if you live in an area that's subject to earthquakes. If neither you nor your partner is comfortable with basic tools like screwdrivers and drills, consider hiring a handyman to install the latches. Someone experienced can probably install all the necessary hardware in just a couple of hours.

Once you've childproofed your cabinetry, the next step is to look for areas of the home that you don't want your baby entering. For example, even if you've installed latches on your cabinets, you may not want your baby coming into the kitchen where he can encounter a hot stove or a hard, tiled floor. Some kind of lockable gate across the entrance to such areas is the answer. Again, there are many styles available. The kind you buy will probably depend on the design of your home. You may need more than one gate, too. If your home has two or more floors, you'll need to install gates at the top and bottom of the stairs; if your home has a basement, be certain to install a gate at the top of that stairwell, or install a latch on the door to the basement.

The bathroom is another area that you will need to childproof. As with any other room, you'll need to install latches on cabinets. Be especially careful, even if various medicines and other substances are in childproof containers, to install a secure latch on the medicine cabinet. You'll be amazed by where little hands go as their owners investigate the world, so don't forget to install a latch on the lid to the toilet!

Finally, keep in mind that once your baby starts taking those first tentative steps, falls are inevitable. Brickwork around fireplaces and the edges of wooden furniture and cabinets can cause serious trauma to little bodies. As a precaution, install padding on any exposed corners, including the lower edges of counters. Such padding may not be aesthetically pleasing, but it can prevent the kinds of injuries that result in frantic trips to the doctor—usually at the most inopportune moments!

No amount of childproofing can completely eliminate the chance that your child will sustain some kind of injury in your home. The bottom line is this: Never leave your baby unattended. Remember that there is no visitor at your front door, no chore, and no phone call that is important enough to justify risking injury to your child.

WORK AND PREGNANCY

If you work outside the home, you will have some decisions to make as your due date approaches. Depending on your job and your employer's policies regarding maternity leave, you will need to decide how much time, if any, you want to take off before and after your baby is born. Your decision must balance your need to recover from the birth and bond with your baby against the satisfaction you get from your job and your need for income.

When to begin maternity leave

One of the more difficult decisions you are likely to face is when to go on maternity leave. Your decision will depend, at least in part, on your employer's policies. A federal law, known as the Family and Medical Leave Act (FMLA) requires most employers to offer 12 weeks of leave for parents-to-be, but if your employer has fewer than 50 employees you may not be entitled to any leave at all. If your employer isn't required to offer maternity leave, you'll need to appeal to your employer's sense of humanity and fairness.

Even if you work for a large company that is covered by FMLA, you will have to consider that the law does not require your employer to pay you while you are on leave. You may be entitled to use accrued vacation time and sick days first and get paid for that time, but once those days are used up you are on your own. If you and your partner have been relying on your paycheck to help maintain your lifestyle, you'll need to consider how long you can do without your paycheck.

What kinds of work are safe for you?

Whether to go on maternity leave, and when, depends in part on what kind of work you do. If your work involves exposure to potentially toxic chemicals or hard physical labor, for example, you may want to reduce the risk to your baby by going on maternity leave early. Keep in mind, though, that the law probably will not protect your job in such a case, since FMLA only requires employers covered by the law to hold your job open for 12 weeks. If you are worried about your baby's safety but cannot afford to give up your job, you should discuss your situation with your boss to see if you can take a different assignment, at least temporarily.

The good news is, there are lots of jobs that are perfectly safe for you. Although there have been concerns in the past about radiation from such workplace items as computer monitors, studies indicate that such fears are unfounded. With rare exceptions, as long as you have the energy and stamina to do your job, there's no medical reason for you to stop. If your job requires standing in one place for long periods, though, you may experience problems caused by reduced circulation. Eventually, the need for frequent trips to the bathroom may make some jobs impractical.

Staying safe on the job

For most pregnant women, keeping themselves and their baby safe on the job amounts to using common sense and good judgment. For example, if your job involves driving a vehicle, you should always wear your seatbelt. (You'd do that anyway, right?) If you need to lift a heavy object, be careful, or ask for help. Be sure to drink plenty of water. In other words, look after yourself. By doing that, you'll also be looking after your baby.

Notes

Checklists

NURSERY

- ❑ Paint/decorate nursery
- ❑ Crib
- ❑ Bassinet
- ❑ Changing table
- ❑ Rocking chair
- ❑ Changing pad
- ❑ Diaper genie
- ❑ Nursing chair/rocker
- ❑ "Onesies"
- ❑ Mitts (to prevent baby from scratching him/herself)
- ❑ Crib sheets (2 or 3 sets)
- ❑ Diapers and wipes
- ❑ Undershirt
- ❑ Socks
- ❑ Booties
- ❑ Receiving blanket
- ❑ Diaper bag
- ❑ Audio monitor
- ❑ Bottles, nipples, plastic liners
- ❑ Bottle warmer
- ❑ Nursing pillow
- ❑ Baby's bathtub

CHILD SAFETY CHECKLIST

- ❑ Install locks on all drawers
- ❑ Install locks on all lower cupboards
- ❑ Install padding on all hard corners/brickwork
- ❑ Install toilet lid locks
- ❑ Install childproof locks on exterior doors
- ❑ Install safety gates on stairwells and kitchen doorways
- ❑ Turn down temperature on the water heater
- ❑ Buy car seat

GETTING READY FOR THE DELIVERY

- ❑ Sign up for birthing classes
- ❑ Pack a bag—include toiletries, change of undergarments, slippers, a robe, a book, videos, music CDs
- ❑ Make practice drives to hospital
- ❑ Interview babysitters/nannies
- ❑ Select pediatrician

MAKING LIFE WITH BABY EASIER

- ❑ Baby carriage with adjustable bed
- ❑ Umbrella stroller
- ❑ Snuggly
- ❑ Backpack baby carrier (for a few months down the road!)
- ❑ Playpen
- ❑ Portable crib
- ❑ Infant's "playground"
- ❑ Stationary play center
- ❑ Motorized swing
- ❑ Vibrating chair
- ❑ Mobile (for over the crib)
- ❑ White noise tapes (for soothing colicky baby)

Lunar Month

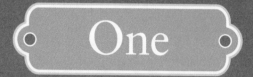

One

PHOTO

Place a photo of you during your first month here

My Monthly Update

Waist Measurement: ____________________

Weight: ____________________

Mood: ____________________

Lunar Month one . . . .

PREGNANCY CHECKLIST

- ❑ Share the good news with your partner
- ❑ Stop smoking and drinking alcohol, and avoid caffeine
- ❑ Avoid water temperatures above 102 degrees, such as in saunas and jacuzzis
- ❑ Schedule your first prenatal care checkup as soon as you think you are pregnant
- ❑ Ask your health care provider what's safe and what to avoid during pregnancy
- ❑ Determine your due date
- ❑ Take a multivitamin with at least 400 micrograms of the B vitamin folic acid every day
- ❑ Begin researching hospitals
- ❑ Choose your OB-GYN or midwife
- ❑ Start thinking about baby names and keeping track of your ideas
- ❑ Familiarize yourself with the changes that will be happening to you during your first trimester
- ❑ Familiarize yourself with the changes that will be happening to your baby
- ❑ Consider beginning a pregnancy journal or scrapbook
- ❑ Connect with women who are due the same month you are

MY PERSONAL CHECKLIST:

- ❑ ....
- ❑ ....
- ❑ ....

MY HOPES FOR THIS MONTH:

....

....

....

Lunar Month One

First Trimester

CONGRATULATIONS ON YOUR PREGNANCY! Though you may have planned this, you are probably experiencing a certain degree of shock. This is perfectly normal! One way to get a handle on what you are facing is to settle down with this book and learn what you can expect over the next 10 months. Indeed, one of the most important things you can do as you begin your first trimester is to educate yourself on have the healthiest pregnancy possible.

Thinking about all of the decisions you will have to make over the next 266 days probably feels overwhelming. Breaking all of the information down into months, weeks, and days will help you to get a handle on what is happening to your body as well as help you to keep track of your baby's development. As you read, keep in mind that the decisions you make during these early weeks are crucial to your developing baby's health.

WHAT TO EXPECT THIS MONTH

Every pregnancy is different, so not every woman will experience the same symptoms. In fact, some women make it through their entire pregnancy with no symptoms. This is rare, however, so expect to experience at least some physical and emotional changes during the next four weeks.

You probably won't look physically different to other people within the first month. This is because your uterus will not expand enough to push your belly out for at least another few weeks, or even months. By the end of the 4th week, you may notice that your pants are snug. Your bra may feel a bit tight. This is mostly related to surging hormones that are preparing your body to house and support your baby. These hormones, as well as pressure on your bladder from your uterus, may also cause you to feel the need to urinate more frequently. Also, you can expect to experience mild to severe nausea this month. It is also possible that you'll be more tired than usual, which can exacerbate emotional changes.

The emotional response to pregnancy is usually mistaken for pre-menstrual syndrome (PMS) at first. You can expect to be irritable, to have mood swings, and to find yourself in tears over just about anything. You can blame these reactions on increased levels of estrogen and progesterone surging through your body.

THINGS TO CONSIDER

You are just starting out on the exciting road to parenthood! Although you have a long way to go, you and partner will be amazed with how fast the time goes. Therefore, now is the time to do some serious planning so you are completely ready on the day you bring your baby home.

It is a good idea to start making to-do lists. These should include everything from home repair to nursery décor to potential names. Keep in mind you may not have time to get to everything on your lists before your baby is born, so it is important to prioritize. Do the most important things first and put off tasks that can wait or can be easily done when the baby arrives. Also, you may want to make a list of all the ways you anticipate your life to change. It will be interesting to revisit it later to see how on the mark you were. Indeed, your lifestyle is about to change dramatically. Remember that you can only anticipate these changes so much, so it is important to be flexible and willing to "go with the flow."

TIPS FOR COPING

Some of the earliest symptoms of pregnancy can also be the most persistent. For example, if you feel nauseated early on, you are getting a preview of what many pregnant women deal with throughout the first trimester (and beyond, for some). There are ways to cope with nausea, however, such as eating smaller, more frequent meals and concentrating on foods that are relatively bland and easy to digest. This means avoiding spicy dishes and foods that are greasy or high in fat.

Another thing you will need to get used to early in your pregnancy is how exhausted you will likely feel. You will probably find it difficult to engage in your normal level of activity. If you do experience fatigue, allow yourself extra rest and get to bed early if you can. Remember, you will get used to these physical symptoms and learn to work around them.

The emotional upheaval you may be experiencing can be trickier to deal with. It is very important to constantly remind yourself that it is natural to feel a little worried, or even ambivalent, about having a baby. Hopefully, knowing these emotions are normal and common might help you feel better. Be sure to discuss your feelings with your partner—he may be experiencing some of the same emotions.

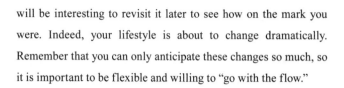

WHAT TO EAT

It is important to eat "smart" when you are pregnant. What you eat will nourish your growing baby. You should eat a varied and healthy diet rich in vitamins and minerals. Some nutrients, such as folic acid are more important than others to your baby's development, particularly in this first month. Folic acid is one of the B vitamins and is crucial to the proper formation of your baby's brain and spinal column. You will probably find it difficult to get all the folic acid you need without a supplement, but taking a good prenatal vitamin in addition to eating green, leafy vegetables and whole grains will ensure that you get the recommended amount (400 milligrams).

In addition to folic acid, you should also consume foods that are high in calcium, vitamin D, and vitamin C. Dairy products are a good source of calcium and vitamin D, but be sure to watch your fat intake. In fact, try to avoid foods that are high in fat, in general. Your priority at this point in time should be to eat a balanced diet.

HOW MUCH WEIGHT TO GAIN

If you are of average weight for your age and height, you should gain anywhere from 25 to 35 pounds over the course of your pregnancy. While you should plan on gaining some weight during your first trimester, it should happen gradually. You probably won't gain very much weight this first month. At most, expect to see a gain of one or two pounds. In fact, many women actually lose a little weight early in their pregnancy due to nausea and vomiting. If you do lose weight, don't worry. You will start to gain it back once your nausea subsides.

EXERCISE TIPS AND ADVICE

It is important to exercise while you are pregnant. If you are already used to exercising, keep it up for as long as your doctor allows. However, if you were not exercising regularly before you became pregnant, you should start out slowly by walking, swimming, or doing prenatal yoga. In general, it is a good idea to engage in exercise that doesn't stress your joints, and it is always important to stay hydrated and cool while working out.

POTENTIAL SYMPTOMS AND HOW TO ALLEVIATE THEM

Some women escape the first month of pregnancy with no symptoms at all. However, if you are like 70 percent of pregnant women in America, you will develop some symptoms that can put a kink in your normal routine.

A very common symptom that women experience this early in their pregnancy is breast tenderness. In fact, many pregnant women have reported knowing they were pregnant because first thing in the morning, their breasts were so sore that simple contact with their sheets and blankets caused discomfort. There is little that can be done about this except to wear a soft sports bra, even to bed. Warm compresses can also help.

Another common symptom that will likely appear this month is nausea. Since pregnancy sickness can strike any time of day, a good way to get a handle on it is to keep your blood sugar even by eating several small meals throughout the day. Make these meals small, bland, and easily digestible—club soda, crackers, and whole wheat pretzels are good choices. Keep them with you at all times.

The third most common ailment early in pregnancy is exhaustion. This can be troublesome if you have to report to work or take care of other children. It is very important that you get plenty of rest at night. Take naps during the day if you can. Also, be sure to sit and rest when you need to and avoid overexerting yourself.

WAYS OTHERS CAN HELP

As your level of fatigue increases, you will need to ask your partner for help. This will probably involve re-dividing household duties. If you have been accustomed to doing most of the grocery shopping or cooking when you get home from work, shift these responsibilities to your partner a few nights a week so you can take a nap before dinner. Additionally, involve your friends and family when you are feeling under the weather. Ask them for help with housework and childcare—and don't be shy. Everyone loves to help a pregnant woman!

"If you want one year of prosperity, grow grain. If you want ten years of prosperity, grow trees. If you want one hundred years of prosperity, grow babies."
~ Chinese Proverb

Week 1

Starting Weight: _________

OVERVIEW

During your first week of pregnancy, you are dealing mostly with your emotional reaction to the news. Though you may have planned this pregnancy, you may still find that the reality of being pregnant has left you feeling a bit shocked. Don't stress out—it can take awhile for you to settle into the idea that you are going to be a mother.

While you adjust to your new reality, your body is hard at work. It takes about a week for your fertilized egg to travel through your fallopian tube to your uterus. As it makes this journey, your uterus thickens with a mucus lining called the endometrium.

When the fertilized egg successfully implants in the endometrium, you will miss your next period, though you may see some light spotting. During this time, your body produces the hormone progesterone, which is essential for your baby's survival. Progesterone has many jobs in your body during pregnancy. It suppresses your immune system just enough so that your body will accept the pregnancy. It also prevents your uterus from contracting while fostering blood vessel growth, which is essential to your baby's nourishment.

DAY 1: Date:____/____/____

MOM - WHAT'S HAPPENING:

Fertilization occurs once your partner's sperm joins with your egg. This causes a single cell called a zygote to form. On Day 1, your fertilized egg is still in the fallopian tube. Though it will be several days before the fertilized egg implants itself in your uterus, your body is producing hormones that will support the implantation process.

BABY - WHAT'S HAPPENING:

At this point the fertilized egg is known as a zygote. The zygote already has its own unique genetic blueprint that is created by the 46 chromosomes passed on from both parents—23 from mom and 23 from dad. The zygote contains all of the genetic information necessary to grow into an adult human being. Neither you nor your partner can tell what it is, but your baby's gender has already been determined. If a sperm cell bearing an "X" chromosome fertilized your egg, you will have a girl; if the sperm that fertilized it bore a "Y" chromosome, you've got a boy on the way.

PREGNANCY FACT: Doctors consider a pregnancy to begin on the first day of your last menstrual period (LMP). However, until a fertilized egg implants itself in your uterus, you aren't actually pregnant. Doctors calculate pregnancy this way for the convenience of time of reference, but you should understand that conception doesn't actually occur until about two weeks later. Therefore, pregnancy lasts 40 weeks according to the LMP timeline, whereas actual pregnancy is 38 weeks. This can seem a bit confusing at first, but you will get used to the weekly counts as your pregnancy progresses.

DAILY JOURNAL

Mood:

Energy:

Cravings:

Symptoms:

Weight:

DAY 2: Date:____/____/____

MOM - WHAT'S HAPPENING:

The inner wall of your uterus is getting ready for implantation. In order to ensure that implantation is successful, the lining of your uterus is thickening with mucus called endometrium. Although it will be another 5 days or so before implantation takes place, your body is already producing the hormones progesterone and estrogen to aid implantation. Progesterone helps suppress your immune system so it does not treat the zygote as an infection and try to attack it.

BABY - WHAT'S HAPPENING:

The zygote has begun its journey into being as cell division, or mitosis, starts. The fertilized egg divides into two cells, which look like two tiny, connected balls. This first cell division is the beginning of what will eventually be more than 100 trillion cells. Each cell has a nucleus in which your little zygote's genetic blueprint is encoded. As mitosis continues, each cell that is produced contains an identical copy of the original cell's DNA.

FOR YOUR HEALTH: If you are a smoker, now is the time to quit (if you haven't already). Smoking is associated with at least 115,000 miscarriages each year in the United States. Additionally, smoking causes low birth weight and can stunt growth in utero. Babies born to women who smoked while pregnant are also 5 times more likely to succumb to sudden infant death syndrome (SIDS) and are much more prone to respiratory illnesses than those born to nonsmokers. You should also stay away from secondhand smoke, as it can contribute to the same health problems.

DAILY JOURNAL

Mood:

Energy:

Cravings:

Symptoms:

Weight:

DAY 3: Date:____/____/____

MOM - WHAT'S HAPPENING:

Thanks to tiny, fine, hair-like cilia, the zygote continues to move toward its destination—your uterus. Cilia are an important part of your zygote's journey. In fact, if cilia don't do their job and push the zygote through the fallopian tube, the mass of cells can get stuck and implant in the fallopian tube. This is called an ectopic pregnancy. If cilia are doing their job, however, your little zygote is getting very close to implantation in your uterus. As the zygote makes it way through your fallopian tube, its cells continue to divide.

BABY - WHAT'S HAPPENING:

Cell division continues, though there is no discernible increase in the size of the embryo. At this point, the zygote is made up of just 16 cells. These cells form a tight unit in the shape of a compact ball. The zygote still has not implanted itself in your uterus, though it will very soon! Around this time your baby is known as a morula, which is Latin for mulberry. The morula stage occurs just before the embryo reaches the blastocyst stage.

FOOD FOR THOUGHT: Many pregnant women report that nausea and heartburn can be eased by eating six small meals instead of three large meals each day. This is because as your uterus grows, it puts pressure on your stomach. This leaves less room for food to sit and wait to be digested. Also, digestive acids are forced upward toward your esophagus, which has slackened thanks to the pregnancy hormone relaxin. Eating smaller meals can help prevent "overflow" of stomach acids and will help to keep your blood sugar even throughout the day.

DAILY JOURNAL

Mood:

Energy:

Cravings:

Symptoms:

Weight:

DAY 4: Date:____/____/____

MOM - WHAT'S HAPPENING:

Today you might experience two of the earliest signs of pregnancy: mood swings and sore breasts. You may find yourself tearing up during commercials for pet food, or notice you are ready to throw a tantrum over small frustrations. Likewise, some women say they knew they were pregnant before they ever took a test because their breasts were so tender. Both emotional upheaval and breast soreness can be attributed to increased levels of progesterone and estrogen.

BABY - WHAT'S HAPPENING:

Your zygote is now made up of approximately 100 cells in the shape of a sphere. This sphere has formed around a fluid-filled pocket. At this point it is called a blastocyst. The blastocyst has entered your uterus by now, but it hasn't yet implanted itself in the uterine wall. It will most likely implant itself within the next several days. Meanwhile, the blastocyst secretes special enzymes that erode a space in your uterine wall in which it will embed itself.

TIPS AND ADVICE: It is a great idea to incorporate prenatal yoga into your daily routine, for a variety of reasons: Yoga increases circulation, which is beneficial to both mom and baby because the increased blood flow provides oxygen. Yoga also promotes relaxation and increases concentration, which help control anxiety related to being pregnant. Flexibility and balance—which can become a problem as your center of gravity shifts throughout your pregnancy—will improve as well. Finally, prenatal yoga can help ease backaches, reduce swelling, and also combat insomnia.

DAILY JOURNAL

Mood:

Energy:

Cravings:

Symptoms:

Weight:

DAY 5: Date:____/____/____

MOM - WHAT'S HAPPENING:

The blastocyst has attached itself to the endometrium, but it has not yet embedded itself in the uterus. Around this time your body starts to produce the human chorionic gonadotropin (hCG) hormone. HCG supports your pregnancy and can be detected in your urine some time between one and two weeks after conception. In fact, some home pregnancy tests can detect hCG in the urine as early as six days after fertilization. HCG levels will double every few days during the first 10-12 weeks of your pregnancy before leveling off.

BABY - WHAT'S HAPPENING:

The inner area of the blastocyst is fluid-filled. This fluid is what will eventually develop into your baby and the amniotic sac. The cells surrounding this cavity are called the trophoblast. This will later become your placenta, which will be your baby's "life raft." The blastocyst will embed itself in your uterine lining, or endometrium, any day now. Meanwhile, it continues to secrete enzymes that will make it possible to fuse with the endometrium.

PREGNANCY FACT: According to a Yale University study, 1 in 5 babies born in the United States are born by Cesarean section. This means that Cesarean rates have quadrupled in the past 20 years! There are several reasons for this increase. One is that doctors began to fear lawsuits, and so wanted to have a more controlled environment in which to deliver babies. Another reason for the increase was that women started planning their births to fit in with work and lifestyle choices. Still, the primary reason for Cesarean delivery continues to be to avert severe health risks to both mom and baby.

DAILY JOURNAL

Mood:

Energy:

Cravings:

Symptoms:

Weight:

DAY 6: Date:____/____/____

MOM - WHAT'S HAPPENING:

At this point, hormonal changes in your body have signaled your ovaries to stop producing eggs. You may be able to get a positive read from an at-home pregnancy test this morning. If you do decide to take a pregnancy test and it does not read positive, don't panic. It can take another 6 days or so to get a positive reading. Odds are at this point, you are starting to feel symptoms similar to those you experience during PMS, such as irritability, exhaustion, swollen and tender breasts, and maybe even some slight cramping. You may even notice some spotting—if so, it is likely that implantation has begun!

BABY - WHAT'S HAPPENING:

It is possible that the blastocyst has begun to embed itself in your uterine wall. If so, you are now the proud carrier of an embryo! No bigger than the point of a pen, your little one is gathering its nutrients from your uterus. He or she will continue to do so until the placenta forms and takes over "life support" duty.

FOR YOUR HEALTH: If you've been trying to get pregnant, you have probably already started taking prenatal supplements. However, if you haven't, now is the time to get started. Folate is necessary for rapid cell production and can be ingested by eating leafy green vegetables such as spinach, beans, peas. It is also found in fortified breakfast cereals. However, since most women are unable to eat enough of these foods to ingest the right amount of folate, it is necessary to get the recommended daily dose (400 micrograms) of folic acid in supplement form, such as from prenatal vitamins.

DAILY JOURNAL

Mood:

Energy:

Cravings:

Symptoms:

Weight:

DAY 7: Date:____/____/____

MOM - WHAT'S HAPPENING:

As implantation continues, you may notice a little spotting. Spotting can occur when the embryo embeds itself in your uterine wall. You may feel some discomfort, and some women feel pressure or the need to urinate. You might even be thinking that you are not actually pregnant, as these symptoms can be mistaken for the beginning of your period. Since your body continues to produce increased levels of hCG, it is possible for you to get a positive result from an at-home pregnancy test.

BABY - WHAT'S HAPPENING:

After implantation, your little ball of cells becomes an embryo. It is building what will become the amniotic sac, which will cushion and protect your baby as she grows. Meanwhile, the embryo continues the implantation process by burrowing deeper into the lining of your uterus. The embryo is still tiny—a mere .006 inches long! Even though it is still very early in your pregnancy, your embryo's brain, spinal cord, and heart have already started to develop.

FOOD FOR THOUGHT: Be sure to start your pregnancy out right by incorporating the following healthy and nutritious snacks. Figs make wonderful snacks, are healthy, and can help you fight the discomforts of first-trimester constipation. If it is not too hard on your stomach, orange juice is a great addition to your mid-morning snack, because it includes vitamin C and is often fortified with calcium. Yogurt is another healthy and easy snack that will give you a mid-afternoon energy boost, since it has protein and is also a great source of calcium.

DAILY JOURNAL

Mood:

Energy:

Cravings:

Symptoms:

Weight:

Week 2

Starting Weight: _________

OVERVIEW

This week, your body is manufacturing high levels of hormones that work together to support your pregnancy. Women who have been trying to conceive hope for high levels of the human chorionic gonadotropin (hCG) hormone. This is because pregnancy tests read hCG in urine and can determine if fertilization has occurred. This week hCG levels will rise, so by day 12 you will be able to get a positive reading from an at-home pregnancy test. HCG is produced by the zygote. It tells the ovaries to continue to produce progesterone. Without hCG, the body would cease progesterone production, and you would shed your uterine lining during menstruation.

Because it has so many jobs during gestation, progesterone is considered the "heavy hitter" of pregnancy hormones. A few things will happen this week due to rising progesterone levels. One is the thickening of your uterine lining, or endometrium. This must occur in order for implantation to "take." Progesterone is also responsible for preventing uterine contractions, which could prematurely expel the zygote.

Thus, due to the many hormonal changes that are occurring in your body this week, you may find yourself experiencing some or all of the following: mood swings, nausea, implantation bleeding, and breast tenderness.

DAY 8: Date:____/____/____

MOM - WHAT'S HAPPENING:

Your endometrium is now thick enough to accept the embryo. As the embryo burrows into your uterine wall, you may notice some yellow or brown discharge. This is a completely normal part of the implantation process. Meanwhile, as implantation continues, your body is producing high levels of progesterone and estrogen. These hormones will be responsible for the many changes to your breasts, cervix, and uterus over the next several months.

BABY - WHAT'S HAPPENING:

The embryo is now attached to your uterine wall by connective tissues called villi (anchoring stem). Villi are responsible for fusing the embryonic cells to the endometrium and for allowing maximum surface area contact between the embryo and the uterus. Your blood reaches the embryo through villi to nourish your growing baby.

FOR YOUR HEALTH: Alcohol and drug consumption can interfere with the implantation process and cause a miscarriage before you even know that you are pregnant. In fact, researchers estimate that between 7 and 10 days after conception is when the embryo is at highest risk for failed implantation. Therefore, it is a good idea to stop drinking before becoming pregnant. Later in your pregnancy, you can discuss with your doctor whether it is OK to have a glass of wine now and then, but it is crucial that you abstain during this critical stage of development.

DAILY JOURNAL

Mood:

Energy:

Cravings:

Symptoms:

Weight:

DAY 9: Date:____/____/____

MOM - WHAT'S HAPPENING:

You may feel some pressure in your lower abdomen. This is normal, and not to be feared! There can be several causes for this sensation. One reason is that you may actually be able to feel when implantation occurs. If so, count yourself lucky to know when your uterus and embryo fused. Other causes may be an increase in blood circulation or your uterus beginning to stretch. If you feel pressure in your lower abdomen, odds are you also find yourself having to urinate more frequently. This is due to an increase in bodily fluids as well as from pressure that your uterus puts on your bladder. Many women, however, have no symptoms at this point, which is also perfectly normal.

BABY - WHAT'S HAPPENING:

The placenta is still forming, and the embryo is now firmly embedded in your uterine wall. The beginning of the umbilical cord, or connecting stalk, also begins to form, while the amniotic sac is in the earliest stage of formation.

FOOD FOR THOUGHT: If you have not yet experienced pregnancy-related nausea, now is a good time to fill your diet with nutrient-rich strawberries. Strawberries, known as "nature's perfect food," contain vitamin C, folate, potassium, calcium, fiber, and even protein. In fact, eating just 1 cup of strawberries provides you with 100 percent of the daily recommended vitamin C intake for pregnant women. Vitamin C is very important for pregnant women since it aids in the body's absorption of iron, which can become deficient as much of your blood is diverted to your growing baby.

DAILY JOURNAL

Mood:

Energy:

Cravings:

Symptoms:

Weight:

DAY 10: Date:____/____/____

MOM - WHAT'S HAPPENING:

You may experience nausea this morning. The degree to which women suffer from morning sickness varies: some have almost none, while an unlucky few experience so much nausea that they have difficulty keeping any food down. Many women also say that morning sickness ought to be called "all-day sickness," since the symptoms are not confined to mornings. You may also be fatigued throughout the day. This is mostly due to your body's around-the-clock effort to build the placenta.

BABY - WHAT'S HAPPENING:

The embryo is busy building its support system. The amniotic bag continues to form and will eventually house your baby. The amniotic bag, or sac, will eventually contain amniotic fluid, which is mostly made up of water. The amniotic sac will protect your baby as he is jostled about as you go about your day. The surface of the amniotic sac is tough. It is big enough to eventually hold your baby and approximately 1 quart of amniotic fluid by the 34th week of your pregnancy.

TIPS AND ADVICE: There are several tricks you can employ to help deal with nausea. For instance, carry around a few lemon slices or lemon-scented candies with you in your purse. This way if you are exposed to odors that cause you to feel sick you can inhale the scent of lemon instead. This has been shown to prevent the escalation of nausea to vomiting. You should also carry around black licorice to nibble on when your stomach is giving you trouble. Sipping peppermint tea also helps, as will inhaling peppermint oil.

DAILY JOURNAL

Mood:

Energy:

Cravings:

Symptoms:

Weight:

DAY 11: Date:____/____/____

MOM - WHAT'S HAPPENING:

If you are waiting to take an at-home pregnancy test, you may be biting your nails with anticipation. However, if you've already confirmed your pregnancy, you may be experiencing anxiety, excitement, or a combination of both. Physically, your breasts continue to change. Your areolas start to spread and darken, and you may even notice small bumps on them—these are sweat glands that become prominent during pregnancy and disappear after delivery. Another breast-related pregnancy sign you may notice is the appearance of blue veins, which are most visible on light-skinned women.

BABY - WHAT'S HAPPENING:

Around this time, two structures develop that feed and eventually house the embryo. They are the yolk sac and the amnion. The yolk sac produces blood cells and will nourish the embryo until the placenta is fully formed. The amnion is a thin membrane that will grow into a sac, which will eventually contain the baby as well as the amniotic fluid.

TIPS AND ADVICE: Once you know you are pregnant, make an appointment with your OB-GYN. Keep in mind that most doctors will not see you before you are 8 weeks pregnant. This gives you plenty of time to prepare a comprehensive list of questions, since your first prenatal visit will probably be the longest appointment you have with your doctor throughout your entire pregnancy. You can expect an internal exam and to have your blood drawn to confirm pregnancy. You will also be tested for anemia and to measure various hormone levels.

DAILY JOURNAL

Mood:

Energy:

Cravings:

Symptoms:

Weight:

DAY 12: Date:____/____/____

MOM - WHAT'S HAPPENING:

You probably feel as if you can never get enough sleep. This is because your body is working hard to create the placenta. Also, as your first trimester progresses, the cells that make up your embryo continue to increase the amount of hCG, which prevents your uterus from shedding its lining (your period). As hCG production increases, so do levels of estrogen and progesterone. All of these changes in your body can make you feel as if you have climbed a mountain by dinner time. Make sure to get extra rest during these early weeks of baby-building. If you haven't already, take an at-home pregnancy test. You should definitely get a positive reading at this point.

BABY - WHAT'S HAPPENING:

It is hard to believe that your baby is only the size of a poppyseed, and yet has developed so much. In fact, the embryo's cells are already poised to do specialized jobs. Some cells will become internal organs, others will become bones or muscles, and still others will form the nervous system.

FOOD FOR THOUGHT: As nausea becomes a daily feature of your pregnant existence, turn to ginger for relief. Ginger root can be grated into soups or cereals. It can be dried and made into tea, or you can buy a pre-made ginger tea. Ginger ale (with real ginger) can help to soothe nausea, and many women find that the bubbles in the soda also help cut down on the severity of feeling sick. It can help to chew on ginger-flavored gum or to suck on ginger candy. Ginger products can be quite spicy, so be careful how much you consume at one time as it can exacerbate heartburn.

DAILY JOURNAL

Mood:

Energy:

Cravings:

Symptoms:

Weight:

DAY 13: Date:____/____/____

MOM - WHAT'S HAPPENING:

Although you won't feel its presence, the placenta is forming. The placenta is an organ that your body creates for the sole purpose of nourishing your growing baby. It is a temporary organ, meaning it will be delivered from your body shortly after you give birth (as afterbirth) when it is no longer needed. It is where nutrients and oxygen from your body are exchanged for waste products from the baby. This amazing organ will grow over the next nine months, and by the time the baby is born will weigh between 1 and 2 pounds.

BABY - WHAT'S HAPPENING:

The embryo and other membranes are enclosed in a two-layered membrane called the chorion, which by now has started to sprout chorion villi. These grow quickly and will cover the entire placenta by the end of your pregnancy. Some chorion villi will attach to the uterine wall. Others are free-floating villi that will attach to the placenta, but not to the endometrium. Their job is to bathe in the mother's blood in order to transfer nutrients and oxygen to your embryo.

FOOD FOR THOUGHT: Although experts generally agree that the amount of caffeine in one 8-ounce cup of coffee probably is not harmful, caffeine in larger amounts may cause miscarriages or result in low-birth weight babies. In some cases, babies born to women who consumed more than 500 milligrams of caffeine per day had breathing problems and faster heartbeats than those born to women who consumed less caffeine or who abstained all together. Thus, experts make a general recommendation that you should limit your caffeine intake to 300 milligrams or less per day.

DAILY JOURNAL

Mood:

Energy:

Cravings:

Symptoms:

Weight:

DAY 14: Date:____/____/____

MOM - WHAT'S HAPPENING:

Due to increases in oil production, you may develop a mild to moderate case of acne. This is normal and should disappear after you give birth. You may also find you frequently feel congested. This is because increased levels of estrogen cause your sinuses to produce more mucus; however, most allergy medications should not be used during pregnancy. If you are really miserable, tell your doctor. He or she will be able to suggest an appropriate remedy.

BABY - WHAT'S HAPPENING:

Today, cells that make up the embryo are flattening into a disc-shape, called the embryonic disc. By now, the primitive streak has started to develop on the embryonic disc. The primitive streak is a ridge on which cells are produced that lay the groundwork for the development of your baby's brain and spinal cord. Also, cells of the embryo have begun dividing into 3 layers: the endoderm, ectoderm, and mesoderm. Each layer has an important developmental job to do.

PREGNANCY FACT: An often overlooked and under-discussed change that your body will go through during pregnancy is the temporary worsening of your vision. Pregnancy-related blurred vision is caused by a temporary thickening of the cornea as well as by a decrease in fluid pressure in your eyes. Other eye-related symptoms include dry eyes and puffy lids. These symptoms are usually normal and will disappear after you give birth. However, a sudden change in vision can be a sign of a serious problem, such as diabetes or hypertension, and should be shared with your doctor immediately.

DAILY JOURNAL

Mood:

Energy:

Cravings:

Symptoms:

Weight:

Week 3

Starting Weight: ________

OVERVIEW

An amazing sequence of events is taking place this week. For instance, by the end of this week, your baby's heart will form into a four-chambered pump and will start beating on or around day 21!

Also, the embryo is firmly embedded in your endometrium and is now developing primitive versions of many of its body systems—a process called differentiation. In particular, this is when the central nervous system, the digestive system, the circulatory system, and the skeleton all begin to form. As your baby grows, you can expect an increase in symptoms as your body changes. By now, you should have confirmed your pregnancy with an at-home test.

It is important to get control of the various symptoms that may settle in this week, such as mood swings, increased nausea and headaches. If you find that any of your symptoms are unbearable, call your health care provider and find out what remedies and medications you may take. In general, it is important to run all medications, even over-the-counter ones, by your doctor. Now is also a good time to cut down or eliminate caffeine and to focus on eating a healthy and balanced diet.

DAY 15: Date:____/____/____

MOM - WHAT'S HAPPENING:

You have now been pregnant for just over two weeks—and you have 251 days left until you deliver your baby! At this point, you may be experiencing headaches with some frequency. Headaches during pregnancy are usually caused by an increase in hormone production and/or by increased blood circulation. Many women also drop their caffeine intake, which can cause intense headaches for four to five days.

BABY - WHAT'S HAPPENING:

Your embryo is still tiny—at 2 weeks and 1 day old, he is just 1/15 inches long. Still, the embryo is hard at work organizing its layered cells for development. The outer layer, or ectoderm, will produce your baby's neural tube from which his spine and brain will form. The middle layer, or mesoderm, is the setting for the growth of your baby's heart and circulatory system, as well reproductive organs and bones. The inner layer, or endoderm, will produce your baby's intestines, lungs, and bladder.

FOR YOUR HEALTH: Your blood volume will increase by up to 50 percent by the time you are ready to deliver your baby. Thus, it is recommended that you increase your water intake to stay hydrated since your heart works 40 percent harder than before you were pregnant. In some cases, the extra weight means that sleeping on your back can put pressure on an artery that can slow or stop blood flow to the lower half of your body. Therefore, it is also recommended that you sleep on your left side to ensure maximum blood flow to your uterus.

DAILY JOURNAL

Mood:

Energy:

Cravings:

Symptoms:

Weight:

DAY 16: Date:____/____/____

MOM - WHAT'S HAPPENING:

Your circulatory system is expanding to allow for the increase in blood volume needed to support your pregnancy. Thus, you may get occasional nosebleeds and your gums might become swollen and bleed when you brush your teeth. Unfortunately, these symptoms can last throughout your pregnancy, but should never result in excessive bleeding. You may also feel dizzy or light-headed and should be careful not to get up too quickly when laying or sitting down. Causes of dizziness include low blood pressure as well as low blood sugar. You can mediate the effects of both by staying well hydrated and eating several small meals a day.

BABY - WHAT'S HAPPENING:

Though still in the shape of a flat disc, your embryo is starting to form its body. By now, a dark line has formed on the top of the embryo—this will eventually be your baby's spine. Also, the earliest form of a heart is starting to develop and will begin beating around the end of the week.

FOOD FOR THOUGHT: Iron is critical to your pregnancy because it is required for hemoglobin production, which carries oxygen in the blood throughout the body. When you lack iron in your blood, you are known as "anemic." In order to avoid becoming anemic during your second or third trimester, the Centers for Disease Control recommends that pregnant women consume 27 milligrams of iron. In addition to eating iron-rich foods, such as red meat, beans, pumpkin seeds, potatoes with skin, and fortified cereals, it is also important to take a prenatal vitamin daily.

DAILY JOURNAL

Mood:

Energy:

Cravings:

Symptoms:

Weight:

DAY 17: Date:____/____/____

MOM - WHAT'S HAPPENING:

If you feel slight tugging or tightness in your lower abdomen, it is probably the ligaments that are attached to your uterus stretching to make room for your expanding womb. As your pregnancy progresses and your uterus continues to expand, you should expect to feel this often. Also, your cervix will begin to swell and may be tender from an increase in blood vessels. This may result in some light spotting after intercourse. There is no need to be alarmed unless you have heavy bleeding and/or cramps.

BABY - WHAT'S HAPPENING:

At this point, the notochord, or soft tissue-supporting rod, rises up out of the mesoderm (middle) layer of the embryo. The notochord is responsible for the early steps that must occur for formation of the central nervous system. Also, around now, the neural plate will form into the neural tube (spinal cord), eventually becoming the brain and the spine. Sometime after your eighth week of pregnancy, the notochord will start to be replaced by your baby's skeletal system.

TIPS AND ADVICE: Consult your doctor before taking any over-the-counter drugs such as acetaminophen, ibuprofen, and cold medicines. If you have a cold or flu, most remedies will unfortunately be off limits. If your doctor prescribes antibiotics or other medications, such as in the case of severe nausea, be sure to ask which letter category the drug falls under. The FDA breaks down drug safety into letter-based categories from A to X. A is the safest, while X indicates that a pregnant woman should not take the medicine under any circumstances.

DAILY JOURNAL

Mood:

Energy:

Cravings:

Symptoms:

Weight:

DAY 18: Date:____/____/____

MOM - WHAT'S HAPPENING:

These days, the same hormones that are necessary for sustaining your pregnancy may be putting you on edge emotionally. You may feel up one minute and down the next. You may even feel so panicked that you fear you've made a mistake by becoming pregnant. If so, don't worry: such self-doubt is normal. However, if you feel depressed for longer than two weeks, consult your physician and/or seek therapy. Keep in mind that 7 out of 10 pregnant women experience mood swings during pregnancy—particularly during the first trimester—thus, you are not alone in what you are feeling.

BABY - WHAT'S HAPPENING:

Your baby is beginning to develop its heart—in fact, the heart will be the first organ to be up and running. By now, though, the embryo has formed heart folds that will later fuse together and become the four chambers of the heart. Your embryo has also developed a cluster of cells called blood islands, which form red blood cells and endothelial cells—both of which line your baby's blood vessels.

FOOD FOR THOUGHT: Vegetarians who eat tofu, eggs, and dairy products should be getting an adequate amount of protein from these foods—though you may need an iron supplement since red meat is a major source of this mineral. However, vegans—who don't eat eggs, honey, or dairy products—must take extra care to make certain they are getting enough protein and iron. All pregnant women can add protein to their diets by incorporating lentils, soy milk, and tofu. Iron can be upped by making sure to eat a diet rich in whole grains, dried beans, and green leafy vegetables.

DAILY JOURNAL

Mood:

Energy:

Cravings:

Symptoms:

Weight:

DAY 19: Date:____/____/____

MOM - WHAT'S HAPPENING:

You may notice a slight increase in your appetite at this point—particularly in the morning. If this is accompanied by nausea, keep some crackers next to your bed so that you may eat a few before getting up. Doing so can soak up pooling stomach acids and help to stabilize your blood sugar, which can control excessive nausea. Also, you may find you are producing more saliva than you can stand to swallow. This is normal but can make nausea worse. Many pregnant women have reported that frequent tooth brushing helps cut down on the undesired side effects of producing excess saliva.

BABY - WHAT'S HAPPENING:

Your embryo has developed neural folds that grow inward to form a type of tunnel, called the neural tube, which will eventually become your baby's spinal cord and brain. It is absolutely critical that you take the recommended dose of folic acid (400 milligrams), as folate is key in the development of your baby's central nervous system.

PREGNANCY FACT: Your employment while pregnant is protected under an amendment to Title VII of the Civil Rights Act of 1964, called The Pregnancy Discrimination Act. Thus, you cannot be fired for pregnancy-related reasons, and your employer may not force you to take leave earlier than you planned to. If you develop limitations during your pregnancy, your employer must accommodate them the same as he would for other types of temporary disabilities. Additionally, no employer may refuse to hire you because you are pregnant. For further information, visit http://www.eeoc.gov.

DAILY JOURNAL

Mood:

Energy:

Cravings:

Symptoms:

Weight:

DAY 20: Date:____/____/____

MOM - WHAT'S HAPPENING:

You may have started experiencing some of the more embarrassing pregnancy symptoms—gas and bloating. Most women report that it "hurts to keep it in," so allow yourself to "let it out." This may be the one time in your life where you can get away with it!

BABY - WHAT'S HAPPENING:

The embryo is in the midst of the most important developmental time in its embryonic life. Inside the mesoderm layer of cells, a bump forms in the center of the embryo—this will become the baby's heart. Indeed, the next 3 weeks are critical to your baby's circulatory development. It is also when she is most susceptible to outside toxins, such as nicotine, alcohol, and caffeine—all of which can negatively impact her cardiac development. Also at this time, cells are coming together to form the beginnings of your baby's lungs, bladder, and intestines. By now, your embryo is just 1/17th of an inch long—about the size of the tip of a pencil.

TIPS AND ADVICE: Constipation is common throughout pregnancy but particularly during the first trimester. This is because when pregnant women experience nausea, they tend to eat starchy products, such as crackers and white bread. Many women also find it difficult to drink water, so instead only drink milk or ginger ale. All of these dietary choices, plus the fact that the uterus is putting pressure on the intestines, can make it difficult to void your bowels. For an easier time in the bathroom, exercise daily, include 25 to 35 grams of fiber in your diet, and drink plenty of water.

DAILY JOURNAL

Mood:

Energy:

Cravings:

Symptoms:

Weight:

DAY 21: Date:____/____/____

MOM - WHAT'S HAPPENING:

You are now five weeks from your last menstrual period, and at the end of the 3rd week of gestational development. You may have started to develop small spider veins. They can appear on your breasts, stomach, and legs. They are harmless and will most likely disappear after you give birth. They are evidence of your expanding circulatory system, and should be seen as a badge of pregnancy rather than a cosmetic flaw.

BABY - WHAT'S HAPPENING:

Your baby is in the most crucial period of heart development. By now, the heart folds have fused together to form a tube and they will soon divide to develop a functional four-chambered pump. Thus, today is the very first day that your baby's heart will start to beat! Though, it will most likely not be audible by you or your doctor, you would be able to see the tiny heart working on an ultrasound. Also, the embryo has developed somites along the sides of the neural tube. Somites will eventually develop into the skin, muscle, and cranial bones.

FOR YOUR HEALTH: Back pain is a very common ailment for pregnant women. There are many causes—weight gain, hormonal surges, and a shifting center of gravity. To ease back pain, it is a good idea to change positions frequently and to stretch several times per day. Purchase a body pillow and sleep with it between your knees while lying on your left side. Though it may be difficult, try to keep good posture, and continue to exercise at whatever level your doctor has approved. Taking action early in your pregnancy can help to mediate extreme lower back pain during and after labor.

DAILY JOURNAL

Mood:

Energy:

Cravings:

Symptoms:

Weight:

Week 4

Starting Weight: _________

OVERVIEW

This week, mom, you can expect to feel exhausted throughout most of your day. A variety of factors could be causing fatigue, but it is likely due to your expanding circulatory system. Over the course of your pregnancy, your body increases its blood volume between 40 and 50 percent. This means that your heart must pump faster and harder to circulate all this extra blood to your organs and extremities. In fact, your resting heart rate will be much higher than it was before you were pregnant. This means that you may become light-headed or dizzy if you get up too fast or bend over for too long. Thus, it is important to be careful when first getting out of bed in the morning. Similarly, use caution while getting in and out of the bathtub. Many pregnant women suffer "head rushes," which are sudden bouts of light-headedness and fuzzy visions. Until you get used to the sensation of experiencing a head rush, take your time when changing positions and also while exercising.

As you are taking it easy and getting extra rest, your embryo is undergoing explosive strides in its development. By the end of this week, your baby will have the earliest formations of her facial features—her eyes, ears, nose, mouth, chin, and neck will all start to develop. As will her liver, gall bladder, arms, and legs. Also, her heart will beat somewhere around 100 beats per minute, and she will be close to 1/3 of an inch long.

DAY 22: Date:____/____/____

MOM - WHAT'S HAPPENING:

Now that you have entered the fourth week of your pregnancy, you should have some idea that you are expecting, even if you haven't already taken a test. In fact, this is the week you will miss your period. If you haven't already, confirm pregnancy with an at-home test or a visit to your doctor. You may even start to have some cravings today—ice cream is a common craving, as are very salty foods. A few pregnant women end up craving strange items such as dirt, copper pennies, or detergent. Never indulge such cravings. They are symptomatic of a condition called pica and should be brought to the attention of your doctor immediately.

BABY - WHAT'S HAPPENING:

Right now, your developing baby is about the size of a bean, and yet she is undergoing some major changes. Around this time, your little embryo has started to develop her facial features, including the earliest versions of her eyes and ears. Additionally, cells are moving around to form her mouth, chin, and neck.

PREGNANCY FACT: The umbilical cord is formed from the same cells that are created when the sperm and egg join together at conception. The umbilical cord is responsible for circulating blood and nutrients between the placenta and the developing fetus, and as the cord develops, it becomes filled with a gelatin-like substance, called Wharton's jelly—named for the doctor who first discovered it. Wharton's jelly protects the blood vessels inside of the umbilical cord and is without nerve endings, so there is no pain associated with cutting the cord after birth.

DAILY JOURNAL

Mood:

Energy:

Cravings:

Symptoms:

Weight:

DAY 23: Date:____/____/____

MOM - WHAT'S HAPPENING:

Around today, some women begin to develop varicose veins. Varicose veins develop when blood pools in a vein and causes it to bulge. Occasionally, this can lead to development of a blood clot. Therefore, varicose veins should always be reported to your physician for monitoring. To prevent or decrease the severity of varicose veins, avoid gaining too much weight during your pregnancy. Also, go for daily walks, avoid crossing your legs while sitting, and wear pregnancy support hose.

BABY - WHAT'S HAPPENING:

If you could see your baby, you would notice a very exciting development has occurred—your baby has formed protruding buds where his arms and legs will be! You would also notice that his head is large in comparison to the rest of him, and he is starting to form nostrils. He has formed two slight indentations on the sides of his head from which his ears will eventually protrude.

PREGNANCY FACT: One out of every 200 pregnant women will develop a condition called hyperemesis gravidarum—severe nausea and vomiting. This is different from normal pregnancy sickness in that "morning sickness" usually begins early in the first trimester, then eases up around the 14th week. Hyperemesis gravidarum, however, often lasts throughout the pregnancy and causes such severe nausea and vomiting that the mom-to-be is unable to consume enough calories and nutrients. Your doctor can provide treatment for this condition should you suffer from it.

DAILY JOURNAL

Mood:

Energy:

Cravings:

Symptoms:

Weight:

DAY 24: Date:____/____/____

MOM - WHAT'S HAPPENING:

Your kidneys are working overtime to help process the extra waste produced by your baby. That's one reason why you feel the need to urinate more frequently. You may find you have trouble sleeping through the night because of those extra trips to the bathroom. It can help to avoid drinking anything within an hour before you go to bed. Also, be sure to completely empty your bladder, because urine left behind can cause painful urinary tract infections. One way to do this is to lean forward while you are on the toilet to help push out all the urine.

BABY - WHAT'S HAPPENING:

Your baby's facial features continue to develop, while some vital organs—particularly the lungs, pancreas, and liver—are also beginning to form. Also, your baby's heart now beats between 100 and 160 beats per minute. This is very fast, considering an adult's heart beats between 70 and 75 times per minute at rest.

TIPS AND ADVICE: As a general rule, a pregnant woman should avoid any activity that raises (and keeps) her body temperature at 102 degrees or more. Studies have shown that it is particularly dangerous to the developing embryo or fetus in the early stages of pregnancy. Thus, you avoid exercising during the hottest part of the day. Also, avoid hot tubs and saunas, both of which make can make you more prone to dizzy spells, fainting, and dehydration. Pregnant women are already at risk for experiencing these symptoms, and don't need more of them.

DAILY JOURNAL

Mood:

Energy:

Cravings:

Symptoms:

Weight:

DAY 25: Date:____/____/____

MOM - WHAT'S HAPPENING:

You are near the end of your fourth week of pregnancy, and at this point your ever-expanding circulatory system is causing your heart to pump faster and harder than before you were pregnant. This allows your body to keep up with the blood volume that is necessary to support both you and your baby. However, because your heart is working so hard, you will most likely discover that you tire easily, have frequent headaches, and get light-headed several times throughout the day.

BABY - WHAT'S HAPPENING:

Your baby is growing fast, and although just a couple of weeks ago he would have been invisible to the naked eye, he is now approximately 1/8 inch long—still tiny, but visible! Right around this time, your baby's brain is rapidly forming differentiated areas and nerves. This is a critical time for brain development. Therefore, it is more critical than ever to avoid exposure to harmful chemicals.

PREGNANCY FACT: Very few women escape stretch marks during pregnancy. In fact, up to 90 percent of pregnant women develop them on their stomach, breasts, upper thighs, and arms. Stretch marks occur when your skin is forced to expand due to weight gain and changes in body shape. Though there are many products that claim to eliminate them, stretch marks do not go away once they develop. They are also hereditary, so if your mother has them, chances are you will, too. As stretch marks develop, your skin may itch. A good lotion with vitamin E can offer some relief.

DAILY JOURNAL

Mood:

Energy:

Cravings:

Symptoms:

Weight:

DAY 26: Date:____/____/____

MOM - WHAT'S HAPPENING:

You may be experiencing an increase in nausea as hormones continue to rage throughout your body. Unfortunately for most women, nausea continues to intensify through the first trimester. Also, your breasts may feel fuller and heavier as glands that will produce milk for your baby continue to expand. For some women, this is a painful process and even putting on a bra hurts, while for others this is just a time to feel more voluptuous.

BABY - WHAT'S HAPPENING:

The embryo has taken on a curvy shape, sort of like a parenthesis. Cells are gathering in blocks along her middle that will eventually form her muscles, ligaments, ribs, and back. If you were able to see your embryo, you might be surprised to see that she has a tail. In fact, at this point, she looks more like a tadpole than a baby. But don't worry, the tail is temporary and will eventually shrink up and disappear.

FOR YOUR HEALTH: Even if you are overweight (BMI of 25 to 29.9) or obese (BMI of 30 or greater) when you become pregnant, do not try to lose weight. Experts advise that rather than trying to shed unwanted pounds, mothers-to-be should eat a healthy diet and get regular exercise. Also, keep in mind that women who are obese when they become pregnant still must consume at least 1,800 calories each day to support their pregnancy. Make those calories count by eating a varied, healthy diet that meets the daily recommendations for protein, calcium, and other vitamins and minerals.

DAILY JOURNAL

Mood:

Energy:

Cravings:

Symptoms:

Weight:

DAY 27: Date:____/____/____

MOM - WHAT'S HAPPENING:

You may find yourself experiencing vivid dreams that wake you up several times during the night. Detailed dreams are very common during pregnancy and an overwhelming majority of women tend to remember them since they often wake up just after having them. During the first trimester it is common to dream of water, fish, and even the sex of your baby. In fact, some women claim the sex of their baby was revealed to them in a dream long before they found out if they were having a boy or girl from their doctor.

BABY - WHAT'S HAPPENING:

By this time, tiny organogenesis has begun. This is the process wherein the ectoderm, mesoderm, and endoderm start to form the organs they are each responsible for creating. This means that your baby's liver and gall bladder are on their way to being developed! These organs are vital to bile production, digestion, and for the processing of toxins that enter the blood stream by crossing the placenta.

PREGNANCY FACT: Ultrasounds are a safe, noninvasive way to monitor your baby's progress in utero. An ultrasound creates a picture by using high-frequency sound waves. Echoes are transformed into black and white images that are viewed on a monitor. The test is performed as needed throughout your pregnancy by your doctor. A topical wand will likely be used on the outside of your pelvis. Occasionally, a probe may be inserted into the vagina, during what is called an "internal ultrasound." This can offer more information if your doctor suspects a problem or wants to confirm your due date.

DAILY JOURNAL

Mood:

Energy:

Cravings:

Symptoms:

Weight:

DAY 28: Date:____/____/____

MOM - WHAT'S HAPPENING:

Although you still have 238 days left until delivery, you may breathe a little sigh of relief, as you have just concluded the first lunar month of your pregnancy! The potential for miscarriage decreases with every week. Because your uterus continues to expand, you are probably noticing that your pants are beginning to get snug. This may be a big reality check for you, as many women report their pregnancy didn't feel "real" until their regular clothes no longer fit.

BABY - WHAT'S HAPPENING:

By the end of his fourth week of development, your embryo may measure up to ¼ inch long, and the cells that make up your baby's body are changing rapidly, becoming more specialized in the jobs they do. For instance, at this point, the brain has developed three major components: the prosencephalon (forebrain), mesencepalon (midbrain) and rhombencephalon (hindbrain), which will further divide during the next week of your pregnancy to set up the senses.

FOOD FOR THOUGHT: Pregnancy is a great time to go organic. Commercially grown foods contain harmful pesticides that can cross the placenta and enter your baby's blood stream. In fact, research has linked these chemicals to cancer and other diseases. Unfortunately, organic products can be quite expensive, so if you have to prioritize, make sure the following items are organic: milk, meat, nectarines, pears, peaches, apples, cherries, strawberries, imported grapes, spinach, potatoes, bell peppers, and raspberries, which often contain the highest levels of chemicals.

DAILY JOURNAL

Mood:

Energy:

Cravings:

Symptoms:

Weight:

Lunar Month

Two

PHOTO

Place a photo of you during
your second month here

My Monthly Update

Waist Measurement: ____________________

Weight: ____________________

Mood: ____________________

PREGNANCY CHECKLIST

- ❑ Drink at least 6-8 glasses of water, juice or milk every day
- ❑ Visit your health care provider for a prenatal care checkup
- ❑ Start eating a healthy and nutritious prenatal diet, including dark green leafy vegetables, whole grains, dried beans and peas, peanut butter, and asparagus
- ❑ Do Kegel exercises to strengthen your pelvic muscles
- ❑ Talk to your doctor about your optimal pregnancy weight range
- ❑ Ask your doctor which prenatal tests you will need
- ❑ Take steps to minimize your morning sickness, such as keeping crackers handy
- ❑ Get another family member to clean your pets' litter box as pets can transmit diseases to pregnant women
- ❑ Avoid foods that cause gas and heartburn
- ❑ Avoid artificial sweeteners — such as those in diet soda — which can upset the stomach
- ❑ Read books on pregnancy and talk to other mothers to alleviate fears and get questions answered

MY PERSONAL CHECKLIST:

- ❑ ....
- ❑ ....
- ❑ ....

MY HOPES FOR THIS MONTH:

....

....

....

....

....

....

Lunar Month

Two

First Trimester

IF YOU ARE LIKE MOST MOMS-TO-BE, you will breathe a sigh of relief as you enter into each new month, because it means your pregnancy is progressing nicely, and that you are getting closer to holding your baby in your arms. As you enter your second month of pregnancy, you should prepare yourself for the many changes that will happen to your own body as well as for the incredible growth that your baby will undergo. For example, during this month, your baby reaches a major milestone—she leaves the embryonic stage and becomes a fetus.

The transition from embryo to fetus brings with it many exciting developments. This month, your baby develops her facial features, including her eyes, nose, mouth, chin, jaw, and ears. With each passing day, she will look more and more like a baby and less like a tiny tadpole. In fact, by the end of this month, your baby will have formed her fingers and toes and her embryonic tail will disappear. Prepare to marvel at your first ultrasound as her body straightens out from the C shape to a nearly erect tiny person!

WHAT TO EXPECT THIS MONTH

The second month of pregnancy is when you can expect to see an increase in the intensity of your symptoms. For instance, you are likely to be more tired than usual, because much of your energy is diverted to growing your baby and to building the placenta. And, due to hormone surges and the pressure of your expanding uterus on your bladder, you can expect to feel the need to urinate more frequently—even waking 2 to 3 times at night after you've gone to bed. Finally, you will probably feel less in control of your emotions this month and nausea will be at its peak. If you find yourself with your head in the toilet wondering how you got into this situation, just keep in mind that though you feel awful, your baby is making massive developmental strides this month.

The next few weeks are critical to the development of your baby's heart. In just a few weeks, your baby's heart will divide into four chambers and begin to form valves. Your baby's heartbeat will be audible by the end of this month by using a handheld ultrasound machine called a Doppler. Her heart will pump very fast—approximately twice as fast as your resting heart rate. Also this month, your baby's brain, spine, kidneys, arms, legs, fingers, and toes will all become functional. Indeed, by the end of the second lunar month of pregnancy, your baby will have grown all the organs she will need to eventually exist outside of the womb. After this month, her organs and body structures will continue to mature as she gains weight and becomes further along in her fetal development.

THINGS TO CONSIDER

As mentioned earlier in this book, it is important to remind yourself in the second month that every woman's pregnancy is different. Try not to compare yourself to other pregnant women you may know. Indeed, even all the pregnancy books are merely outlines of what may happen over the course of gestation. Thus, you may experience symptoms not covered in this or any other book, or you may have minimal or even no symptoms at all.

The second month of pregnancy is very exciting, because you will have your first visit with your doctor or health care provider. This visit often includes an ultrasound, during which you will get the first glimpse of your baby! It is a good idea for both you and your partner to come prepared to the appointment with information about your family medical history. And of course, bring a list of questions to ask your doctor, as you will likely forget some of what is on your mind.

TIPS FOR COPING

You may be experiencing the same symptoms as last month, though more intensely. Therefore, continue last month's strategies for coping and begin to employ a few new ones. Make going to bed early a priority, take naps during the day if you can, and be sure to go for a brisk walk in the fresh air each day—even if you don't feel like it. Though it is true that you may notice your motivation plummet this month, getting outside each day is good for your overall health and disposition.

You may also notice that your appetite has either increased or decreased this month—either way, it is a good idea to always be prepared with a snack to either take the edge off sudden hunger, or to avert nausea. It can also help to carry around slices of lemon in a plastic bag so you can put the fruit up to your nose to cover any offending odors—pregnant women swear by this little trick!

WHAT TO EAT

As you did in the first month, continue to eat a variety of nutrient-rich foods. Calcium becomes very important this month since your baby's heart and bones are on the developmental fast track. Overall, virtually every nutrient that is considered important for human health should be increased so you can meet the needs of your changing body and those of your developing baby—and this includes fat!

You might be surprised to learn that fat is something that you should be including in your diet now that you are pregnant. Fats are important during pregnancy because they contribute to a well-rounded and varied diet, and help your body absorb nutrients. For example, research has shown that certain vitamins (A, D, E, and K) are fat- soluble, meaning that the body can use them only if they are eaten with a certain amount of fat. Note, however, that this does not justify adding unhealthy saturated or trans fats to your diet. Instead, focus on monounsaturated and polyunsaturated fats—known as "good fats," that lower LDL (bad) cholesterol and increase HDL (good) cholesterol. Avoid fat-free products entirely, as they are often filled with chemicals your body does not need.

Indeed, there are several foods that pregnant women should avoid altogether. These include lunch meats, raw fish, unpasteurized dairy products, and soft or blue-veined cheeses. These products can be contaminated with bacteria that are hazardous—even deadly—to your growing baby.

HOW MUCH WEIGHT TO GAIN

Over the coming month, aim to gain only another pound—two at the most. As your pregnancy advances, you will probably notice an acceleration of weight gain, but at this point it is a good idea to gain slowly. Excessive weight gain can intensify the symptoms of pregnancy, such as joint and back pain. Also, studies have shown that women who overeat during pregnancy have more trouble losing the excess weight after their baby is born.

EXERCISE TIPS AND ADVICE

If you haven't begun an exercise regimen already, this is a good time to start. It is important, though, to consult with your health care provider to make certain that any proposed fitness program is appropriate for the individual needs of your pregnancy. This is especially true if you are not in the habit of exercising already, because a workout routine that is too strenuous can result in injury to both you and your fetus. Women who are already in the habit of exercising regularly can continue those same workouts with their doctor's approval, even if they are quite rigorous. A safe bet for nearly every pregnant woman, though, is to go for a 20- to 30-minute walk each day.

POTENTIAL SYMPTOMS AND HOW TO ALLEVIATE THEM

This month you will probably find that the toilet has become your closest friend. This is because you will likely spend lots of time in the bathroom either vomiting or clearing your bladder. Unfortunately, these symptoms are likely to get worse before they get better, which is usually around week 14. In the meantime, it is a good idea to keep bland snacks handy to prevent stomach acids from accumulating and stirring up nausea. You may also want to wear panty liners in case you have an accident while waiting for the bathroom. Leaks happen—it is nothing to be ashamed of, and being prepared will help you ward off embarrassing situations.

WAYS OTHERS CAN HELP

If you have other children, it will be important to ensure that their needs are met, even as you deal with the increasing symptoms of your pregnancy. If you need help tending to your other children, involve your family members. Ask grandma to take your toddler to the park or out to lunch on a Saturday afternoon—make it special and individual for each child. Also, encourage your partner to start spending extra time with the children. There's a good chance that the kids will appreciate having Dad to themselves while you catch an extra hour of sleep in the morning or nap during the afternoon.

"Before you were conceived I wanted you, Before you were born I loved you, Before you were here an hour I would die for you, This is the miracle of Mother's Love."
~ Maureen Hawkins

Week 5

Starting Weight: _________

OVERVIEW

This week you will probably notice some vaginal discharge, called leukorrhea. It is usually white or light yellow and will be with you for the duration of your pregnancy. Another symptom you may experience is extreme soreness in your breasts. You may even feel a tingling sensation that makes any contact unbearable. This is a normal side effect, and occurs as a result of your breasts preparing themselves to feed your baby after he is born. You may also find that your bra is uncomfortable—not quite too small, but not the right fit. If you haven't already, it is a good idea to purchase a few soft sports bras that can stretch as you grow.

As you continue to grow, so does your baby. This week he will start to form the early stages of his facial features. His eyes will start to develop, though their final color will not be set until a week or so after birth. Your baby's brain will undergo rapid development this week as it forms its three main sections. His arms and legs will appear, as will his feet and hands—though they are webbed. Also this week, your baby's embryonic tail will continue shrink. By the end of this week, your baby will have a heartbeat that is visible on an ultrasound, and though you will not be able to feel it, he will be testing out his new limbs by moving and kicking inside the amniotic fluid.

DAY 29: Date:____/____/____

MOM - WHAT'S HAPPENING:

By now your body secretions have created a mucus plug that seals off your cervix. This helps protect you and your growing baby from infection. Also, your cervix continues to soften and may start to have a blue tint. Softening of the cervix occurs over the course of your pregnancy to prepare it for effacement, which is the thinning or shortening of the cervix. This must occur in order for the cervix to dilate, or open, so your baby can pass through during birth.

BABY - WHAT'S HAPPENING:

At the beginning of this week, your baby's facial features begin to form. Her eyes are starting to develop lenses and a little color. She is beginning to look more recognizable as a human as her arms, hands, legs, and feet become more prominent. Meanwhile, the umbilical cord is well-established and visible at the point where it is connected to your uterus. It houses a large vein and two arteries that work together to circulate blood and nutrition to your baby.

PREGNANCY FACT: In vitro fertilization (IVF) is a procedure used to bypass blocked fallopian tubes. IVF is done by removing a healthy egg from a woman and combining it with healthy sperm in a fluid medium. Once the egg is fertilized and has undergone cellular division, the blastocyst is implanted in the woman's uterus. It was considered quite a miracle when Louise Brown became the first "test tube" baby. She was the first successful IVF birth, born by Cesarean section on July 25, 1978, weighing 5 pounds, 12 ounces. Since Brown's birth, the procedure has become fairly common.

DAILY JOURNAL

Mood:

Energy:

Cravings:

Symptoms:

Weight:

DAY 30: Date:____/____/____

MOM - WHAT'S HAPPENING:

As your body settles in to being pregnant, you may find you are in the apex of nausea, irritability, and breast soreness. One symptom that starts to become particularly troublesome this week is the frequent need to urinate. This is because your uterus has nearly doubled its size and is putting additional pressure on your bladder. It is important to void your bladder whenever you feel the urge to urinate. Holding urine in can lead to urinary tract infections and will definitely make you feel bloated and uncomfortable.

BABY - WHAT'S HAPPENING:

Your little ½-inch, raspberry-sized embryo now has hands and feet. Though visible at this point, they do not really look like hands and feet, but rather resemble tiny paddles, since the fingers and toes are webbed. His arms and legs are getting longer, and he even has shoulders. Your baby's tailbone still has the appearance of a tail, but it will continue to shrink and will eventually disappear.

PREGNANCY FACT: If you have a cat, it is time to pass kitty litter duty to your partner. In fact, you should have limited contact with your cat until your pregnancy is over. This is because cats can carry the toxoplasmosis virus. This virus is very dangerous to your developing baby and is found in cat feces. Keep in mind that indoor cats who use litter boxes can track the virus all over the house, so it is important that your partner keep the house extremely clean by vacuuming and mopping daily. Consider moving the litter box to a part of the house you rarely visit, such as the basement or boiler room.

DAILY JOURNAL

Mood:

Energy:

Cravings:

Symptoms:

Weight:

DAY 31: Date:____/____/____

MOM - WHAT'S HAPPENING:

Today your feelings of dizziness or faintness may be accompanied by hot flashes. This is due in part to your ever-expanding circulatory system. Because your heart is pumping harder and faster, you can expect to continue to feel dizzy. If you find you are fainting frequently or experiencing vertigo, be sure to speak to your doctor. Emotionally, you may feel mild to severe anxiety about becoming a parent—this, too, is normal, and it can help to discuss your fears with your partner or other women who have been pregnant.

BABY - WHAT'S HAPPENING:

Your baby's face continues to form, and the nose, mouth, and jaw are now visible. Also, the inner ear is connecting to the middle ear, getting her closer to being able to hear your voice through the womb. Her brain has divided into its three main sections—the hindbrain, midbrain, and forebrain. Each of these areas is responsible for several body functions and will continue to mature as your pregnancy progresses.

FOR YOUR HEALTH: During the early stages of pregnancy, the cervix swells with extra blood and becomes very sensitive to touch. Thus, bleeding after the insertion of a gynecological instrument or after intercourse is common and not cause for alarm. In fact, light spotting or bleeding throughout pregnancy is normal. However, if you notice you are bleeding heavily, or if it is accompanied by cramps and fever, call your doctor immediately, as this could indicate a serious problem. Your doctor may restrict your activity and ask you to abstain from intercourse for the duration of your pregnancy.

DAILY JOURNAL

Mood:

Energy:

Cravings:

Symptoms:

Weight:

DAY 32: Date:____/____/____

MOM - WHAT'S HAPPENING:

By now, you may start to notice a thick, whitish vaginal discharge called leukorrhea. This is caused by high levels of estrogen and increased blood flow to the vaginal area. It is a normal pregnancy symptom and should not worry you. If, however, the discharge has a foul odor or is green or yellow, be sure to let your doctor know about it, because that could indicate an infection or STD. Wearing panty liners can decrease the unpleasant side effects of leukorrhea, but avoid using over-the-counter creams and definitely do not douche.

BABY - WHAT'S HAPPENING:

If you could see your embryo, you would find that she is about the size of your pinky nail. You would also notice that her eyelids have crept down her eyes and will eventually be sealed shut and appear as two slits. Also, your baby's digestive system continues to build itself, and she has likely developed her pancreas and appendix by now.

TIPS AND ADVICE: You should completely avoid most herbal products while you are pregnant. Certain herbs, such as St. John's wort and black cohosh, can stimulate uterine contractions and cause a miscarriage. Essential oils made from herbs can also be dangerous. These include rosemary, cinnamon, fennel, oregano, and sage. Since the Food and Drug Administration does not regulate herbal remedies, one can never be sure what is in an herbal product. If you feel unsure about whether a particular herb could threaten your pregnancy, play it safe and avoid it.

DAILY JOURNAL

Mood:

Energy:

Cravings:

Symptoms:

Weight:

DAY 33: Date:____/____/____

MOM - WHAT'S HAPPENING:

Thanks to surging levels of hCG, estrogen, and progesterone, you may be experiencing occasional headaches. These should be similar in intensity to headaches that you would get if you skipped your morning coffee or before you get your period. If you suffer from migraines, you may find that they go away completely, get much worse, or stay the same. Before taking anything to relieve your headaches, it is very important to consult your doctor.

BABY - WHAT'S HAPPENING:

At this point, your baby's liver is producing red blood cells. Later in her development, bone marrow will take over this very important job. Also, at this point, her final set of kidneys have formed, but are not yet processing urine. Meanwhile, her facial features continue to become more prominent, as does the definition of her hands and feet. Additionally, another exciting brain development has occurred by now—your baby's hypothalamus is formed.

FOR YOUR HEALTH: It is a great idea to start doing Kegel exercises early in pregnancy, because they will strengthen the muscles at the bottom of your pelvis, which will help with several pregnancy-related complications, such as urinary incontinence and hemorrhoids. Kegels will also strengthen muscles that do much of the work during labor and delivery. Kegel exercises are simple once you identify the correct muscle group. To do to this, stop urination midstream and take note of the muscles you use to do this. Once you have done identified the correct muscles, flex and release several times a day.

DAILY JOURNAL

Mood:

Energy:

Cravings:

Symptoms:

Weight:

DAY 34: Date:____/____/____

MOM - WHAT'S HAPPENING:

By now, you've probably burst into tears at work and was asked to "be rational" by your partner. Though it can be incredibly frustrating to feel out of control of your emotions, know that you are not alone. In fact, most women report feeling like a stranger to themselves while pregnant, because of mild to wild mood swings. Take comfort in knowing that this is temporary, and you will feel like yourself again once you have your baby.

BABY - WHAT'S HAPPENING:

Your baby's brain is working overtime to develop all of the nooks and crannies in which spinal fluid and blood will circulate. Interestingly, his skull is transparent, and the cranial bones that will protect his head have not yet formed. This means that if you were able to look at your baby's head, you would probably be able to see straight through to his brain. Meanwhile, the hypothalamus continues to mature, and is responsible for the regulating of body temperature, emotions, hunger, and thirst.

FOOD FOR THOUGHT: Consider steaming, blending, and then freezing a large batch of broccoli puree to add nutrition to sauces, baked goods, and salads. There may come a point at which your nausea prevents you from eating this powerhouse vegetable, and so disguising it in other foods you can tolerate is a great way to get the same nutritional benefits. Broccoli contains vitamins C, K, A, E, B1, B3, B5, as well as folate, fiber, protein, iron, calcium, and omega 3s—plus much more. Be creative with recipes, and make foods that are easy to tote, like muffins and breads.

DAILY JOURNAL

Mood:

Energy:

Cravings:

Symptoms:

Weight:

DAY 35: Date:____/____/____

MOM - WHAT'S HAPPENING:

With 231 days left to go in your pregnancy, you might feel a bit overwhelmed, especially if you are experiencing moderate to severe pregnancy sickness. You may also be feeling nervous about the condition of your baby and anxious to talk to your doctor. This final week before your first prenatal appointment can feel like it is dragging on forever—but rest assured, your emotions will turn to awe and excitement once you see your tiny babe on the ultrasound monitor.

BABY - WHAT'S HAPPENING:

At the end of the fifth week of development, a groove has formed in your baby's throat where her voice box, or larynx, will be. Her face also continues to take shape, and her mouth seems huge compared to the rest of her face. And though you won't be able to feel it, your baby has begun to swim and kick inside the amniotic sac.

PREGNANCY FACT: If you haven't already done so, you will probably be given the option to see a genetic counselor at or around the time of your first prenatal appointment. Genetic counselors ask you many questions about your family medical history and may also take blood and tissue samples from both you and your partner to find out if either of you has specific genes that carry diseases such as cystic fibrosis, sickle cell anemia, and Tay-Sachs—all three of which both parents must carry in order for it to be passed on to your baby.

DAILY JOURNAL

Mood:

Energy:

Cravings:

Symptoms:

Weight:

Week 6

Starting Weight: _________

OVERVIEW

Though other people likely have no idea that you are pregnant, you will probably notice that your midsection has grown just enough to make your clothes feel tight across your belly. You are certainly not ready to buy maternity clothes yet, but you may want to wear pants and skirts that have an elastic or stretchy waste so that you can breathe easier. Also, forcing yourself into tight pants will make heartburn and gas more intense as these symptoms start to make regular appearances in your day. Indeed, gas and heartburn will increase this week and get progressively worse as your stomach is crowded out by your expanding uterus. Also, you may find you have developed aversions to some foods—meat is often a big turn off when pregnant. Don't worry if this happens to you—just be sure to get protein from other sources, such as tofu, nuts, and beans.

As you adjust to your expanding belly and digestion issues, your baby is busy building her lungs. Indeed, this is a big week for her respiratory system. Though the lungs will not finish forming until very late in the last trimester, by the end of this week they will have their basic structure and resemble a tiny version of a fully functional set of adult lungs. Also, by the end of this week, your baby will graduate from the embryonic stage of development into the fetal stage.

DAY 36: Date:___/___/___

MOM - WHAT'S HAPPENING:

Your uterus has doubled in size and your expanding circulatory system has added extra fluids to your system. As a result, you have started to grow out of your clothes and may feel increasingly bloated or gassy as pressure mounts on your intestines. Additionally, your breasts are probably feeling fuller and heavier than normal. Keep in mind that as your pregnancy progresses, you will likely go up a size or two in bras. Also, after you have your baby, you may still go up another size once your milk comes in.

BABY - WHAT'S HAPPENING:

Facial definition continues as your baby's features become more prominent. His nose, nostrils, eyes, and lips are recognizable. Exciting things are happening inside his mouth, as well. Today, your little baby has a tongue and approximately 20 buds line the gums where his teeth will be.

FOR YOUR HEALTH: Hip and joint pain often accompany pregnancy—and if steps are not taken to manage your joint health early on, it can become very painful later in your pregnancy. Therefore, it is a good idea to get in the habit of stretching, walking, and resting every single day. A sample itinerary is to do some simple yoga stretches in the morning before you get out of bed. If you have time, take a brisk walk in the morning or during lunch. At various points in the day, be sure to get some rest and to change your positions often.

DAILY JOURNAL

Mood:

Energy:

Cravings:

Symptoms:

Weight:

DAY 37: Date:___/___/___

MOM - WHAT'S HAPPENING:

You may start to have the sensation that food "sits like a brick" in your stomach after you eat, only to suddenly feel ravenous and desperate to fill your stomach again. This is a common pregnancy complaint. In fact, many women report that they go from starving to full and straight back to starving again with no gradation. This is because increased levels of progesterone cause your stomach and intestines to become sluggish, slowing digestion. This causes the sensation that food is not moving.

BABY - WHAT'S HAPPENING:

If you could see into your uterus, you would notice that your baby's fingers and toes are starting to form. Though they are still webbed, their definition as individual digits is apparent. Also, the process of ossification, or the hardening of the bones, has begun. In fact, tiny bones have likely grown to meet the first joint in your baby's fingers and toes.

TIPS AND ADVICE: You may develop carpal tunnel syndrome as your wrists swell, because fluid puts pressure on the nerve that runs from the arm to the hand. This can be quite painful, especially if you had carpal tunnel syndrome before you were pregnant or if you work at a computer. Many drugstores sell splints that will help relieve the pain by keeping the wrist supported. It is also a good idea to wear soft splints while you sleep so that your wrists are protected throughout the night. Luckily, this type of carpal tunnel syndrome usually goes away after the first week the baby is born.

DAILY JOURNAL

Mood:

Energy:

Cravings:

Symptoms:

Weight:

DAY 38: Date:___/___/___

MOM - WHAT'S HAPPENING:

Around this time your placenta becomes responsible for producing another important pregnancy hormone called human placental lactogen (HPL). HPL is the hormone that is most responsible for the growth of your baby. It also breaks down sugars and proteins so that your baby is able to digest them. HPL is also in charge of stimulating milk production in your breasts so that your baby may feed immediately after delivery.

BABY - WHAT'S HAPPENING:

Your baby's digestive system is developing quickly, and her intestines are actually protruding into the umbilical cord, rather than being located inside her lower abdomen, which isn't yet large enough to accommodate them. This is because her kidneys, liver, and pancreas take up most of the space in her lower abdominal area. Also, though you still cannot tell the sex of your baby, cells are aligning to form your baby's external reproductive organs and nipples.

FOOD FOR THOUGHT: Cranberries are a wonder food when it comes to staving off urinary tract infections (UTI), which can be common during pregnancy. Indeed, drinking 8 ounces of sugar-free cranberry juice per day can help protect your bladder from the contaminating Escherichia coli, which is the most common bacteria found in UTIs. Researchers believe that tannins in cranberries may prevent Escherichia coli from attaching itself to the bladder, thus flushing it before causing infection.

DAILY JOURNAL

Mood:

Energy:

Cravings:

Symptoms:

Weight:

DAY 39: Date:___/___/___

MOM - WHAT'S HAPPENING:

You are in the middle of your sixth week of pregnancy, and eight weeks from your last period. Thus, you may be feeling anxious about your first prenatal visit. Keep in mind your fears about the health of the baby are natural and should be alleviated by the reassuring sight of seeing your baby's heart beating on the ultrasound. Many women say that seeing the heartbeat for the first time was when they felt a connection to their baby. If this does not happen for you, don't fret—there will be some other marker that connects you to the baby.

BABY - WHAT'S HAPPENING:

Your baby's lungs continue to develop, and by now he should have formed two primitive tubes called main stem bronchi that connect his throat to his lungs. As time goes on, each bronchus will branch out into smaller bronchi forming a kind of upside down tree in each of his lungs. The smallest bronchi are called bronchioles, and your baby will eventually have 30,000 of them when his lungs reach maturity.

TIPS AND ADVICE: There are a few reasons you become more prone to hemorrhoids while pregnant. One is that high levels of progesterone causes the outer part of your veins to relax, which allows them to swell. If you are troubled by hemorrhoids, try adding more fiber to your diet to make moving your bowels easier, since straining can result in hemorrhoids. You should also make sure to get plenty of exercise as the increased blood circulation can prevent blood from pooling in the lower half of your body—another reason why veins tend to swell.

DAILY JOURNAL

Mood:

Energy:

Cravings:

Symptoms:

Weight:

DAY 40: Date:___/___/___

MOM - WHAT'S HAPPENING:

By now your uterus has expanded from the size of a pear to about the size of a grapefruit. This would account for any additional pressure you may feel on your bladder. You may also have a tightening sensation in the area between the top of your pubic bone and your belly button. This means that the skin is either starting to—or getting ready to—stretch. If you are very thin, you may also notice that your skin is itchy and dry as a result of early stretching. Cocoa butter can offer relief; unfortunately, it cannot prevent stretch marks.

BABY - WHAT'S HAPPENING:

Your baby's first set of 20 teeth—called primary, baby, or milk teeth—form in utero beneath her gums between six and eight weeks of development. Thus, by this time, your baby's gums house the tiny structures that will produce her teeth. She will likely be born with smooth, shiny gums, unless she is among the very small percentage of babies who are born with one or two neonatal teeth.

PREGNANCY FACT: Braxton Hicks are uterine contractions that can start up as early in your pregnancy as six weeks. You won't be able to feel them yet, of course, but sometime in the middle of your pregnancy, you may start to notice a slight sensation of tightening and releasing in your lower abdomen. Some women feel them as early as the second trimester, though they are more common during the third. If you experience Braxton Hicks contractions with any intensity before 37 weeks, however, you should immediately let your doctor know.

DAILY JOURNAL

Mood:

Energy:

Cravings:

Symptoms:

Weight:

DAY 41: Date:___/___/___

MOM - WHAT'S HAPPENING:

By now, you've probably developed a superhuman sense of smell. Odds are you can smell a cup of coffee four or five cubicles away from you. Or perhaps your husband's once alluring cologne now sends you reeling, even when he's on the other side of the room. This very normal pregnancy side effect is due to the additional estrogen that is surging through your body. An old wives' tale states that it is nature's way of alerting mom to possible toxins long before they come near her and her growing baby.

BABY - WHAT'S HAPPENING:

Your baby's body is starting to uncurl and straighten out. She is moving around in the amniotic fluid and makes reflexive movements in response to outside stimuli—such as if you put headphones to your belly or push on your pelvis. These reflexive movements will be visible to you when you have your first ultrasound. If you've already had one, you know how exciting it is to see your baby move for the first time!

FOR YOUR HEALTH: If you are having trouble sleeping at night, try to eliminate any conditions that disturb sleep. For instance, avoid drinking caffeinated beverages or eating chocolate in the evening. Even a small amount of caffeine can affect your sleep when you are pregnant. Experts recommend you to engage in relaxing activities before bed—take a bath, ask your partner for a massage, or meditate. Unwinding can make a world of difference in the quality of your sleep, since you are likely stressed much of your day about becoming a parent.

DAILY JOURNAL

Mood:

Energy:

Cravings:

Symptoms:

Weight:

DAY 42: Date:___/___/___

MOM - WHAT'S HAPPENING:

You have reached the end of your eighth week of pregnancy, according to the LMP calculation. Your baby has completed six weeks of incredible development. Right around now, you will miss your second period. That, coupled with your first prenatal visit, may have you settling into the reality that you are, in fact, pregnant. This can be both an exciting and anxious time for you and your partner. This reality check along with increasing fatigue, nausea, and mood swings may make you feel crazy, but you're not—just pregnant!

BABY - WHAT'S HAPPENING:

Your baby is no longer an embryo as he now begins his journey through fetal development. His tiny body has formed all the organs and other components that he will have when he is born. From now until the end of your pregnancy, the structures and organs that he already has will simply be maturing. With each passing day, the fetus will look more and more human as his features continue to sharpen and take shape.

FOOD FOR THOUGHT: It can be difficult to consume enough protein while you are pregnant. This is especially true during the first trimester when nausea often prevents you from eating meat and other good protein sources. Keep in mind that the FDA recommends pregnant women consume 60 grams of protein each day—just 10 grams more than before you were expecting. If you are turned off by meat , or if you are a vegetarian, you can easily get the recommended daily dose of protein by eating eggs, lentils, dried beans, cheese, tofu, tempeh, and seitan (wheat gluten).

DAILY JOURNAL

Mood:

Energy:

Cravings:

Symptoms:

Weight:

Week 7

Starting Weight: _________

OVERVIEW

This week you will find yourself feeling hot, tired, and cranky. All these symptoms can be blamed on surging levels of hormones. Indeed, the increased levels of estrogen and progesterone are likely to wreak havoc on your moods. You may find yourself in tears at work or cursing everyone in front of you while driving home. Hopefully, your partner is reading this book with you and, therefore, knows what to expect as well, since he will likely receive the brunt of your whirlwind mood swings. It is important to recognize, however, if you are experiencing unmanageable depression, particularly if you suffered from bouts of depression before you were pregnant. If you find that you are unable to perform your normal daily tasks for more than 2 weeks, it is time to alert your doctor, as you may need treatment for depression.

Meanwhile, your little babe is looking more human each day. This week, his embryonic tail will completely disappear, and his skeleton will begin to form. His fingers, toes, arms and legs will be wiggling around in the amniotic fluid. Your baby is well into his fetal stage of development and is starting to form his very individual characteristics. For instance, this week the swirls of your baby's one-of-a-kind fingerprints will appear on his fingers. Also, the beginning stages of the development of your baby's external sex organs occur this week, making it just a matter of weeks before you can find out if you are having a boy or a girl.

DAY 43: Date:___/___/___

MOM - WHAT'S HAPPENING:

You are now nine weeks from your last period and may find yourself feeling overheated much of the time. This is due to estrogen production and an increase in blood volume, which forces your heart to pump extra beats every minute. Thus, walking up a single flight of stairs may leave you feeling sweaty and winded. Take it easy when you can and dress in layers. Many pregnant women end up wear tanks tops indoors most of the time—even in winter—because their internal thermostat is so high.

BABY - WHAT'S HAPPENING:

By now, your fetus has developed nerves and muscles throughout his body. Additionally, cartilage and bones continue to form, giving your baby bendable joints and expanded mobility. Your baby also has the tiniest kernel of external sex organs, though you can't see anything or tell whether you are carrying a boy or a girl just yet; however, the sex was determined at the moment of conception.

TIPS AND ADVICE: Due to fluctuating estrogen levels and increased cardiac output, between 50 and 70 percent of pregnant women experience hot flashes at some point in their pregnancies. For some women, hot flashes occur mostly at night while in bed and are called night sweats. A simple solution is to wear very little clothing to bed (or none at all) and have a fan nearby in case it gets bad enough to wake you. Hot flashes are often accompanied by excessive thirst. So, keep ice water on your nightstand for a late-night refreshment.

DAILY JOURNAL

Mood:

Energy:

Cravings:

Symptoms:

Weight:

DAY 44: Date:___/___/___

MOM - WHAT'S HAPPENING:

It is important to be mindful of what you consume, as your baby has begun to drink the amniotic fluid. It is OK to eat a varied diet, of course, and some mothers swear their babies end up having a taste for the foods they ate while pregnant. However, any over-the-counter medications, herbal teas, alcohol, and nicotine will be ingested by your baby through the placental connection as well as through the amniotic fluid. When your baby's kidneys begin producing sterile urine in the next week or so, he will urinate in the very same amniotic fluid that he drinks.

BABY - WHAT'S HAPPENING:

Around today, your baby's abdomen expands to make room for his intestines, which have begun moving out of the umbilical cord and into his abdominal cavity. The placenta continues to mature and produces hormones that suppress ovulation and menstruation. Also, your baby now has tiny earlobes, and his eyeballs are formed. Another exciting characteristic has developed—your baby's fingerprints!

PREGNANCY FACT: The natural birthing technique known as the Lamaze method was first introduced in 1951, by the French physician Ferdnand Lamaze. Dr. Lamaze had studied the technique in Russia. He then began to teach this new approach to giving birth, which included breathing exercises, coaching from the partner, childbirth classes, and relaxation techniques. The method was popularized in the late 1950s after Dr. Lamaze helped Marjorie Karmel give birth. She wrote a book called, Thank You, Dr. Lamaze, and became a Lamaze instructor, co-founding what is now Lamaze International.

DAILY JOURNAL

Mood:

Energy:

Cravings:

Symptoms:

Weight:

DAY 45: Date:___/___/___

MOM - WHAT'S HAPPENING:

Your biggest complaint these days is likely to be extreme exhaustion. This is partially due to the construction zone in your pelvis that is building your placenta. Also contributing to fatigue is the fact that your body's metabolism has sped up and your blood pressure and your blood sugar are lower than before you were pregnant. This has your system operating on overdrive.

BABY - WHAT'S HAPPENING:

Your baby is now about the size of a cherry. Her hands can open and close and she may even "grab" her nose, umbilical cord, or anything else she can get her hands on. Also, your baby's skeleton is shaping up and hardening as her bones are forming by maturing cartilage and her joints become usable. At this point, your baby has pronounced elbows and is probably moving around quite a bit, testing out her new body. If you haven't had your first ultrasound yet, prepare to be dazzled by your tiny baby's acrobatics.

FOOD FOR THOUGHT: It is important to consume 1,000 milligrams of calcium each day to support your growing baby. She needs calcium to form strong bones and teeth and to develop healthy organs. Indeed, calcium is necessary for your baby to establish a normal heart rhythm and to perform healthy blood clotting. Therefore, include 4 servings of calcium-rich foods each day, such as low-fat dairy products, tofu, calcium-fortified orange juice, cereal, and whole grain bread. If your baby does not get enough calcium she will absorb it from your bones, causing problems for you later on.

DAILY JOURNAL

Mood:

Energy:

Cravings:

Symptoms:

Weight:

DAY 46: Date:___/___/___

MOM - WHAT'S HAPPENING:

Today you might be suffering from heartburn. Heartburn is caused by stomach acids rising up into the esophagus. Because the esophagus slackens during pregnancy, you may feel a burning sensation from your throat all the way down into your stomach. Heartburn affects 1 out of 4 pregnant women. To minimize the discomfort of heartburn, eat several small meals each day. Do not lay down immediately after eating. Have your last meal 2 to 3 hours before you go to sleep. Add an extra pillow so that you are not lying flat. Avoid food and drinks that increase stomach acids, such as orange juice, caffeinated beverages, chocolate, and fatty foods, and ask your doctor if it is OK to take antacids.

BABY - WHAT'S HAPPENING:

Your baby is now about 1½ inches long from the top of his head to the base of his bottom. His heart has now clearly divided into four chambers. At this point, his heart has also started to form its valves.

FOR YOUR HEALTH: The Centers for Disease Control recommends that women who will be pregnant during flu season—October through March—have a flu shot. The flu shot is considered safe during pregnancy since it does not contain a live virus, and though it cannot protect you against every strain of the flu, it increases your odds of making it through flu season without getting sick. It is important that you do not use flu vaccines that are inhaled through the nasal passages, as these are live vaccines and can cause you to become ill.

DAILY JOURNAL

Mood:

Energy:

Cravings:

Symptoms:

Weight:

DAY 47: Date:___/___/___

MOM - WHAT'S HAPPENING:

With 219 days to go and pregnancy symptoms on the rise, you may feel as though you will never make it through your pregnancy. Take heart knowing that you are halfway to 14 weeks, the point that some women consider the "honeymoon" phase of pregnancy. However, if you are feeling defeated by the many pregnancy side effects, know that you are not alone.

BABY - WHAT'S HAPPENING:

Your baby's joints are formed and working, which allows him increased mobility within the amniotic sac. His knees, elbows, wrists, shoulders and ankles are all formed and moving. When viewed on an ultrasound, your baby probably looks like he is swimming the doggy paddle in the amniotic fluid. This wonder fluid protects him from everything outside your body, including bumps to your expanding belly.

TIPS AND ADVICE: Acne breakouts tend to come on in pregnant women as a result of dry skin. When the body produces excess oil on the face to compensate, you end up with acne. If you suffer from pregnancy-induced acne, check with your health care provider before taking any medications for it. Some medications—particularly Retin-A and Accutane—can cause birth defects and even miscarriage. The best way to get control of increased oil production is to wash your face with a mild cleanser a few times a day and to moisturize often.

DAILY JOURNAL

Mood:

Energy:

Cravings:

Symptoms:

Weight:

DAY 48: Date:___/___/___

MOM - WHAT'S HAPPENING:

You may notice you have more digestive problems than you've had before, including a sense of being bloated and the urge to pass gas. This kind of digestive upset is caused by pregnancy hormones, which relax many of your muscles, including those in your digestive system. In addition to passing gas, relief also comes from avoiding foods that cause bloating, such as greasy food, raw vegetables, and beans.

BABY - WHAT'S HAPPENING:

Your baby is getting all the oxygen that she needs through blood that circulates through the umbilical cord as her body continues to mature. Her body will continue to elongate and straighten out. Her head may seem huge compared to the rest of her body, but as time goes on her growth will even out and her body and head will become proportional to each other.

PREGNANCY FACT: Amniotic fluid, also known as the "bag of waters," collects in the amniotic sac over the course of your pregnancy. By the time your uterus has expanded to its full capacity, you will be carrying approximately 800 ml of amniotic fluid that is made up mostly of water, but also contains proteins, carbohydrates, and electrolytes for your baby's growth. Sometime toward the end of your third trimester, your amniotic fluid level may drop to 600 ml. Your doctor will monitor you closely to be sure it never gets too low, though.

DAILY JOURNAL

Mood:

Energy:

Cravings:

Symptoms:

Weight:

DAY 49: Date:___/___/___

MOM - WHAT'S HAPPENING:

Perhaps you are finding that your energy level continues to plummet and keeps you in bed most of the day, causing you to miss work or rendering you unable to perform other duties. If so, mention it to your doctor who will test you for anemia at your first prenatal visit and again around 18 weeks. In the meantime, be sure you are getting enough iron from food sources as well as from your prenatal vitamin. Your blood production will increase up to three times what it was before, and your red blood cells need the additional iron in order to produce enough energizing oxygen.

BABY - WHAT'S HAPPENING:

If your baby is in the right place in your uterus, you will be able to hear his heartbeat on a handheld device called a Doppler. Your doctor will use this wand to amplify the sound of your baby's heartbeat. However, if you are unable to hear the heartbeat, don't panic. It may just be that your baby is out of range of the Doppler's ability to pick up the sound.

FOR YOUR HEALTH: If possible, avoid having X-rays while pregnant. Though harm to the fetus is unlikely given the specificity of modern X-ray equipment, it is always better to err on the side of caution. However, if you had an X-ray before you realized you were pregnant, don't worry—the odds of a single X-ray damaging the fetus are extremely low. Of course, your health is of utmost importance, and if you require X-rays while pregnant, you should follow your doctor's orders and do what is necessary to ensure your own well-being.

DAILY JOURNAL

Mood:

Energy:

Cravings:

Symptoms:

Weight:

Week 8

Starting Weight: _________

OVERVIEW

It won't be long now before your close friends and family members will begin to suspect that you are pregnant. Consider that before you were pregnant, your uterus was about the size and shape of a pear. By this week in your pregnancy, your uterus is the size and shape of a grapefruit! Thus, if you are thin, your belly may protrude and others may start to ask if you are pregnant. Also, due to the size of your uterus, you will be making even more trips to the bathroom this week. You might also see a dramatic increase in your fatigue. Keep in mind these symptoms tend to peak over the next few weeks and then subside around week 14 until you begin your last trimester.

This week your baby's heartbeat can be heard at your prenatal visit. For many moms, this is the first major reality check of pregnancy. Hearing your baby's heart beat for the first time can be very emotional, so be sure to bring tissues with you to your appointment. By the end of this week all your baby's vital organs will be in place and will even start to function. Your baby's yolk sac is receding and will eventually completely disappear and give way to the functioning of the placenta and your baby's liver.

DAY 50: Date:___/___/___

MOM - WHAT'S HAPPENING:

Due to your expanding circulatory system, you are probably starting to notice that the veins in your hands and feet are bulging. Like the rest of you, your veins must stretch to make room for the increase in blood flow. It is likely that by now you have also noticed blue veins appearing on your breasts and perhaps on your lower abdomen. Bulging veins are a distinct part of pregnancy and will go away after your baby is born—though if you intend to breast-feed you will be host to veiny breasts until you wean your infant.

BABY - WHAT'S HAPPENING:

Your baby is approximately 1.8 inches long and about the size of a small slice of dried apricot. The kidneys are producing urine that is circulated through the amniotic fluid and back through the fetal system again. Due to your good health, though, your baby is not exposed to toxins from its urine. Your baby's stomach has also begun to produce stomach acids will which aid in digestion.

FOOD FOR THOUGHT: Research shows that almonds are the most nutritionally dense nut, which makes it an indispensable pregnancy snack. Just one almond contains vitamin E, magnesium, protein, potassium, calcium, phosphorous, and iron. Almonds are also an excellent fiber source and are chock full of heart-healthy monounsaturated fat. Another bonus is that a 1-ounce serving of almonds is just 160 calories. Almonds are versatile and can be added to cereal, salads, or eaten as-is. Almond milk is also a great substitute for dairy if you are turned off by milk.

DAILY JOURNAL

Mood:

Energy:

Cravings:

Symptoms:

Weight:

DAY 51: Date:___/___/___

MOM - WHAT'S HAPPENING:

In addition to growing your baby and placenta, your body is already starting to prepare to feed your baby after he is born. Thus, you may notice several tiny bumps appear around the surface of your darkening areolas. These bumps are called Montgomery Glands. When mature, they will secrete a tiny bit of lubricant to keep the areola and nipple supple and moist, protecting it from dryness or cracking during breast-feeding. You may also find that your nipples protrude out farther than before you were pregnant. If you are shy about this, consider adding an extra layer of clothing.

BABY - WHAT'S HAPPENING:

Your baby's forehead is bulging out to make room for his growing brain—in fact, this week your baby's brain will produce around 250,000 neurons every single minute! Your baby's face is filling out and the outer part of his ears is starting to take its final shape. Also, if you are having a boy, his little testes will have started producing testosterone this week.

PREGNANCY FACT: In the case of a normal or low-risk pregnancy, sexual intercourse is perfectly safe, and even recommended in some cases for stress reduction and to foster intimacy between partners. You may find that you have some cramping in your abdomen and lower back after having an orgasm. Though uncomfortable, this is perfectly normal, and should go away on its own after a few minutes. You may also have some light spotting after intercourse. If cramping continues or becomes severe and is accompanied by heavy bleeding, call your doctor right away.

DAILY JOURNAL

Mood:

Energy:

Cravings:

Symptoms:

Weight:

DAY 52: Date:___/___/___

MOM - WHAT'S HAPPENING:

You may start noticing a darkening of your skin pigmentation on various parts of your body. This is known as the "pregnancy mask" and is very common. In fact, according to the American Academy of Dermatology, 70 percent of pregnant women develop this condition, called melasma, which is characterized by dark, blotchy areas of skin. Melasma occurs due to increased levels of the hormone melanin. It most commonly develops on the upper lip, cheekbones, and along the brow. Sun exposure will darken these areas, so use a good sunscreen and wear a hat when you plan to be outdoors.

BABY - WHAT'S HAPPENING:

Your baby's arms are now about the size of this typed "l," and they house the necessary arteries and veins to circulate blood and oxygen. If a baby girl is growing inside your uterus, her clitoris is starting to form from the same cells that the penis will develop from if you are having a boy.

TIPS AND ADVICE: If you prefer that people do not call your baby by name while in utero, don't discuss potential names with anyone other than your partner. People have a tendency to latch onto a name that is pleasing to them and go with it. Some mothers-to-be find this maddening. Avoid becoming the receptacle for everyone's opinions on what you should name your child. Nip it in the bud by saying, "My partner and I have a few names picked out, but we're not going to decide until after the baby is born."

DAILY JOURNAL

Mood:

Energy:

Cravings:

Symptoms:

Weight:

DAY 53: Date:___/___/___

MOM - WHAT'S HAPPENING:

By now, you may be starting to look pregnant, even if you are still managing to fit into some of your regular clothes. There's also a good chance that the extra blood circulating through your veins will give you a slightly rosy complexion, and the extra hormones will cause your skin to be a bit oilier, making it smooth and shiny. People may even tell you that you appear to glow! Some women may find that they have never looked better, even though they feel terrible. So, if your partner tells you that you look beautiful, avoid the urge to deflect the compliment—take it and smile!

BABY - WHAT'S HAPPENING:

Your baby's liver is producing red blood cells as the yolk sac shrinks and starts to give way to the liver's functioning. Your baby may also start to be covered by fine hair called lanugo. Lanugo's function is to insulate the fetus until it has developed enough fat. As your baby accumulates fat stores, he will shed the lanugo.

FOOD FOR THOUGHT: The omega-3 polyunsaturated fatty acid known as DHA (docosahexaenoic acid) is considered a must-eat for all of its nutritive properties. DHA is necessary for eye development, brain growth, and functioning in utero and during the first three months of your baby's life. A diet rich in DHA-foods have also been linked to a decrease in postpartum depression, which is great news. So, include oily fish in your diet, such as wild salmon. And if you are a vegetarian, DHA-rich eggs, walnuts, and flaxseeds are great options.

DAILY JOURNAL

Mood:

Energy:

Cravings:

Symptoms:

Weight:

DAY 54: Date:___/___/___

MOM - WHAT'S HAPPENING:

You may start to notice that you are not as light on your feet as you once were. In fact, you may be downright clumsy. This is a normal pregnancy side effect, but it can be surprising when you take your first fall or drop your first glass. It is important to be careful, because your ligaments and joints respond to the hormone relaxin by loosening up in preparation for birth. Thus, it is a good idea to trade heels in for flats until after your baby is born, since your ankles or knees can give way at the most unexpected moment. If you do fall, however, don't worry—your baby is protected by the amniotic fluid filled sac.

BABY - WHAT'S HAPPENING:

By now, your baby's fingers and toes are each separated digits. On an ultrasound, it may look like he is counting off his fingers, as he can't seem to resist moving everything that wiggles. Your baby's spine continues to elongate and his skeleton is replacing cartilage with bone.

TIPS AND ADVICE: The sciatic nerve runs from your lower back, down the back of your legs to your feet. When pressure is put on the nerve (as during pregnancy) the nerve can become inflamed and cause acute back pain, pins and needles, and even numbness. This condition is called sciatica. To manage sciatic pain, try alternating hot and cold compresses. Consider getting a massage or seeing an acupuncturist. Unfortunately, sometimes sciatica does not go away until after you give birth, but speak to your doctor about remedies if the pain is severe.

DAILY JOURNAL

Mood:

Energy:

Cravings:

Symptoms:

Weight:

DAY 55: Date:___/___/___

MOM - WHAT'S HAPPENING:

Today you might experience changes in your vision. As your body continues to fill with fluid and extra blood, pressure is mounting behind your eyes. Also, your corneas will become 3 percent thicker than before you were pregnant. The side effects of these changes are peaking right about now, and thus you may find that your vision has become blurry. Also, if you wear contact lenses, they may no longer fit, and so you might have to go back to wearing glasses for awhile. These changes usually last until about 6 weeks after you have your baby. They subside when fluid levels return to normal.

BABY - WHAT'S HAPPENING:

Your baby's eyes are nearly fully formed, with irises and pigmentation, though his eyelids will remain fused shut until about week 25 or 26. Your baby's ears are starting to move up the side of his head to their final placement. Your baby's head is taking on a more rounded shape and it now separated from his body by his newly formed neck.

TIPS AND ADVICE: It is just as important to wear a seatbelt during pregnancy as it is at any other time in your life. A properly positioned belt should be worn low across your pelvis and high across your chest. If you were to have an accident, the seatbelt would not harm the fetus, because your baby is protected by layers of your fat as well as by the amniotic fluid-filled sac. However, serious injury to you and your baby are likely if you do not wear a seatbelt because of the impact of your body hitting the steering wheel.

DAILY JOURNAL

Mood:

Energy:

Cravings:

Symptoms:

Weight:

DAY 56: Date:___/___/___

MOM - WHAT'S HAPPENING:

By now, you may have noticed that you get nosebleeds for no apparent reason. Nosebleeds are caused by increased production of estrogen and progesterone, which cause the mucus membranes to swell. This will also result in congestion. As long as you do not have frequent, gushing nosebleeds you need not be concerned. When you get a nosebleed, put gentle pressure on the bridge of your nose with a cold washcloth. Avoid over-the-counter medications (especially medicated nasal sprays) to treat congestion unless you have permission from your doctor. You may use saline nasal sprays, however, for they are considered safe during pregnancy and can offer relief by lubricating nasal passages.

BABY - WHAT'S HAPPENING:

By today your baby's legs have completed their major development. They will stay where they are as they continue to fatten and lengthen.

FOR YOUR HEALTH: When it comes to food safety, it can literally be a matter of life and death for your baby. Thus, to avoid bacterium called listeria monocyotogenes, the FDA recommends that pregnant women avoid eating hot dogs, smoked seafood, unpasteurized dairy products, and soft cheeses. It is also recommended that all perishable foods be stored at or below 40°F. If you contract the bacteria, it can lead to an infection called listeriosis, which can lead to miscarriage or still-birth.

DAILY JOURNAL

Mood:

Energy:

Cravings:

Symptoms:

Weight:

Lunar Month

Three

PHOTO

Place a photo of you during
your third month here

My Monthly Update

Waist Measurement: ____________________

Weight: ____________________

Mood: ____________________

Lunar Month three . . . .

PREGNANCY CHECKLIST

- ❑ Time to share the good news with your friends!
- ❑ Shop for a new bra if your old ones are feeling tight and uncomfortable
- ❑ Start a prenatal exercise routine, but consult your healthcare provider to learn what is safe
- ❑ Speak with your doctor about getting a flu shot
- ❑ Familiarize yourself with what to expect from early screening tests
- ❑ If your doctor recommends it, have chorionic villus sampling (CVS) testing done
- ❑ Stock up on moisturizer and pamper your pregnancy skin
- ❑ Stop coloring your hair, or ask about a chemical-free alternative
- ❑ Involve your partner in your pregnancy by talking about your hopes and fears
- ❑ Have your breasts checked for nursing
- ❑ Find out if you're having twins (and plan accordingly)
- ❑ Schedule a prenatal massage
- ❑ Stay hydrated. Drink 8 to 12 glasses of water a day

MY PERSONAL CHECKLIST:

- ❑ ....
- ❑ ....
- ❑ ....

MY HOPES FOR THIS MONTH:

....

....

....

Lunar Month Three

First Trimester

WELCOME TO THE LAST MONTH of your first trimester! By now, you are nearly one-third of the way done with your pregnancy and that much closer to meeting your new baby. The third month of pregnancy is significant, because it is a transition from feeling terrible to (hopefully) feeling much better. Toward the middle of this month your hormones will level off as both the placenta and your baby take on some of the hormone-production duty, which gives your ovaries a bit of a break (though they do continue to produce hormones as well).

Since your body is adjusting to being pregnant, you will probably still experience many of the same symptoms that you suffered during the first and second months—some, like constipation and fatigue may even peak this month. And though you will still have to contend with nausea, exhaustion, and heartburn, the first two should decrease considerably soon after you begin the second trimester. In other words, relief is on the way!

WHAT TO EXPECT THIS MONTH

This month you can expect to see your doctor who will check your baby's heartbeat by using the Doppler. This will become a regular and exciting feature of your appointments. Your doctor will also perform an external exam where she places his or her hands on your lower abdomen and uses pressure to measure both the size of your uterus as well as the height of your fundus (the top of the uterus). These examinations inform your doctor about both your estimated due date (EDD) and confirm that your baby is growing at the expected rate. If measurements appear below or above what is expected, your doctor may change your EDD. Your doctor will also weigh you, take your blood pressure, and check your ankles for swelling—all of which will become a regular feature of your prenatal appointments from now on.

THINGS TO CONSIDER

This is a big month for both mom and baby. By the end of this month, you will definitely notice that your clothes are tighter, so you may want to set aside some money to purchase more comfortable clothing or maternity outfits. It will be more cost-effective to buy just a few versatile pieces for the upcoming month, because if you buy too far ahead, you may find that you are either much larger or much smaller than you planned and that what you bought won't fit.

Meanwhile, your baby is on the fast track to growing a body that is in proportion to her head. At the start of the month, her organs are mostly formed and are in their final positions. Her lungs and brain, however, will continue to develop, and her lungs will not be complete until close to delivery. By the end of this month, your baby will be nearly 4 inches long and approximately the size of a peach. Though the critical period for development is ending, it is still crucial that you take excellent care of yourself and that you are careful about what you put in your body, since many substances can cross the placenta and be toxic to your baby.

TIPS FOR COPING

Since much of what you are experiencing is reminiscent of previous months, coping largely consists of continuing to do what works and stop doing what doesn't. You should find that eating smaller, more frequent meals will help you manage indigestion and nausea and that getting as much rest as you can help alleviate fatigue. Despite this, it is somewhat necessary to accept that pregnancy makes you tired—your body is completely renovating itself to accommodate its new tenant, after all!

Along those lines, it can really help your overall state of mind to surrender yourself to the process of pregnancy. Trying to fight the changes and symptoms will cause you a great deal of anxiety and potentially increase the likelihood of complications. So, write out a mantra similar to, "I trust my body to handle my pregnancy. My baby is healthy and growing. Pregnancy is happening to me just the way it's supposed to." Repeat your mantra several times each morning when you first get up and at night before you go to bed—in fact, repeat it any time you find yourself start to panic about your health or that of your baby.

WHAT TO EAT

If you are eating a balanced diet of complex carbohydrates, vegetables and fruits, lean protein, and limited fat, keep up the good work. In other words, healthy eating during pregnancy is mostly the same as healthy eating when you are not pregnant. Although you need to be taking in an additional 300 calories each day to support your baby's growth, sweets or fatty foods should be eaten only in moderation. Instead of snacking on a chocolate chip cookie, which can have as much as 275 calories and few nutrients, enjoy 8 ounces of yogurt with fruit, which has roughly 250 calories and also supplies calcium, vitamins, and even a little fiber.

Since it is difficult to get enough folic acid and other vitamins through diet alone, you should also be taking a multivitamin that is specially formulated for pregnant women. Don't let the prenatal vitamin do the heavy lifting, though—food is still the best source for vitamins, minerals, and overall nutrition. So even though you are taking a dietary supplement, continue to eat a wide variety of fruits and vegetables. In addition to vitamins and minerals, these foods (along with whole grains) are excellent sources of fiber, which will help alleviate constipation.

HOW MUCH WEIGHT TO GAIN

This month, your weight gain should remain modest since your baby, despite enormous developmental progress, will still only weigh 1½ ounces by the end of the month. So, over the course of the coming month, you should expect to gain about a pound or two. However, if you find that you are gaining more or less than 2 pounds per month in the first trimester, don't panic. Or, if you've lost some weight, that's OK, too, because many women actually lose a pound to nausea and vomiting. And if you've gained 10 pounds, don't berate yourself. It is very important to refrain from dieting, since that could be harmful to your baby. Try to relax, eat well, and realize that eventually your weight will even out and you will get into a groove.

EXERCISE TIPS AND ADVICE

As in the past 2 months, listen to your body when you exercise. Avoid overheating, since it may cause your body to shift blood supplies to your skin to help you cool off, which could, in turn, reduce the blood supply to your uterus. Stay well hydrated, and if you begin to feel faint or notice pain of any kind, stop what you are doing immediately.

It's also important to remember that your body is manufacturing hormones that relax your joints. This will serve you well when the time comes to deliver your baby but right now it puts you at increased risk for injury. For this reason, you should be wary of participating in exercise that requires quick starts and stops or sudden changes of direction. For example, tennis may not be the best sport for you, unless you are already an avid player and in excellent physical condition.

One type of exercise that's especially appropriate at this point in your pregnancy is Kegel exercises. These exercises concentrate on strengthening the muscles in the pelvic floor by flexing the very same muscles that you would use to stop the flow of urine. These muscles will be stretched greatly during labor and delivery and keeping them strong now will help you prevent urinary incontinence after the baby is born.

POTENTIAL SYMPTOMS AND HOW TO ALLEVIATE THEM

As mentioned earlier, you are likely to see a slight increase in nausea at the beginning of the month, but it should start to wane by the time you enter your second trimester. The big symptom this month, though, is heartburn. So, continue to eat several small meals per day. Also, avoid drinking liquids with your food. This can add to the feeling of fullness and add product to an already sluggish digestion system, giving your stomach more fuel for heartburn. Instead, drink water, juice, and milk between meals so that your stomach doesn't become overfull and bloated.

WAYS OTHERS CAN HELP

Your partner can help by doing the grocery shopping and preparing meals, since many pregnant women find they are unable to eat meals they've prepared for themselves. This usually comes about as a result of inexplicable and sudden aversions to specific foods and odors. This is also a good time to pass on other chores that may cause your stomach to churn, such as cleaning the toilet (of which you've seen enough!) or filling the car up with gasoline. In fact, you should ask your partner to take on all chores that involve chemicals that could be inhaled or absorbed by you and the baby.

"A babe in the house is a well-spring of pleasure, a messenger of peace and love, a resting place for innocence on earth, a link between angels and men."
~ Martin Fraquhar Tupper

Week 9

Starting Weight: _________

OVERVIEW

At the beginning of this week, your baby's organs are developed and in their permanent spots. With the exception of your baby's lungs and brain, the organs will start to perform their duties with some regularity this week. The lungs and brain will continue to develop throughout your pregnancy, however. In an exciting development, your baby's external sex organs should be fully developed by the end of this week, though they may not be seen on an ultrasound if your baby is facing in the wrong direction.

Sometime this week the placenta will take on hormone-production duties, giving your ovaries a bit of a break. You will likely continue to feel nauseous and may see an increase in the symptom known as round ligament pain. This occurs when the ligaments attached to the uterus are forced to stretch as the uterus expands. One way to prevent sudden sharp attacks is to move slowly when getting up from lying down or sitting—quickly doing so can cause sharp pain on either side of your pelvis.

This week is a good time to get ready for your next prenatal visit. Make a list of questions for your doctor and mention any symptoms that persist or seem out of the ordinary. Also, in preparation for this next appointment, read up on prenatal testing options and be prepared to make decisions about which ones to participate in.

DAY 57: Date:___/___/___

MOM - WHAT'S HAPPENING:

Pain you feel in your pelvic region is caused when the ligaments that are attached to your uterus stretch. Avoid getting up too fast after sitting or lying down. You may also feel this pain when you cough or sneeze. Keep in mind that these pains will likely increase as your uterus outgrows your pelvic area, and are normal. But if the pain is persistent or accompanied by fever, chills, or bleeding, call your health care provider right away.

BABY - WHAT'S HAPPENING:

Your baby's organs are all formed and in their correct positions. From this point on, her organs will continue to grow and take on their specific functions. In fact, this week kicks off a major growth spurt, and to accommodate your baby's growth the placenta is producing larger blood vessels that will be able to keep up with your baby's increasing nutritional needs.

FOR YOUR HEALTH: Approximately 20 to 25 percent of pregnant women have genital herpes. Of those with the condition, less than 1 percent of them pass the infection on to the baby. Though these percentages are low, it is very important that you let your doctor know if you do have genital herpes, because if you have an outbreak around the time you are supposed to deliver, you may pass it on to your baby. Herpes can have devastating consequences for babies, including neurological damage, mental retardation, and even death.

DAILY JOURNAL

Mood:

Energy:

Cravings:

Symptoms:

Weight:

DAY 58: Date:___/___/___

MOM - WHAT'S HAPPENING:

This week represents the last week where your ovaries are doing most of the work when it comes to hormone production. By the end of next week, the placenta will take over most of the work when it comes to producing estrogen and progesterone. In the meantime, and over the next few weeks, you are likely to still feel exhausted, nauseous, and downright irritable. However, you will probably find that others compliment your skin as it continues to look plump and shiny.

BABY - WHAT'S HAPPENING:

Your baby's fingers and toes are fully formed by now and nail beds have started to appear. Your baby's face is filling out, and his profile is distinctly like that of an infant. At this point, his eyes are nearly finished developing. If you were to peek inside your uterus, you would find that your baby's movements appear to be deliberate and that he is moving whatever he can!

FOOD FOR THOUGHT: Consider making sweet potatoes a regular feature of your pregnancy diet. Not only are they versatile and delicious, but they are full of important nutrients. Researchers have found that sweet potatoes contain proteins with antioxidant properties and have classified them as an "antidiabetic" food. This means sweet potatoes have been shown to stabilize blood-sugar levels and decrease insulin resistance. Sweet potatoes are also a powerhouse for nutrients. Just one serving is packed with vitamin A, C, B6, as well as copper, dietary fiber, potassium, and iron.

DAILY JOURNAL

Mood:

Energy:

Cravings:

Symptoms:

Weight:

DAY 59: Date:___/___/___

MOM - WHAT'S HAPPENING:

The continuing changes in your circulatory system probably have you feeling tired throughout most of the day. If you are unable to take a nap in the afternoon, try to set aside 15 minutes of quiet time to just zone out. This can give you just enough rest to keep you going until dinner. You may also find that you feel light-headed with some frequency. The sudden shift in fluids can cause you to lose your balance, and though your baby would probably be fine if you fell, you are at risk for injury, so be careful when moving around.

BABY - WHAT'S HAPPENING:

Your baby's external sex organs continue to develop and should be visible on an ultrasound by the end of this week. Also, your baby's head makes up about half of his 1-inch length—over the next few weeks, though, his body will lengthen and will eventually be in proportion to his seemingly giant head. Meanwhile, your baby's irises are developing and hair follicles make an appearance on his scalp.

TIPS AND ADVICE: Make an appointment for an evaluation with your dentist at least once while you are expecting. This is because during pregnancy, hormones cause your gums to swell, and they may even split and bleed during a meal or when you brush your teeth. Your gums also become more vulnerable to bacteria and plaque, gingivitis, and even periodontitis, which can lead to low-birth weight or premature delivery. As with everything, prevention is the best defense, so limit sweets, brush and floss after meals, and get plenty of calcium and vitamin C.

DAILY JOURNAL

Mood:

Energy:

Cravings:

Symptoms:

Weight:

DAY 60: Date:___/___/___

MOM - WHAT'S HAPPENING:

The soreness in your breasts could be starting to decrease as your body adjusts to all the changes it is experiencing. By now, you may have gone up an entire cup size or perhaps underwire bras have become too uncomfortable to wear. Keep up with the changes in your breast size by purchasing soft cup or sports bras. Forcing yourself into tight, lacy bras will only increase your misery as your breasts continue to grow. Also, many women experience itching as their breasts fill out and their skin stretches—cocoa butter and moisturizing baths can help ease this discomfort.

BABY - WHAT'S HAPPENING:

Your baby is nearly 2 inches long by now and weighs just under one-third of an ounce. Her bones are hardening, and her skin is still transparent—thus, your baby's skeleton would be visible through her skin if you could see her. Her body continues to lengthen and straighten out, and she is almost constantly moving, though you still cannot feel it.

FOR YOUR HEALTH: If you are suffering from pregnancy-related symptoms, try acupuncture. Studies show that acupuncture can offer relief from many of the side effects and symptoms of pregnancy. One study showed that acupuncture during the first trimester significantly reduced morning sickness and hyperemesis gravidarum (severe vomiting) when participants received regular treatments. In the second trimester, women saw relief from hemorrhoids, heartburn, and headaches. In the third trimester, women experienced a decrease in sciatica and other aches and pains.

DAILY JOURNAL

Mood:

Energy:

Cravings:

Symptoms:

Weight:

DAY 61: Date:___/___/___

MOM - WHAT'S HAPPENING:

Between weeks 8 and 11 of pregnancy (according to the LMP calendar) your health care provider will offer to do a screening test called chorionic villus sampling (CVS). This test can determine whether your baby is at risk for certain developmental abnormalities. It could reveal a predisposition toward Down syndrome, though it will not tell you if your baby actually has the condition. If you have the CVS test and there is some indication of a birth defect, your doctor will probably recommend having amniocentesis around week 16 to confirm the CVS test indications.

BABY - WHAT'S HAPPENING:

By now your baby's kidneys produce urine, which becomes part of the amniotic fluid. The addition of urine causes the volume of amniotic fluid to increase and is a good indicator for your doctor of whether your baby's kidneys are functioning. Your baby's urine is sterile and though some of it will be swallowed, much if it will be filtered out.

PREGNANCY FACT: Ectopic pregnancy is a serious condition in which the fertilized egg implants itself in an organ other than the uterus. This occurs most often in the fallopian tube, thus it is also called a "tubal pregnancy." Symptoms of ectopic pregnancy include severe pain on one side of the lower abdomen, vaginal bleeding, low blood pressure, fainting, and extreme lower back pain. If you experience any of these symptoms, call your doctor—immediately if they occur simultaneously—because an untreated pregnancy inside the fallopian tube may result in rupturing of the tube.

DAILY JOURNAL

Mood:

Energy:

Cravings:

Symptoms:

Weight:

DAY 62: Date:___/___/___

MOM - WHAT'S HAPPENING:

You may be frustrated with how you look these days, because though you've put on a few pounds, you don't quite look pregnant. Also, by this time you may be bloated thanks to water retention and constipation. Your face may be broken out, and you probably have dark circles under your eyes due to lack of sleep. Odds are that other people probably still don't notice any difference in your figure, but if your appearance bothers you, try pampering yourself. Buy clothes that fit more comfortably, for example, or visit a day spa and get a massage. It's important to take care of yourself and to keep stress levels as low as possible.

BABY - WHAT'S HAPPENING:

By now your baby's upper lip, tongue, tooth buds, and diaphragm are formed. In fact in the next week or so, she will start to hiccup now and then and you may even be able to feel it as a slight flutter in your belly. Some women feel this before they feel traditional kicks.

FOR YOUR HEALTH: According to the American Diabetes Association, gestational diabetes affects 4 percent—or 135,000—of pregnant women in the United States every year. Thus, it is important that you take the glucose screening test when your doctor recommends it, which is usually around 28 weeks. Left unchecked, gestational diabetes can cause your baby's pancreas to work overtime to produce enough insulin to process the excess sugar in his body. This can lead to a very fat baby, which can cause delivery complications for you and health problems for him after he is born.

DAILY JOURNAL

Mood:

Energy:

Cravings:

Symptoms:

Weight:

DAY 63: Date:___/___/___

MOM - WHAT'S HAPPENING:

You will start to look pregnant as your uterus expands upward and outward, pushing your belly out once your uterus can no longer fit inside your pelvic area. This puts additional pressure on your bladder. It may also start to crowd your stomach, which is another reason to eat several small meals each day.

BABY - WHAT'S HAPPENING:

At the end of your baby's ninth week of development, she is just 2 inches long and weighs just about 1/3 of an ounce. The external sex organs are nearly visible, though a penis will be easier to detect on an ultrasound than a clitoris. Your little babe is doing somersaults and waving his or her arms and legs, and would even be able to close his or her hand around an object, making a fist.

PREGNANCY FACT: Approximately 1 out of 8 known pregnancies end in miscarriage during the first trimester. Miscarriage is the loss of a pregnancy within the first 20 weeks of gestation. However, once the baby's heartbeat is detected and the mother is 12 weeks pregnant, the risk of miscarriage drops to about 1 percent. If you miscarry during the first trimester and it is your first miscarriage, the odds of you having a full-term pregnancy next time around are just as good as they were before you first became pregnant. In fact, if you've been pregnant, you know you can get pregnant again.

DAILY JOURNAL

Mood:

Energy:

Cravings:

Symptoms:

Weight:

Week 10

Starting Weight: _________

OVERVIEW

This next week can be a doozy in the dizzy department. This is because increased levels of progesterone divert extra blood to your baby, while slowing the return of blood flow back to your upper extremities and brain. This may lead to dizziness or feeling faint—both of which are normal, with some exceptions. If you actually faint, be sure to call your doctor and let him know about the episode and what you were doing just before. Stabilizing your blood sugar, resting often, and staying well-hydrated can help to lessen the frequency of dizzy spells. Also, move more slowly than you normally would, since fast, jerky movements can cause fluid shifts in the body that can exacerbate light-headedness.

Some good news to look forward to this week is that your uterus will expand just enough to move slightly higher in you pelvic region, thus alleviating some of the pressure on your bladder, which should give you a break from feeling the constant need to urinate.

This week, your baby is growing longer and starting to put on a bit of weight. He is also developing facial features, and his ears are moving up the sides of his head to their final position. This week also marks the development of your baby's larynx, or voice box, as well as the continued maturation of his digestive tract.

DAY 64: Date:___/___/___

MOM - WHAT'S HAPPENING:

You are nearing the end of your first trimester, and though it is an exciting milestone, you probably are preoccupied with your symptoms, which may peak around now. Your uterus is about the size of a grapefruit and so it is probably time to purchase some underwear with a little extra room. You will be surprised at how quickly your waistline expands over the next few weeks. You may wake up one morning to find none of your regular undies and bottoms fit, so plan ahead.

BABY - WHAT'S HAPPENING:

Your baby is now slightly larger than the size of an apricot, meaning he has more than doubled in size over the past few weeks. He still has plenty of room in your ever-expanding uterus, though, and will continue to practice his acrobatics unnoticed (except by ultrasound) for several more weeks. At this point, your baby has developed his pituitary gland at the base of his brain, which secretes hormones responsible for growth and blood pressure.

PREGNANCY FACT: The fundus of the uterus is the opening at the top of the uterus that is opposite the cervix. When you visit your doctor each month for your prenatal checkup she will press her hand gently into your lower abdomen to find the fundus, and measure from it to the top of your pubic bone. This measurement helps determine if your baby is on target with his growth. Measurement of the fundus can help identify problems in the pregnancy if the growth is deemed too little or too much when compared with the gestational age of the baby.

DAILY JOURNAL

Mood:

Energy:

Cravings:

Symptoms:

Weight:

DAY 65: Date:___/___/___

MOM - WHAT'S HAPPENING:

If you haven't been to the doctor yet this month, you may become worried that something is wrong. Most mothers live from ultrasound to ultrasound or from Doppler to Doppler—fearing that something is wrong until they can once again hear the sweet sound of their baby's heartbeat. Work to get control over stressing about the health of your baby. As long as you are eating well and taking care of yourself, chances are that your baby is doing just fine.

BABY - WHAT'S HAPPENING:

Your baby's voice box, or larynx, is formed by this time. Amazingly, although your baby is unable to make sound in utero, she will immediately know how to cry the minute she is born and her throat and mouth are cleared of fluid. Also, by now, your baby's ears have moved up to their final position on her head and are ready to hear you talk and sing to her, or play your favorite music by putting headphones against your abdomen.

FOOD FOR THOUGHT: It is necessary to consume enough dietary fiber while you are pregnant. This is because many women experience mild to severe constipation at some point during their pregnancy. Though severe cases of constipation may be solved by a mild laxative prescribed by your doctor, a simpler solution is to increase your fiber intake. Thus, in addition to drinking at least 10 cups of water each day, it is a good idea to add several servings of fiber-rich foods to your diet, including bran, lentils, split peas, beans, and prunes.

DAILY JOURNAL

Mood:

Energy:

Cravings:

Symptoms:

Weight:

DAY 66: Date:___/___/___

MOM - WHAT'S HAPPENING:

By this time in your pregnancy, your enlarged uterus and growing baby are probably putting a strain on your back. Paying attention to your posture and concentrating on keeping your back and shoulders aligned can help avoid soreness. It will also do you a world of good to stretch a few times a day and walk for at least 30 minutes. Another tip to relieve a sore lower back is to sleep on your side with a pillow between your knees. If the pain is particularly bad, alternate heat and ice and get plenty of rest.

BABY - WHAT'S HAPPENING:

Your baby's digestive tract is busy maturing. Today, his intestinal walls might be practicing contractions—called peristalsis—that will be necessary to push food through his intestines when he is older. Also, your baby's pancreas has begun to produce insulin, which will help digest sugars. It is a good idea to keep your sugar consumption low so your baby's pancreas isn't forced to work overtime to make enough insulin to match your sweet tooth.

FOOD FOR THOUGHT: If nausea is preventing you from eating a variety of vegetables, consider drinking a few servings a day instead. Indeed, many women find they can quickly drink down a serving of greens much easier than trying to chew and swallow a plate full of spinach. There are several good organic vegetable juices on the market—but be sure that you purchase only juices that are pasteurized. Another option is to purchase a juicer and make your own. If you do this, make only as much as you plan to drink and drink it right away.

DAILY JOURNAL

Mood:

Energy:

Cravings:

Symptoms:

Weight:

DAY 67: Date:___/___/___

MOM - WHAT'S HAPPENING:

As your uterus moves up from the bottom of your pelvis, the pressure on your bladder is eased somewhat. As a result, you may find some relief from constantly needing to visit the bathroom. However, dizziness will increase as progesterone levels rise, sending more blood to your baby and placenta, with less blood returning to your brain, which results in a drop in blood pressure. Dizziness can be stabilized if you stay hydrated and keep your blood-sugar levels even.

BABY - WHAT'S HAPPENING:

Your baby is still so small that you probably cannot feel her movements. But at your next ultrasound, you may be lucky enough to see your baby sucking her thumb. This is because she has developed the sucking and rooting reflex. These will help guide your baby to breast or bottle once she is born. A slight brush against your baby's cheek or mouth will kick off this miraculous reflex and your baby will turn in the direction the touch came from, seeking something to suck.

TIPS AND ADVICE: Check your company's policy on paid leave, and find out your state's rules governing the federal Family and Medical Leave Act (FMLA). FMLA typically allows for up to 12 weeks of unpaid leave either during your pregnancy or after the birth of your child. It also protects you from losing your job while on leave—though some states also pay a percentage of your income. FMLA is unique in that it may be taken anytime during the first year after your child is born. After that, you are no longer eligible for benefits, so be sure to take advantage of it while you can!

DAILY JOURNAL

Mood:

Energy:

Cravings:

Symptoms:

Weight:

DAY 68: Date:___/___/___

MOM - WHAT'S HAPPENING:

Today you might notice a decrease in your nausea and may want to munch between meals. It is true that many women see an increase in their appetite as their nausea subsides. You may even have the urge to binge in celebration! Just be sure to limit sugars and saturated fats, because these are empty calories that offer little nutrition to you and your baby. Also, bingeing on sugary foods will exacerbate late afternoon fatigue with a sugar crash. So, instead, keep healthy but satisfying snacks on hand, such as carrot sticks, granola bars, almonds, yogurt, and bananas.

BABY - WHAT'S HAPPENING:

Your baby's bone marrow has begun producing white blood cells. These are key to his health because they are his first line of defense against infections. When faced with an invading germ, white blood cells fight it by either producing antibodies or attacking the bacteria.

FOOD FOR THOUGHT: If you can stomach them, make brussels sprouts part of your pregnancy diet. These tiny power foods have a bad rap, but the fact is these cabbage cousins are jam-packed with the nutrients necessary for a healthy pregnancy. Just one serving of brussels sprouts contains vitamin C, vitamin A, folate, and lots of fiber! A great and healthy way to prepare brussels sprouts is to roast them in a little bit of olive oil and broth. This should remove the stinky odor produced when they are steamed.

DAILY JOURNAL

Mood:

Energy:

Cravings:

Symptoms:

Weight:

DAY 69: Date:___/___/___

MOM - WHAT'S HAPPENING:

You may have noticed that your sex drive has taken a nosedive. This is common during the first trimester and, for some women, lasts throughout pregnancy. Several factors influence this change, including weight gain, exhaustion, nausea, and fear of hurting the baby. For your own emotional health and that of your partner, be sure to communicate your issues but don't let physical intimacy fall by the wayside. Studies show that physical closeness with your partner reduces stress hormones and increases blood circulation—as well as the disposition of everyone involved!

BABY - WHAT'S HAPPENING:

Because your baby's organ systems are complete, the risk of birth defects is greatly reduced. However, that doesn't mean that you should let your guard down in relation to toxic substances. Your baby's organs—particularly the brain and lungs—still need to mature and toxins like secondhand smoke and alcohol could compromise healthy development.

PREGNANCY FACT: Placenta previa is when the placenta grows low in the uterus and either partially or completely covers the cervix. Placenta previa usually will not cause any problems early in your pregnancy. And even if it is discovered during your second trimester on an ultrasound, there is still time for it to migrate up and away from the cervix as your uterus expands, taking the placenta with it. However, in some cases, the placenta stays put and may cause bleeding. In that case, you will be carefully monitored until your baby is born by Cesarean section.

DAILY JOURNAL

Mood:

Energy:

Cravings:

Symptoms:

Weight:

DAY 70: Date:___/___/___

MOM - WHAT'S HAPPENING:

By now, you've probably gained between 2 and 4 pounds. Your head is probably swimming with to-do lists for when the baby arrives. In order to prevent stress overload, take an evening to sit down and put those lists on paper. There is much to be said for developing a plan with steps that you can check off as each is accomplished. However, do only what you can manage and never push yourself to the point of exhaustion to get tasks done.

BABY - WHAT'S HAPPENING:

By now your baby's external sex organs are developed enough that they would be visible on an ultrasound. If you are having a boy, his testes and penis will be prominent. If you are having a girl her clitoris and labia majora will visible. Being able to determine your baby's sex, however, is dependent on which way he or she is facing when you have the ultrasound.

FOR YOUR HEALTH: If you were treated for depression before you became pregnant, now is not the time to drop your treatment plan. It is true that if you are taking antidepressants for mild depression, your doctor may advise you to go off them while pregnant. However, women who suffer from major depression may be at higher risk for complications. The doctor may recommend that you continue taking antidepressants. Wherever you may fall on the depression spectrum, don't try to manage it on your own. Continue with therapy and be sure to keep your OB-GYN in the loop.

DAILY JOURNAL

Mood:

Energy:

Cravings:

Symptoms:

Weight:

Week 11

Starting Weight: ________

OVERVIEW

This week you will might notice you are going through as many panty liners as you would during menstruation. This is due to the increase in the vaginal discharge known as leukorrhea. If your discharge is milky and thin, your body is doing what it is supposed to: cleansing the birth canal and keeping infection out. Similarly, you will likely notice an increase in congestion and may develop a persistent runny nose. Though annoying, it too, means that your body is sealing all the passageways to keep harmful bacteria and illness away from your baby.

Meanwhile, inside your womb your baby is continuing on her path to looking like a person. By now, she's doing what looks like the jitterbug with some regularity, though you will not be able to feel her movements for another several weeks. Also, this week, your baby's intestines will continue the slow migration out of the umbilical cord and into her abdomen. This process will last as long as it takes for her abdomen to grow large enough to accommodate her intestines. Meanwhile, if you are having a girl, her ovaries now contain approximately 2 million eggs, and if you are having a boy his penis will be clearly visible on an ultrasound if he is facing in the right direction.

DAY 71: Date:___/___/___

MOM - WHAT'S HAPPENING:

You might be secreting the white, sometimes creamy, mild-smelling discharge vaginal discharge called leukorrhea. Though it can be a nuisance, it has a very important job: leukorrhea, increases in response to higher levels of estrogen. Its job is to keep your birth canal free of infection. It also maintains the proper pH balance in the vagina. If, however, you experience any pain or itching or find that the discharge is slightly chunky, be sure to see your doctor—you may have a yeast infection. It is OK to wear panty liners but never wear tampons or douche while pregnant.

BABY - WHAT'S HAPPENING:

Your baby has grown considerably and is now approximately 3 inches long! Her entire body is about the size of a small nectarine, with her head still making up most of her mass. Her tiny body is still covered in transparent skin, and if you could look at her in the light, you'd be able to see a vast network of veins, as well as her bones and organs.

TIPS AND ADVICE: The vast majority of pregnant women have vivid dreams when they are expecting—particularly during the first trimester. It is theorized that hormone surges are responsible for this sleep-cinema. In fact, many women report that they dreamed they were pregnant before they ever took a test, and even more pregnant women claim to have dreamed their baby's gender very early on. Whatever messages your dreams are sending, take the time to write them down. Keeping a pregnancy dream journal is cathartic and an incredible keepsake to pass down to your child.

DAILY JOURNAL

Mood:

Energy:

Cravings:

Symptoms:

Weight:

DAY 72: Date:___/___/___

MOM - WHAT'S HAPPENING:

If this is not your first pregnancy, or your breasts are very full, they may have already started to produce colostrum—the fluid that feeds your baby for the first few days after birth until your milk comes in. At this stage, colostrum is clear and may leak a little from one or both nipples, causing wet marks on your shirt. This is easy to handle by purchasing nursing pads and inserting them into your bra. Consider it a sneak-peek into life with leaky breasts after your baby is born!

BABY - WHAT'S HAPPENING:

By now, your baby has developed a thin set of nails that have grown in the nail beds on his fingers and toes. His teeny baby nails will grow fast and become surprisingly sharp after birth, considering how pliable and thin they are. In utero, your baby continues to flex his hands and may even grab the umbilical cord or stick his thumb in his mouth. A few lucky parents get to see their baby "wave" during the next ultrasound.

TIPS AND ADVICE: Some women find that drinking liquids makes them feel nauseated. If you have trouble drinking, be sure to eat foods that contain water, like fruits and squash. It is also helpful to drink water, milk, or juice between meals instead of during. Fluids with food tend to increase nausea, bloating, and discomfort. Thus, saving your daily servings of low-fat drinks and water for between meals will increase the likelihood of it staying down. It is very important to stay hydrated, so if you find you are unable to keep any liquid down, alert your doctor right away so action can be taken.

DAILY JOURNAL

Mood:

Energy:

Cravings:

Symptoms:

Weight:

DAY 73: Date:___/___/___

MOM - WHAT'S HAPPENING:

As your circulatory system continues expand, your body is producing more blood than ever before. At this point, it is mostly the liquid component called plasma. Red blood cells are not manufactured fast enough to keep up with the increase in plasma, thus you may develop anemia if you do not get enough iron. This, plus the fact that your respiratory system really picks up the pace this week, may have you feeling out of breath and tired throughout the day. In order to get enough oxygen to you, the placenta, and your baby, your lungs are now taking in 30 to 40 percent more air with each breath.

BABY - WHAT'S HAPPENING:

By now, your baby's intestines should have moved out of the umbilical cord and into her abdomen. Her digestive tract will continue to practice contracting and releasing the walls of her intestines. Meanwhile, the placenta—weighing in at just about an ounce—continues to develop and grow to keep up with your baby's nutritional needs.

FOR YOUR HEALTH: As long as your pregnancy is progressing normally, receiving oral sex is a safe and healthy way to exchange intimacy with your partner. It is important, though that your partner does not blow air into your vagina. This could introduce an air bubble into your bloodstream, which could have potentially fatal results for you and for the fetus. This is rare, however, and should not be cause for concern. If, however, you are experiencing early contractions, it is a good idea to speak to your doctor about how having an orgasm can affect these.

DAILY JOURNAL

Mood:

Energy:

Cravings:

Symptoms:

Weight:

DAY 74: Date:___/___/___

MOM - WHAT'S HAPPENING:

Your uterus is expanding to make room for all of its contents—the placenta, your baby, and amniotic fluid. And as the uterus expands, it puts pressure on the veins that return blood from your legs back up to your heart. This can cause leg cramps, especially when you are lying down for long periods of time. If you experience these, avoid the urge to bring your heel in toward your calf, because this will intensify the cramp. Instead, push your toes up as if you are trying to make them touch your knees. This stretch can help pull you out of a cramp and, if done regularly, may lessen the intensity before an attack.

BABY - WHAT'S HAPPENING:

Your baby's vocal cords are formed by now. This development positions her to be ready to cry her little head off after she is born to let everyone in the room know that she is breathing and missing the perfect environment of your womb.

PREGNANCY FACT: Amniotic fluid, also known as the "bag of waters," collects in the amniotic sac over the course of your pregnancy. By the time your uterus has expanded to its full capacity, you will be carrying approximately 800 ml of amniotic fluid that is made up mostly of water, but also contains proteins, carbohydrates, and electrolytes for your baby's growth. Sometime toward the end of your third trimester, your amniotic fluid level may drop to 600 ml. Your doctor will monitor you closely to be sure it never gets too low, though.

DAILY JOURNAL

Mood:

Energy:

Cravings:

Symptoms:

Weight:

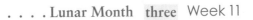

DAY 75: Date:___/___/___

MOM - WHAT'S HAPPENING:

Once again, increased levels of progesterone are wreaking havoc on your digestive system. As your smooth muscles relax, you will find it takes longer for food to break down and leave your stomach. This is to your baby's benefit in that it allows more time for nutrients to be absorbed by your blood and to be passed on to your baby. However, this likely has you feeling miserable. Again, the solution is to eat small meals and to never allow yourself to overeat, which can make discomfort linger longer than normal.

BABY - WHAT'S HAPPENING:

Your baby's body is busy trying to catch up to the growth of his head. Don't, worry, it will—and in the meantime your baby's head is forming what will become the bones of his skull. Your baby's skull is amazing in that the bones that make it up don't fuse in utero, but after birth. This allows for the molding or reshaping of the baby's skull as it fits through your pelvis during delivery.

FOOD FOR THOUGHT: Though you can certainly benefit from the omega-3s in oily fish, such as salmon, be sure to limit your intake of fish that may contain high levels of mercury. This is because your fetus is vulnerable to mercury toxicity. In fact, the FDA and the EPA recommend that pregnant women limit their fish intake to just 12 ounces per week of shrimp, salmon, catfish, Pollock, or canned light tuna (tuna steaks have higher levels of mercury than the canned variety). Due to high mercury levels, pregnant women should completely avoid shark, swordfish, king mackerel, and tilefish.

DAILY JOURNAL

Mood:

Energy:

Cravings:

Symptoms:

Weight:

DAY 76: Date:___/___/___

MOM - WHAT'S HAPPENING:

Progesterone is causing your body to relax, yet your mind is probably racing, wondering if the fact that you have urinate for the 15th time today means that you have a urinary tract infection. Progesterone causes the tubes (called ureters) that urine pass through on its way from your kidneys to your bladder to relax, which slows the urine flow. That, plus the fact that your uterus is crowding your bladder, may make it impossible for you to completely empty your bladder. If it burns when you pee or if you have a fever, let your doctor know right away, because urinary tract infections left untreated can lead to a more serious kidney infection.

BABY - WHAT'S HAPPENING:

Although the baby's eyes and ears are basically formed, they still have some fine-tuning to do. In fact, as your baby's skull grows, her eyes will continue to move toward their final, forward-facing position. Meanwhile, your baby's digestive tract continues to develop and today marks the day when her liver begins to produce bile.

TIPS AND ADVICE: As your pregnancy progresses, you will find that your feet and ankles will swell, especially when you sit for long stretches. This condition is called edema and is due to poor circulation and fluid that pools in the bottom of your legs and ankles. A great solution is to invest in a good pair of compression hose. Compression hose work by putting a gradual amount of pressure from the ankles (most pressure) up the leg (least pressure), increasing the flow of blood back up to the upper half of your body, thus relieving leg cramps and swelling.

DAILY JOURNAL

Mood:

Energy:

Cravings:

Symptoms:

Weight:

DAY 77: Date:___/___/___

MOM - WHAT'S HAPPENING:

The increased blood volume and pressure of your expanding uterus is likely to cause some very unwelcome additions to your anatomy: hemorrhoids. You can alleviate some of the discomfort by taking warm baths, but if you notice severe itching or bleeding, allow your doctor to prescribe an appropriate treatment. Other than that, you may be feeling slightly less nauseous and have a bit more energy these days. You might even fear something is wrong, due to the absence of symptoms. These are all signs that you are getting very close to the "honeymoon" period of your pregnancy, so enjoy it while it lasts!

BABY - WHAT'S HAPPENING:

Around this time, your baby's first 20 teeth have formed under his gums and will remain there until approximately 6 months after he is born. Your baby is swallowing amniotic fluid with frequency now, which is great practice for when he is either at the breast or bottle and must swallow milk or formula.

FOOD FOR THOUGHT: Approximately 3 percent women are pregnant with either identical or fraternal twins each year—and the numbers are increasing as moms wait into their 30s and 40s to conceive and are aided by fertility drugs. Twins are conceived in one of two ways: Fraternal twins develop when two separate eggs are fertilized by two separate sperm and implanted in the uterus, while identical twins form from the same divided egg. Fraternal twins are as genetically similar to each other as they are to any other siblings, while identical twins have identical genetic composition.

DAILY JOURNAL

Mood:

Energy:

Cravings:

Symptoms:

Weight:

Week 12

Starting Weight: ________

OVERVIEW

You may start to show this week. Your uterus is starting to outgrow your pelvic area and push up and out, forcing your belly to protrude. In fact, now is a great time to purchase a few inexpensive, stretchy garments that will allow you to breathe easier and feel less constricted. Also this week, you may feel extreme fatigue as your circulatory system continues to expand. In fact, its superhuman output of plasma (the liquid component of blood) far exceeds your body's ability to produce red blood cells. Thus, if your energy level is plummeting you may want to ask your doctor to test you for anemia (low iron).

As for your baby's progress, this week is big for the reproductive system. If your baby is male, his prostate gland starts to develop. If you are having a girl, her ovaries start to migrate down into her pelvis. Additionally, your baby's thyroid gland is formed and begins functioning and producing hormones that will regulate his or her metabolism. The thyroid gland depends on iodine to function properly, so include iodine-rich foods in your diet.

Speaking of diet, this week should bring about a decrease in nausea, so take advantage and load up on those nutritious foods you've been avoiding. If you are feeling uninspired to cook, just throw together a plate of varied and vibrant-colored fruits and vegetables, and you can't go wrong!

DAY 78: Date:___/___/___

MOM - WHAT'S HAPPENING:

Your hormones are starting to stabilize, and you should notice a decrease in the amount you are vomiting. You still may get nauseous now and then, especially if you are hungry or right when you wake up in the morning. But overall, you should not be vomiting midday anymore. However, there is a small percentage of women who are afflicted with hyperemesis gravidarum—excessive vomiting—throughout their entire pregnancy. If you are still unable to keep food or liquids down this week, ask your doctor about treatments for this condition.

BABY - WHAT'S HAPPENING:

Your baby's body is growing quickly now to catch up to her head size. She is also straightening out and becoming more erect. Her neck is longer, and there is a clear separation between her shoulders and her head. Her movements are more controlled and graceful. If you are scheduled for an ultrasound, you may get to see her sucking her thumb.

TIPS AND ADVICE: Traveling while you are pregnant is fine as long as you have the OK from your doctor. Most women feel better in their second trimester, so it might behoove you to wait until you are 15 or 16 weeks along before you take a trip. Keep in mind that no matter how you get where you are going—by car or plane—you should move your body as often as you can, even if you just make circles with your feet or walk up and down the aisle. This will help prevent fluid accumulation in your ankles and feet.

DAILY JOURNAL

Mood:

Energy:

Cravings:

Symptoms:

Weight:

DAY 79: Date:___/___/___

MOM - WHAT'S HAPPENING:

Experts advise against sleeping on your back during pregnancy since doing so can put pressure on the artery that supplies blood to the lower half of your body. Now is a good time to get used to sleeping on your side, which will probably be the only comfortable position anyway. Purchase a body pillow and put it between your knees while you sleep. Later, when your belly is huge, you can slide the pillow under your belly for extra support. Hopefully, you are able to find some sleeping positions that are more comfortable than others.

BABY - WHAT'S HAPPENING:

Your baby is nearly 3½ inches long and is starting to use his facial muscles. In fact, he may go from smiling to frowning to squinting to sucking his thumb all in under a minute. In fact, the little guy rarely stops moving, except when you sleep at night, since he is getting in tune with your sleeping and waking patterns.

FOOD FOR THOUGHT: A doula is a person who can provide you with support throughout your pregnancy, during birth, and postpartum. Doulas are not medical professionals, though they are well educated about childbearing and delivery. Their role is to provide emotional support and information without supplanting the partner—in fact, many husbands find that having a doula frees them up to focus on mom during delivery. Having a doula present for the birth can help communicate your wishes to your doctor while keeping you as comfortable as possible.

DAILY JOURNAL

Mood:

Energy:

Cravings:

Symptoms:

Weight:

DAY 80: Date:___/___/___

MOM - WHAT'S HAPPENING:

You may be feeling down if you have gained more weight than you'd intended this trimester. But keep in mind that many women do not fall within the typical 3-to-5-pound weight gain during the first trimester. This is more of a recommendation or guideline issued by medical doctors. The fact is some women actually lose weight during the first trimester due to nausea and vomiting, while others gain upwards of 10 pounds. However your weight gain starts out during pregnancy, it is likely to even out during the second trimester, so don't be too hard on yourself.

BABY - WHAT'S HAPPENING:

Your baby's external reproductive organs are formed and in place and, as your pregnancy progresses, either the penis or the vagina will become more prominent, making it easier to determine—by ultrasound—whether you are having a boy or a girl. Meanwhile, if you are having a boy, his prostate gland continues to develop, and if you are having a girl, her ovaries are still moving into position in her pelvis.

FOOD FOR THOUGHT: Low-fat yogurt is a great pregnancy snack because it is loaded with nutrients and easy to transport. A serving of plain, low-fat yogurt contains just 155 calories and a host of vitamins and minerals, such as iodine; calcium; phosphorus; vitamins B2, B5, and B12; potassium; and zinc. Yogurt also offers an excellent protein boost and can be substituted for sour cream in many dishes. Finally, yogurt contains probiotics (healthy bacteria) that help maintain the pH balance in your vaginal area and ward off yeast infections.

DAILY JOURNAL

Mood:

Energy:

Cravings:

Symptoms:

Weight:

DAY 81: Date:___/___/___

MOM - WHAT'S HAPPENING:

As your uterus swells, it will move up and out of your pelvic area. This often results in a break from the need to urinate frequently, and may even help with constipation. However, this development can cause a different problem. It is common around this time to feel short of breath. This is partially because your lungs are breathing for two and also because the upward movement of your uterus puts pressure on organs near your diaphragm. Those reasons, plus the fact that your heart is beating much faster than you are used to, may have you feeling out of breath while doing simple tasks.

BABY - WHAT'S HAPPENING:

Your baby's thyroid gland is functioning by now, which means she is able to produce hormones that help to regulate her growth. The thyroid gland is one of the largest endocrine glands, and it develops just below your baby's larynx, in the center of her neck. The hormones produced by your baby's thyroid glands will eventually regulate her metabolism and the remainder of her brain development.

FOOD FOR THOUGHT: The thyroid gland has an important role in your baby's growth and brain development, and it depends on sufficient levels of iodine to do its job properly. Thus, it is important that you include the following foods in your diet to ensure that your thyroid gland is functioning properly, as well as your baby's. Foods with concentrated levels of iodine include: yogurt, sea vegetables, milk, mozzarella cheese, strawberries, and eggs. Table salt is often iodized but should be used in moderation, since sodium can increase blood pressure and exacerbate swelling.

DAILY JOURNAL

Mood:

Energy:

Cravings:

Symptoms:

Weight:

DAY 82: Date:___/___/___

MOM - WHAT'S HAPPENING:

Though the nausea you experienced during the past several weeks is probably waning by now, it has likely been replaced with frequent (maybe even constant) heartburn. For a lucky few, heartburn doesn't make an appearance until the third trimester, but most women experience some degree of acid indigestion from the earliest weeks of pregnancy until after their baby is born. If you are unable to sleep or you find that you are getting a mouthful of regurgitated food, check with your health care provider about taking antacids.

BABY - WHAT'S HAPPENING:

At this point, taste buds are forming on your baby's tiny tongue—when he has a complete set, your baby will have 10,000 taste buds! It is a good idea to eat a variety of foods, because it is presupposed that when it comes time to feed table food to babies, they tend to be more willing to accept foods that they "tasted" in their mom's diet while in utero. So, bring on the garlic bread and taco sauce!

TIPS AND ADVICE: Pay attention to your partner, because he may feel left out of the pregnancy experience. Women are lucky in that they are able to form an immediate attachment to the baby by being responsible for its nourishment. Thus, impending parenthood may feel more real and magical to you than it does to your partner. So, include him. Ask him to read or sing to your belly. Let him have "alone time" with your belly, where he can talk to the baby while you listen to headphones. You can also purchase books written specifically for expectant fathers that he might find interesting.

DAILY JOURNAL

Mood:

Energy:

Cravings:

Symptoms:

Weight:

DAY 83: Date:___/___/___

MOM - WHAT'S HAPPENING:

You may be amazed at how different your breasts look this early in your pregnancy, because by now, your areolas are probably starting to spread and darken. It is likely that you've either gone up a cup size or are just large enough that your regular bras are no longer an option. If you haven't already purchased some soft cup or sport's bras, now is the time, because your breasts are only going to get larger, fuller, and heavier. A good, supportive bra is an invaluable asset in your constant effort to help reduce back pain—so once you find one that works, buy a few and pack away your smaller, underwire bras for after you are done nursing.

BABY - WHAT'S HAPPENING:

By now, your baby is between 3½ and 4 inches long and weighs approximately 1½ ounces. The placenta has taken over the job of nourishing your baby. Therefore, find out what substances and over-the-counter drugs are able to cross the placenta and be ingested by your baby, and avoid them.

FOR YOUR HEALTH: You will probably be asked if you want to store the blood from your baby's umbilical cord after she is born. This blood is very special, as it contains stem cells, which are used to increase immune system functioning and grow new tissue. Banking your baby's cord blood can be a lifesaver should someone in your family develop a serious condition such as leukemia, sickle cell disease, Hodgkin's disease, or breast cancer. If you decide to store your baby's cord blood, be sure the banking facility is accredited by the American Association of Blood Banks (AABB).

DAILY JOURNAL

Mood:

Energy:

Cravings:

Symptoms:

Weight:

DAY 84: Date:___/___/___

MOM - WHAT'S HAPPENING:

Congratulations! This is the last day of your first trimester. When you wake up tomorrow, you will be one-third of the way to holding your baby in your arms. This may cause you to feel relief, excitement, and/or panic—all of those reactions are normal. You will also see an increase in your energy as hormones level off. However, you may notice that your ears feel clogged and that your nasal passages are congested—your body is desperately trying to keep infections out, thus is constantly sending fluids out of your body.

BABY - WHAT'S HAPPENING:

Keep in mind that your baby's hearing is probably fairly well developed about now. As a result, your baby might respond by moving if you are exposed to loud sounds. But even the soothing sound of your voice has an impact—studies show that just 5 seconds of hearing mom's voice or classical music pumped into the womb via headphones can affect your baby's heart rate and pattern of movement.

FOR YOUR HEALTH: You may have noticed that unwanted hairs have begun to pop up in unexpected places, such as on your upper lip, down the sides of your face, on your chin, belly, toes or elsewhere. Hair growth is fairly common at this stage of pregnancy. Avoid depilatories, since it is unknown whether the chemicals used are absorbed by the body. For the same reasons, bleaching of body hair is not recommended while pregnant. Instead, remove unwanted hair by plucking or waxing. Many women buy several pair of tweezers and keep them in their car, office, and purse.

DAILY JOURNAL

Mood:

Energy:

Cravings:

Symptoms:

Weight:

Lunar Month

Four

PHOTO

Place a photo of you during your fourth month here

My Monthly Update

Waist Measurement: ____________________

Weight: ____________________

Mood: ____________________

PREGNANCY CHECKLIST

- ❑ Your belly is beginning to show, so start shopping for maternity clothes
- ❑ Check with your doctor to see if you need to take iron supplements
- ❑ Revise your budget to make room for baby
- ❑ Sign up for childbirth classes
- ❑ Get your baby's first picture — the ultrasound
- ❑ Find sleeping positions that are comfortable
- ❑ Prepare for and record your pregnancy dreams
- ❑ If you're RH negative, ask your doctor about a RhoGam shot
- ❑ Take pictures of your growing belly
- ❑ Get your partner involved — look into parenting classes
- ❑ Plan a babymoon — one last getaway together before the baby comes!

MY PERSONAL CHECKLIST:

- ❑ ....
- ❑ ....
- ❑ ....

MY HOPES FOR THIS MONTH:

....

....

....

....

....

....

....

....

....

Lunar Month Four

Second Trimester

WELCOME TO THE SECOND TRIMESTER of your pregnancy! This month is an exciting milestone for many women because it marks the beginning of a reduction in pregnancy-related symptoms. For baby, the second trimester also marks a dramatic decrease in the likelihood for developing birth defects. In addition, you can breathe a sigh of relief today, as the odds of miscarriage at this point are less than 1 percent.

Since the odds of miscarriage are so low, many women choose to share their good news with friends, family, and coworkers at this point. For some, this can be the moment they've waited for all of their lives, while others find that telling people they are pregnant opens the door to unsolicited advice. Both scenarios are often true, and so expect that you will be the recipient of pregnancy-related tales that run the gamut from the very touching to the absolutely tragic. Set limits with people who share only horror stories, though, since these are likely to increase your anxiety.

WHAT TO EXPECT THIS MONTH

This month you can expect to feel markedly less nauseous and fatigued. In fact, many women see a steady increase in their energy level this month, so take advantage of your renewed sense of motivation. Though many symptoms should wane this month, other symptoms will either intensify or make an initial appearance. In general, though, you can expect to feel much better during this trimester than you did in the first or will in the third.

You can also expect to see your OB-GYN again this month. Many women look forward to seeing their doctor each month, because they find it reassuring to hear the baby's heartbeat on the Doppler and find their doctor's ease and confidence in how the pregnancy is progressing to be quite comforting. It is a good idea to always come to your appointment prepared with questions and detailed information regarding any unusual symptoms.

THINGS TO CONSIDER

Though you may be anxious to feel your baby's kicks, swats, and flutters, keep in mind that it is rare to feel movement this early in the second trimester—especially if this is your first baby. So, if you are concerned at the lack of movement, don't be—rest assured that your baby is moving, you just can't feel it yet. In fact, though most women don't feel the first movement until 20 weeks, there is a slight chance that you will feel movement in the form of "butterflies" at the end of this month or early next month.

While you're waiting for that first kick, take some time to think about what you would like to do during the next few months' respite from nausea, fatigue, and the need to urinate frequently. The lightening of the load of these symptoms often makes the second trimester a great time for travel. Consider a weekend getaway with your partner because finding time for such things will be difficult once baby has arrived.

TIPS FOR COPING

This month you may find that your coping skills have more to do with the emotional side of pregnancy than the physical. Indeed, it is common to experience everything from fear to elation when you consider what it means to be a parent. In addition, you are probably also adjusting to your new physique, and it may be hard for you to deal with gaining weight from week to week—especially if you started your pregnancy very thin. The fact is that gaining weight is a necessary part of pregnancy, and if you're gaining steadily, eating well, and exercising, then you should have little trouble getting back down to your pre-pregnancy weight and figure. A good way to cope with weight gain is to immediately recognize when garments no longer fit and start wearing clothes that do fit. Trying to stuff yourself into pants or shirts that are clearly too small will only cause you to feel bad about yourself.

In general, it is beneficial for your disposition, and thus for the health of your baby, for you to engage in activities that make you feel good about yourself. Focusing on weight gain and other changes in your appearance that displease you may eventually lead to depression. So, be sure to wear clothes that fit comfortably and to spend a little time each day focusing on positives, such as the health of your baby. Additionally, practicing prenatal yoga can help to make you feel strong and limber, which can cut down on the negative side effects of weight gain.

WHAT TO EAT

Since it is likely that you will be feeling quite a bit better this month, now is a great time to increase your intake of vegetables and other foods you may have been avoiding. In fact, if you've lost some weight due to pregnancy sickness, you will probably catch up on calories this month—just be sure to make them count.

The best way to make calories count is by starting the day off with a healthy breakfast. Front-load your day with high-quality calories; a great breakfast, for example, is whole grain oatmeal with egg whites or tofu with steamed zucchini and brown rice. This may seem more like a lunch and it can be, but starting your day with high-quality protein and vegetables can help your body maintain blood-sugar levels for longer than a sugary cereal or muffin. Also, keep in mind that you should always have a midmorning snack while pregnant. Additionally, you should never skip a meal to cut down on calories.

HOW MUCH WEIGHT TO GAIN

Starting with the first week in your second trimester, you should expect to gain about 1 pound per week until the end of your pregnancy, or 4 pounds per month. If you're gaining a bit more than this guideline, don't panic. Just continue to eat well and be sure to walk for at least 20 to 30 minutes each day, and if your doctor has given you the green light to exercise, go for it. But don't overdo it. Of more concern to you and your baby is gaining less than 4 pounds per month—3 or 3½ pounds is OK, but any less and you are going to have to either increase your caloric intake or cut down on your exercise regimen to be sure your baby is getting enough nutrition.

EXERCISE TIPS AND ADVICE

As long as your pregnancy is progressing normally, continue the exercise regimen you have already established for yourself. However, if you find you are unable to jog comfortably or that you have difficulty maintaining your balance doing other exercises, now is a great time to take up swimming laps. Most large gyms have indoor heated pools and may offer day rates or reduced fees for pool use only. Swimming is an excellent exercise to do while pregnant because it does not put stress on loosening joints and it utilizes nearly every muscle in your body. If you're new to the pool, let the lifeguard know that you are pregnant so he or she can keep an eye on you in case you get tired and need some help mid-lap.

POTENTIAL SYMPTOMS AND HOW TO ALLEVIATE THEM

This month you should see a decrease in nausea, which may be accompanied by an increase in appetite. This rediscovered hunger may have you wanting to eat everything in sight. While it is OK to indulge in a hot-fudge sundae now and then, you will feel better and do more for your baby's nourishment by maintaining your healthy diet. Overindulgence of your sweet tooth can cause other problems this month as well.

Many women see an increase in dental problems this month. Swollen, bleeding gums can make it painful to brush your teeth, so purchase a soft toothbrush and toothpaste for sensitive teeth and gums. You may even want to buy a child's toothbrush, as they tend to have softer bristles. Since you're less likely to brush as vigorously as you did before you were pregnant, limit your intake of sweets, as your teeth may become prone to cavities at this point.

WAYS OTHERS CAN HELP

As you check off the weeks on your calendar, you may start to feel like you will never get everything done in time for your baby's arrival. Though this is probably true, you should enlist the help of your friends with kids when you make your to-do lists. Other people with kids can be a great resource for moms-to-be, because they can tell you exactly what they needed for their babies' arrivals and also what you can save until later.

"Before you were born I carried you under my heart. From the moment you arrived in this world until the moment I leave it, I will always carry you in my heart."
~ Mandy Harrison

Week 13

Starting Weight: ________

OVERVIEW

This week can go one of two ways for you. If you are lucky, you will see a dramatic decrease in nausea, fatigue, and the frequent need to void your bladder. However, some women do not see any relief this week and wonder where the heck this idea of the "honeymoon" phase of pregnancy came from. The majority of women, though, should experience an increase in energy this week. And some women may notice the appearance of a few new symptoms.

Around the 13th week of your baby's development you may start to experience back pain in a place that is lower than where you've become used to it. This is due to excess weight and added pressure on your coccyx, (tailbone). In fact, some women find that sitting for too long causes their tailbone to feel like it is going to press through the skin. As your pregnancy progresses, this condition may worsen, so it is a good idea to purchase a donut pillow, which will allow for some open space between your coccyx and the seat.

DAY 85: Date:___/___/___

MOM - WHAT'S HAPPENING:

Due to an increase in estrogen and progesterone production the glands inside your breasts that are responsible for producing milk might expand today. If so, you're probably feeling quite heavy on top. All of that extra weight can start to put a strain your lower back. Good posture can help alleviate some of the symptoms associated with lower back pain. Remember, however, that if you're experiencing back pain at this point in your pregnancy, it will probably worsen as you head into your third trimester. Thus, it is important to exercise in order to strengthen and support your abdominal and lower back muscles.

BABY - WHAT'S HAPPENING:

Your baby's bones are gradually hardening as he absorbs calcium supplied by your diet through the placenta. His bone marrow continues to mature as well, and his muscles are becoming more substantial. He is long and lean and his body is starting to catch up to his head proportionally.

TIPS AND ADVICE: If you're feeling up to it, the second trimester is a great time to start registering for gifts for your baby. It is a good idea to register at just one or two stores so that your items don't overlap. Also, be sure to register for items that are practical—it may not seem like fun to register for diapers, for example, but you'll be glad you did once you've gone through 70 diapers in your baby's first week of life. Keep in mind that you can update your registry as your pregnancy progresses, so don't feel locked in by decisions made at this point.

DAILY JOURNAL

Mood:

Energy:

Cravings:

Symptoms:

Weight:

DAY 86: Date:___/___/___

MOM - WHAT'S HAPPENING:

By now you've probably gained close to 5 pounds. If you've gained more or less, it's OK. Remember that dieting can be harmful to your developing baby, so avoid the urge to cut calories if you're gaining more than expected. Just be sure to eat enough calories from a variety of foods and continue to walk or do some form of daily exercise. Since your baby's bones are in the process of ossification, you should increase your calcium intake from food sources (rather than from supplements) so that she doesn't start to pull calcium from your bones and teeth.

BABY - WHAT'S HAPPENING:

The lanugo that's protecting your baby's skin is made up of a very thin layer of fine downy hair. His skin is also very thin—like tracing paper. In fact, if you could see your baby now, you'd be able to see the blood vessels beneath his skin. And if you were to have an ultrasound this week it would be possible to see the outline of your baby's skeleton.

PREGNANCY FACT: Amniocentesis is a test that can detect abnormalities in your baby's development. It is usually offered between weeks 16 and 20 if you are 35 or older, if your family history includes a condition the test covers—such as Down syndrome or Tay-Sachs—or if you have another child with a genetic disorder. Amniocentesis is performed by your doctor. She will insert a long hollow needle into your uterus and remove about 2 tablespoons of amniotic fluid. The test carries a small risk to the fetus, but complications are rare and the test is 99 percent accurate in its detection abilities.

DAILY JOURNAL

Mood:

Energy:

Cravings:

Symptoms:

Weight:

DAY 87: Date:___/___/___

MOM - WHAT'S HAPPENING:

Odds are that by this time you may have noticed some extra darkening on the skin above your eyebrows, on your cheeks, or across the bridge of your nose. As mentioned earlier, this "pregnancy mask" will darken with exposure to sun, so be sure to wear sunscreen and a hat if you will be outside for long periods of time. There are several treatments that claim to lighten the skin, but none of these are recommended during pregnancy.

BABY - What's Happening:

Your baby is starting to develop hair along his eyebrows and hair has also begun to appear in a unique pattern on his scalp. Unless he is genetically predisposed to very dark hair, though, the color will not yet be visible. In fact, your baby's hair color and texture may be very different when he is born from when he was in utero. Also, by now the three bones inside the middle ear have begun to harden, further developing his hearing.

FOOD FOR THOUGHT: Research shows that babies born to parents who suffer from allergies are likely to inherit an allergy—though not necessary the same one as his parents. This is especially true if mom eats highly allergenic foods while pregnant or nursing, such as peanuts and dairy products. If you currently have allergies or did as a child, consider limiting your intake of high allergen foods—especially peanuts. Peanut allergies affect 1.3 percent of the population, making it the number one food allergy in America. Allergy to peanuts is also one of the most severe of the food allergies.

DAILY JOURNAL

Mood:

Energy:

Cravings:

Symptoms:

Weight:

DAY 88: Date:___/___/___

MOM - WHAT'S HAPPENING:

By now, the placenta should be fully functional, which means it has taken on the majority of progesterone production to sustain your pregnancy. It is also responsible for getting nutrients and oxygen to your baby while filtering out waste. The umbilical cord connects the baby to the placenta, which grows against your uterine wall. Thus, the placenta is made up of both fetal and maternal components. Your blood and the food you eat (as well any medications and toxins) are filtered through the placenta before they reach your baby.

BABY - WHAT'S HAPPENING:

If you're dying to find out your baby's sex, it is possible at this point to tell by ultrasound. However, it is still early in your pregnancy, thus there is a certain amount of error possible when deciphering the baby's sex in this way. If you are scheduled for an amniocentesis, though, this test will be able to tell with accuracy whether you are carrying a boy or a girl.

FOR YOUR HEALTH: Exercising can cause slight uterine contractions. Though this can be scary the first time it happens, it is usually not cause for alarm. Many women fear they are in premature labor when they feel a tightening sensation in their lower abdomen, so it helps to know what premature labor actually is. It is signified by painful uterine contractions that don't stop after you've ceased exercising, or contractions accompanied by vaginal bleeding and/or a rush of discharge, cramping, backaches, and pelvic pressure.

DAILY JOURNAL

Mood:

Energy:

Cravings:

Symptoms:

Weight:

DAY 89: Date:___/___/___

MOM - WHAT'S HAPPENING:

Thanks to pregnancy-induced congestion, you have probably become a bit of a snorer at night. This is a common pregnancy side effect, and if you were not one to snore before you were pregnant, you will probably stop once you have your baby. If your snoring is disrupting you or your partner's sleep, try using saline drops in your nose before bed (avoid medicated nasal sprays while pregnant) or nasal strips that drape across the bridge of your nose and force the nasal passages to stay open while you sleep.

BABY - WHAT'S HAPPENING:

Your baby is able to make several different facial expressions as the nerves and muscles in her face become more fully developed. Her eyes are nearly in their final position on her face, and her eyelids remain fused shut. Meanwhile, on the sides of her head, her ears are continuing on with their migration up to be even with her nose. This facial activity is adding to your baby's increasingly human appearance.

TIPS AND ADVICE: Headaches are common during pregnancy for many reasons—hormones, caffeine withdrawal, congestion, and stress can all cause mild to severe headaches. Though it is usually OK to take Tylenol while pregnant, there are some other tips that may help as well. As soon as you feel a headache coming on, retreat to a dark room and put a soft ice pack on your head. Stay well hydrated, and when feeling particularly stuffed up, spend time in the bathroom while running the hot shower. The steam will help break up the congestion and relieve pressure that causes headaches.

DAILY JOURNAL

Mood:

Energy:

Cravings:

Symptoms:

Weight:

DAY 90: Date:___/___/___

MOM - WHAT'S HAPPENING:

If you are over the age of 35 or are at risk of having a baby with any of a number of genetic abnormalities, your health care provider will schedule you for an amniocentesis around this time. This test is extremely useful in learning whether a fetus will be born with genetic disorders, such as Down syndrome, Hunter's syndrome, Fifth disease, or sickle cell anemia. Amniocentesis is also able to clarify the results of a problematic CVS result and an irregular ultrasound image.

BABY - WHAT'S HAPPENING:

By now your baby is about 4½ to 5 inches long and weighs about 2½ ounces. He is about the size of a softball and is constantly wiggling his fingers and toes. He is able to make an impressive fist, which he waves around in the amniotic fluid as if he was boxing. He is also practicing his breathing and swallowing, which prepares him for life on the "outside."

FOR YOUR HEALTH: Many moms-to-be turn to artificial sweeteners while pregnant to cut down on caloric intake. The problem, however, is that there is not enough research available to know what effects they have on babies in utero. Scientists advise pregnant moms against ingesting saccharin, as there is evidence it can potentially increase baby's risk for bladder cancer. Aspartame, a more common sweetener, is considered safe is small amounts, but it is advisable to limit your intake of the sugar substitute as there are conflicting reports about its safety when used regularly.

DAILY JOURNAL

Mood:

Energy:

Cravings:

Symptoms:

Weight:

DAY 91: Date:___/___/___

MOM - WHAT'S HAPPENING:

Around this time, approximately 50 to 70 percent of moms-to-be develop pregnancy gingivitis. As mentioned earlier, high levels of the hormone progesterone cause gums to swell and bleed, leaving them susceptible to bacteria. It is important that you be sure to brush your teeth at least twice a day, floss, and use an antimicrobial rinse (being careful not to swallow any). Occasionally, a large lump develops at the top of the gum, called a pregnancy tumor. But this is rare, benign, and will go away after the baby is born.

BABY - WHAT'S HAPPENING:

It is likely that by now the roof of your baby's mouth is completely formed. Thus, the rest of her taste buds have developed on the roof of her mouth, giving her a complete set. She is also beginning to respond to the foods that you eat—especially to particularly spicy or sweet flavors.

PREGNANCY FACT: Prenatal massages are growing in popularity. Prenatal massage can be done with you lying on your side or on your stomach with a specially designed cut out so your belly is not pressed against the table. It is important to see a practitioner who is experienced in pregnancy massage as there are special considerations. Research conducted by the University of Miami School of Medicine shows that getting a massage while pregnant greatly reduces stress hormones while increasing circulation—which is great for both mom and baby.

DAILY JOURNAL

Mood:

Energy:

Cravings:

Symptoms:

Weight:

Week 14

Starting Weight: ________

OVERVIEW

Try to relax this week, if possible. Odds are you're feeling less fatigued and nauseated than you were in your first trimester, so it's great time to do something special to celebrate.

Something else you may want to celebrate is that people will start to notice that you look pregnant instead of thinking you've developed a potbelly. In fact, by the end of this week, you should be able to feel the top of your uterus by pressing down midway between your pubic bone and your belly button. It is also likely that you will need to trade in your button-fly jeans for some stretchy pants as your belly has popped out just enough to make last month's pants feel tight. Unfortunately, your sinuses will continue to cause you even more trouble this week as your nasal passages swell from increased blood circulation and congestion. If you haven't already purchased a humidifier—now is the time. Be sure to avoid warm-mist humidifiers, though, as they require quite a bit of maintenance in order to avoid bacteria growth—which can be harmful to both you and the baby.

Speaking of baby—this is the time to sing, talk, and read to your little one while in utero as her ears are mature and will be able to detect and remember sounds from the outside. Studies have shown that infants recognize the sounds they hear while in utero—such as songs sung repetitively and the voices of their parents.

DAY 92: Date:___/___/___

MOM - WHAT'S HAPPENING:

Today you should see some relief from breast pain—it may even disappear completely, though you will continue to see an increase in breast size over the course of your pregnancy and while you are breast-feeding. Count yourself lucky if you have escaped the effects of swollen nasal membranes thus far, though you could experience them any day—nosebleeds are a common and usually harmless side effect of high levels of estrogen production.

BABY - WHAT'S HAPPENING:

If you could see into your womb it might appear that your baby is making deliberate, almost coordinated movements. This is because her skeleton and connective tissue have developed enough to make fluid, less jerky motions. Also, your baby continues to make a variety of facial expressions—though she is not aware of them, so smiles do not equal happiness nor do frowns indicate sadness. In addition, as your baby's skeleton hardens, her neck becomes stronger, causing it to straighten out.

PREGNANCY FACT: It is likely that you will come down with at least one cold while you are pregnant. Unfortunately, you will not be able to knock it out with high doses of vitamin C or other medications (though acetaminophen should be OK for aches and pains). So, if you find yourself with a cold, the best course of action is to get plenty of rest, continue to eat well (even if you don't have an appetite, it's important to eat), stay hydrated, gargle with warm salt water to relieve a sore throat, use a humidifier to ease breathing, and prop yourself up on a couple of pillows when you sleep.

DAILY JOURNAL

Mood:

Energy:

Cravings:

Symptoms:

Weight:

DAY 93: Date:___/___/___

MOM - WHAT'S HAPPENING:

There's a good chance that you're feeling better than you have in weeks, so this is the time to enjoy being pregnant—especially because you should be much less anxious about something going wrong with the pregnancy. Perhaps today you and your partner might begin shopping for the nursery. If you decide to paint, let your partner do the job: inhaling paint fumes is not healthy for you or your baby.

BABY - WHAT'S HAPPENING:

Your little one is about the size of a small pear and weighs around 3½ ounces. Her eyes are starting to move a little beneath her eyelids, and if you were to aim a powerful beam of light into your uterus, your baby might react to it by turning away. This is because her eyes are now nearly face-forward and able to see light through her thin, fused eyelids.

FOOD FOR THOUGHT: It is common for women with morning sickness to avoid tomatoes during their first trimester. Now that you are feeling better, consider adding them to your sandwiches, salads, or just eating them on their own. The USDA has found that in addition to having high levels of vitamins A, C, and K, tomatoes contain the carotenoid lycopene, a powerful antioxidant that can help protect the body from breast, pancreatic, and intestinal cancers. Because it is fat-soluble, in order to get the most out of lycopene, tomatoes ought to be eaten with avocados, olive oil, and nuts.

DAILY JOURNAL

Mood:

Energy:

Cravings:

Symptoms:

Weight:

DAY 94: Date:___/___/___

MOM - WHAT'S HAPPENING:

Most doctors will recommend that you have the triple screen blood test between (LMP) weeks 16 and 18. The triple screen test lets doctors analyze AFP protein produced by your baby's liver and excreted into your blood stream. This test also measures the hormones hCG and estriol (estrogen produced by the placenta). Doctors use the information to detect neural tube disorders as well as Down's syndrome. Like all pregnancy diagnostics, the triple screen is controversial in that its results may not actually indicate a problem, or point to defects that don't actually exist. At the end of the day, you and your partner must decide whether you see value in this screening.

BABY - WHAT'S HAPPENING:

Your baby's circulatory system is working hard today, pumping up to 25 quarts of blood through his tiny 4½-inch body each day. With each day, his heartbeat gets stronger and more pronounced.

FOR YOUR HEALTH: Thanks to pregnancy hormones, you are more prone to yeast infections while you are expecting. Researchers believe these hormones change the pH balance in the intestines and vagina, which can promote excess growth of yeast. To help restore the chemical balance, you should eat plenty of yogurt and cut down on your sugar intake. If you develop symptoms related to a yeast infection, such as foul-smelling discharge and itching, tell your doctor. Treatment will likely be the same as if you were not pregnant.

DAILY JOURNAL

Mood:

Energy:

Cravings:

Symptoms:

Weight:

DAY 95: Date:___/___/___

MOM - WHAT'S HAPPENING:

The increasing size and weight of your uterus may start to put more of a strain on muscles and joints in your mid-section, causing pain in your abdomen and lower back. This is also due to the thickening and lengthening of the ligaments attached to your uterus. Round ligament pain can be managed through slow and careful movements combined with warm compresses, while yoga and/or meditation might help cut down on backaches by strengthening muscles and relieving tension.

BABY - WHAT'S HAPPENING:

Your baby's movements are quite impressive for such a little one. At this point he can open and close his mouth, which is how he is able to swallow the amniotic fluid. He can also turn his head from side to side and up and down. These moves are unconscious, but if you were to watch him, your baby might look like he is looking around and talking.

TIPS AND ADVICE: As your pregnancy progresses you will find you have trouble sleeping for a variety of reasons. During your second trimester, this has less to do with having to get up during the night to go to the bathroom and more to do with your racing mind and growing belly. Battling pregnancy-induced insomnia is possible by getting enough exercise during the day, avoiding meals too close to bedtime, and by establishing a bedtime routine that includes relaxing activities such as taking a warm bath, meditating, and journaling about your major stressors.

DAILY JOURNAL

Mood:

Energy:

Cravings:

Symptoms:

Weight:

DAY 97: Date:___/___/___

MOM - WHAT'S HAPPENING:

You uterus is now approximately 3 inches below your belly button. You should be able to feel the top of your uterus, or fundus, when you press in and down on your lower abdomen. Also, today you might find that the increased blood flow to the lower half of your body has made the swelling in your feet and ankles more pronounced. Your doctor will check this swelling at each visit, but be sure to call her if it seems excessive. Too much swelling can be a sign of preeclampsia, or pregnancy-induced hypertension.

BABY - WHAT'S HAPPENING:

Your baby has not yet developed fat layers to add weight and warmth, though she will grow at an extremely rapid pace over the next several months. Consider that today your baby weighs just 3½ ounces and by the time she is born she will probably weigh between 7½ and 8½ pounds. This means over the next several months your baby's weight must increase considerably in order to be of average birth weight.

PREGNANCY FACT: If you have opted for the triple screen test to check for neural tube defects, you may be awaiting results this week. Waiting for tests results can be nerve-wracking. While you wait, discuss with your partner how you will handle the results of the test. Practice deep breathing exercises to stay calm. Also, remember that even if your test is positive, your baby may still be fine, since false positives are fairly common. Usually, a second test will be done, and if the results are still positive, your doctor will suggest an ultrasound exam and/or amniocentesis to clarify the diagnosis.

DAILY JOURNAL

Mood:

Energy:

Cravings:

Symptoms:

Weight:

DAY 97: Date:___/___/___

MOM - WHAT'S HAPPENING:

Bulging veins can be painful, so it is important to pay attention to their appearance and size. Often, the veins that appear on your breasts and stomach do not swell enough to bulge or cause pain. However, it is common to develop one or two painful varicose veins on your legs or even your vagina. Wearing support hose designed for pregnant women can help keep veins in check as can keeping your legs elevated whenever possible. Also, switch positions frequently, and avoid crossing your legs while sitting.

BABY - WHAT'S HAPPENING:

Today you might want to sing, talk, and read to your little one—her ears are mature and will be able to detect and remember sounds from the outside. Studies show that infants recognize the sounds they hear while in utero—such as songs sung repetitively, the family dog's bark, and the voices of their parents. Also today, she can flex her feet and toes, and she is bending and straightening her legs at the knee.

FOR YOUR HEALTH: It is a great idea to stretch a few times every day even if you are unable to exercise. Two great stress-relieving exercises are shoulder and leg stretches. The shoulder stretch is done by standing with your feet hip-length apart. With your knees slightly bent, grab your arm just below the elbow and pull your arm toward the other shoulder as you exhale. To perform the leg stretch, hold on to the back of a chair and grab the top of your foot with the hand that is on the same side. Hold your back straight and pull your foot toward your bum and hold. Repeat.

DAILY JOURNAL

Mood:

Energy:

Cravings:

Symptoms:

Weight:

DAY 98: Date:___/___/___

MOM - WHAT'S HAPPENING:

In addition to pain in your lower back, you may start noticing pain in your neck and upper back. The causes of this pain are stress, the new distribution of weight, and the increased size of your breasts. Wearing a good, supportive bra should help ease upper back pain, but there are other things you can do as well. Stretching exercises that target your neck muscles and upper back are best, as these areas are where most of your tension builds up, causing muscles to tighten and become painful.

BABY - WHAT'S HAPPENING:

Your baby may be performing somersaults by now! As he discovers his mobility his moves will become more aggressive and pronounced but, for now, they are still very light and probably not detected by you just yet. Your baby will begin to develop fat deposits next week and soon his weight and strength will keep you up at night as he kicks and tumbles and karate-chops his way around your uterus.

PREGNANCY FACT: It is true that most women who start their pregnancies overweight give birth to healthy babies with little complications. However, it is necessary to understand that if you were overweight before becoming pregnant, you are at higher risk for complications, such as developing gestational diabetes. It may also be difficult for your doctor to feel the height of the fundus or hear the baby's heartbeat with the Doppler. Don't panic if you are overweight—just practice healthy eating habits, exercise at an appropriate level, and follow your doctor's instructions.

DAILY JOURNAL

Mood:

Energy:

Cravings:

Symptoms:

Weight:

Week 15

Starting Weight: _________

OVERVIEW

This is an exciting week for your baby's development, because this is the week that she will start developing fat stores under her skin. This is an important step in your little one's growth. Babies must accumulate enough fat before they are born to sustain them for a little while until mom starts nursing (or until the first bottle). The fat your baby develops in utero will also help to regulate her body temperature after she is born. Your baby will also start to store up stool in her intestines, called meconium. Meconium is made up of debris in the amniotic fluid, such as shed lanugo, digested amniotic fluid and discarded cells. This is all part of the process of your baby's major growth spurt this week, which will also have an impact on your body.

As your baby enters a growth spurt this week, your uterus will expand to about the size of a cantaloupe. This will bring the top of your fundus to just about 2 inches below your belly button. You will also probably notice that although your appetite is increasing, your ability to eat large meals is on the decline. This is because your uterus is starting to crowd the organs above it, including your stomach. So, it's a good idea to eat even smaller meals than you have been, and to eat these more frequently. In fact, it helps to carry a variety of snacks around with you all day long, as many women find that they are much more comfortable grazing than eating meals.

DAY 99: Date:___/___/___

MOM - WHAT'S HAPPENING:

As your circulatory system continues its massive output and your body continues to get heavier, today you might find you are sweating frequently and having hot flashes. In addition to sweating, you will likely see an increase in the aforementioned leukorrhea. These may have you feeling swampy and gross most of the day. Reduce this feeling by freshening up midday and carrying a change of underwear and panty liners with you. Dress in layers, hydrate, and rest after climbing stairs or engaging in any form of exercise.

BABY - WHAT'S HAPPENING:

The baby's digestive system is already operating by today. His bowels now contain a substance called meconium. This stool is unusual in that it is sterile, since it is only made up of lanugo and other materials that are digested by your baby when he swallows the amniotic fluid. Meconium is usually emptied from your baby's intestines within the first few days after birth.

FOOD FOR THOUGHT: Contrary to what many believe, sodium is a necessary mineral for pregnant women to help regulate their body fluids. Thus, it is not recommended to go on a low-sodium diet when you are pregnant. However, there is a difference between sodium and salt. Sodium is only 40 percent of the composition of table salt, and should be limited. Sodium found naturally in foods is an important component of the pregnancy diet. Be sure to read food labels and keep in mind that you should consume around 2,400 milligrams of sodium each day while pregnant and nursing.

DAILY JOURNAL

Mood:

Energy:

Cravings:

Symptoms:

Weight:

DAY 100: Date:___/___/___

MOM - WHAT'S HAPPENING:

Your uterus is now about the size of a small melon, and it is between 1½ and 2 inches below your belly button. Your expanding womb may have you feeling achy and sore, so take it slow, especially when getting in and out of the car as these motions can exacerbate round ligament pain. By now you have probably gained between 5 and 10 pounds. If you've gained more or less than this, remind yourself once again that every woman's pregnancy is different.

BABY - WHAT'S HAPPENING:

Your baby is a giant today compared to his size 14 weeks ago! Weighing in at just about 5 ounces, your baby's body is busy accumulating fat stores under his skin during this week's major growth spurt. Fat is a necessary part of your baby's ability to regulate his body temperature after he is born. Fat also helps to stabilize your baby's metabolism and gives him enough energy to survive the first few shaky hours (or days) of breast-feeding.

TIPS AND ADVICE: If you happen to be involved in a car accident while pregnant, see your doctor right away or go to the emergency room. Even if the accident was minor and you feel fine, it is important to have a thorough exam. Even though your baby is protected by the amniotic sac and fluid, there is a chance that the placenta can become dislodged. This can be very dangerous and could lead to preterm labor or even miscarriage. Thus, a thorough exam, including ultrasound, is necessary to make sure everything is as it should be.

DAILY JOURNAL

Mood:

Energy:

Cravings:

Symptoms:

Weight:

DAY 101: Date:___/___/___

MOM - WHAT'S HAPPENING:

An amazing feature of pregnancy is your body's ability to adapt to the many changes to your physical being. For example, as the uterus expands, it simply moves other organs out if its way. In fact, it will push the intestines over to the side of your abdomen. This can make constipation number one on your symptoms list. Thus, now is a good time to increase your fiber intake and add a few prunes to your snack mix each day. Naturally relieving constipation is the best way to avoid straining on the toilet, which can lead to hemorrhoid development.

BABY - WHAT'S HAPPENING:

As your baby grows, so do the placenta and the umbilical cord. Today, in fact, the placenta should be about 5 inches long and weight approximately 5 ounces—the same as your baby. Your baby will weigh between 6 and 9 times more than the placenta at the time of birth.

FOOD FOR THOUGHT: Eat several servings of complex carbohydrates each day. These unrefined carbs are rich in fiber and full of B vitamins, minerals, and protein. Examples include whole grain breads and cereals, dried beans, potatoes with skin, brown rice, and fresh vegetables and fruit. A diet that includes these goodies will reduce the risk of developing gestational diabetes and reduce incidences of constipation and nausea. However, diets that include lots of refined carbs, such as white bread, white rice, and sugary snacks, increase your risk of developing gestational diabetes.

DAILY JOURNAL

Mood:

Energy:

Cravings:

Symptoms:

Weight:

DAY 102: Date:___/___/___

MOM - WHAT'S HAPPENING:

Today you might feel dizzy, which is normal. The further along you get in your pregnancy, the more likely it is that blood will pool in your legs and feet, depriving your brain (if only slightly) of oxygen. Try to sitting or reclining with your feet elevated. Or, walk in place or flex your ankles—moving the muscles in your legs will put pressure on your veins and force blood upward.

BABY - WHAT'S HAPPENING:

Your baby's face continues to develop its character. If you could see your baby's face up close, you would see the arch of his eyebrows and the slightest bit of soft, downy hair. Likewise, his scalp continues to fill in with hair in a predetermined pattern. Also, around today, your baby's reflexes are becoming more frequent, and he may be startled by loud noises outside the womb. Thus dogs barking, alarms, and your sneezes may send your baby into surprised somersaults!

PREGNANCY FACT: The Bradley Method of childbirth was developed in the 1940s by a doctor who believed that months of preparation could lead to a natural, drug-free labor and delivery. The classes are broken down into 12 sessions and include: diet and nutrition; the importance of exercise; symptoms of pregnancy and how to manage them; relaxation techniques for labor and delivery; coaching skills for your partner; coping with the different stages of labor; avoiding medical interventions; making a birth plan; and finally, bringing baby home, which includes information on breast-feeding.

DAILY JOURNAL

Mood:

Energy:

Cravings:

Symptoms:

Weight:

DAY 103: Date:___/___/___

MOM - WHAT'S HAPPENING:

Because your circulatory system is still expanding at a rapid rate, avoid taking hot showers. The dramatic change in temperature can cause you to become so light-headed that you actually pass out. In fact, take only warm showers and baths that are close to your own body temperature. At this point, low blood pressure may cause symptoms when you lay on your back. This puts pressure on the vena cava, which sends blood from your legs back up to your heart. The additional weight of your uterus can slow this return of blood when you lie on your back, so lie on your side instead.

BABY - WHAT'S HAPPENING:

As you will quickly learn after you give birth, babies have their own internal clocks that tell them when to sleep or wake up. That clock is developed even now, telling your baby to sleep and then wake up. As his or her movements become more noticeable, you'll get a sense of that internal clock's setting.

FOR YOUR HEALTH: If you live in an apartment or home built before 1978 and have the urge to scrape and paint the nursery, pause to consider the following: Most homes built before 1978 were decorated using paint containing lead. It was eventually discovered that lead residue can cause miscarriage, low birth weight, and mental retardation in children, and was banned in homes after 1978. If you live in an older house, you should not scrape paint off the walls. If paint is chipping on its own, visit www.epa.gov for information about how to test for and remove lead.

DAILY JOURNAL

Mood:

Energy:

Cravings:

Symptoms:

Weight:

DAY 104: Date:___/___/___

MOM - WHAT'S HAPPENING:

Around today you might start experiencing a decrease in the natural moisture produced by your eyes. Thus, your eyes are probably red, irritated, itchy, and very dry. As mentioned earlier, the best way to deal with this condition is to use over-the-counter lubricant. By now you may also have to officially retire your contact lenses as your eyeballs have changed shape. Glasses are more comfortable at this point, and can offer some protection against the additional drying effects of wind and debris in the air.

BABY - WHAT'S HAPPENING:

By now your baby is close to 5½ inches long and her body is getting plump with fat as each day comes and goes. As your baby gets bigger, so does her appetite. In fact, her digestive tract is maturing and continues to practice its skills by engaging the amniotic fluid. At this point, your baby is swallowing so often, she's likely to have the hiccups several times a day. If this is not your first pregnancy, you have probably felt these tiny flutters by now.

PREGNANCY FACT: The very first time you feel your baby move is called quickening. If this is your first baby, you can expect to feel him move for the first time between 15 and 22 weeks. If this is not your first pregnancy, you will probably feel it sooner. Many women describe this sensation as butterflies, gas, or bubbles. It can often be attributed to baby's hiccups or somersaults. Kicking usually isn't felt until later, when the baby is heavy enough to be able to kick or slap with some force. Quickening is an exciting and beautiful moment for both you and your baby, one that you will never forget!

DAILY JOURNAL

Mood:

Energy:

Cravings:

Symptoms:

Weight:

DAY 105: Date:___/___/___

MOM - WHAT'S HAPPENING:

Today you might feel overcome with anxiety over the financial responsibility involved in raising a child. It is common to switch your focus to post-pregnancy concerns as your attention is no longer on dealing with the immediacy of nausea. Today is a great time to sit down with your partner and come up with a strategy. A good first step would be to see a financial planner who can cater a financial plan to your specific needs. At the very least, express your concerns to your partner. He is assuredly experiencing financial anxiety as well, and just talking about it can help take the edge off.

BABY - WHAT'S HAPPENING:

Today, your baby is exploring the outside world with his ears. Researchers have discovered that babies who are exposed to many different sounds in utero are less likely to be startled by these same noises after they are born. Thus, a fetus who hears the family dog's bark on a regular basis will be more likely to sleep through that same dog's barking when born.

FOOD FOR THOUGHT: Be sure to incorporate a variety of legumes into your diet. Peas, lentils, and beans are low in fat and high in folate and potassium. They also contain elevated levels of fiber, iron, magnesium, and protein. Legumes are a great substitute for meat and can be added to nearly any dish, including soups, salads, and stews. They are also tasty with rice, tortillas, cottage cheese, and vegetables. Consider purchasing dry beans and soaking them—it is more time-intensive than opening a can of ready-made beans but the dried variety contains more nutrients and less salt.

DAILY JOURNAL

Mood:

Energy:

Cravings:

Symptoms:

Weight:

Week 16

Starting Weight: _________

OVERVIEW

Give yourself a pat on the back and breathe a sigh of relief! You are now in the 16th week of your baby's development. Not only have most of your symptoms stabilized, but this is also an exciting time for your baby. Over this next week, her nervous system begins to further specialize its functions—especially those of the five senses. In fact, as your baby's hearing gets more tuned in to her surroundings she will become used to familiar sounds and even start to react to them through her movements. Also, this week your baby will grow to be more than 6 inches long, and she will continue to accumulate fat stores under her skin.

Your baby's increasing size will make it possible for you to feel movement this week. Her constant kicking, swatting, hiccupping, and somersaults are bound to give you butterflies. Unfortunately for your partner, it will still be another few weeks (or months) before he can feel these movements from the outside. Even so, it is a wonderful bonding exercise for the whole family to have dad to talk to baby and spend time with his ear and hands on your abdomen. If you are due for an ultrasound this week, make sure that your partner comes along with you, because neither of you will want to miss the debut of your baby's new trick—yawning. That's right, this week your baby will add this sleepy pantomime to her repertoire of facial movements.

DAY 106: Date:___/___/___

MOM - WHAT'S HAPPENING:

Thanks to an increase in appetite, you are likely in the midst of a growth spurt, as is your baby. You may find yourself more drawn to carbohydrates as your energy needs increase. Also today you may notice a thin, dark line appear anywhere from just above your stomach all the way down to the top of your pubic bone. This is a common side effect of hormones and will likely increase as your pregnancy progresses.

BABY - WHAT'S HAPPENING:

Your baby's neurons are being covered by a white insulating substance called myelin. Myelin coats neurons in a sheath that allows for efficient transfer of electrical impulses throughout the body. Myelin is composed of 20 percent protein and 80 percent fat, which makes for a strong protective layer. Myelination is important in your baby's development. In fact, damage to the myelin sheath, called demyelination, results in disruption of signals that the brain sends to the rest of the body, which can have serious results.

TIPS AND ADVICE: For some women, pregnancy is a time of anxiety rather than joy—particularly if this is your first baby or if you do not have a partner to share the experience with. Thanks to the age of online message boards, you do not have to go through pregnancy alone. If you find that you're up at 2 in the morning wishing for someone to talk to, try joining a chat room for pregnant women. Online chat rooms and message boards are a great resource for tips on everything from how to manage symptoms to product suggestions, exercise tips, and emotional support.

DAILY JOURNAL

Mood:

Energy:

Cravings:

Symptoms:

Weight:

DAY 107: Date:___/___/___

MOM - WHAT'S HAPPENING:

Today you may notice a shift in your center of gravity. As your uterus grows and pushes out your belly, you may start to walk with your feet slightly farther apart. It may feel sort of like someone is pushing into your lower back with their knee. A good way to stabilize this off-balance feeling is to hold onto a chair or other stable surface and squat down. This allows your back to straighten out while being supported.

BABY - WHAT'S HAPPENING:

Today your baby might be practicing yawning! The yawning reflex is another skill in a series of in utero behaviors that your baby will carry with him into the world. Your movements throughout the day will likely lull him to sleep, so he might yawn as he gets ready to sleep the day away while you're at work.

FOR YOUR HEALTH: Consider treating yourself to a facial at least once or twice while you are pregnant. Having a facial is a great way to clear out pores that may become more clogged than usual due to excess oil from to pregnancy hormones. When making an appointment, be sure to tell the spa that you are pregnant and that you want either an oxygen-based facial or hydrating facial—these are both safe while you are pregnant. However, it is important to avoid microdermabrasions, aromatherapy, and chemical peels, as they are not recommended for pregnant women.

DAILY JOURNAL

Mood:

Energy:

Cravings:

Symptoms:

Weight:

DAY 108: Date:___/___/___

MOM - WHAT'S HAPPENING:

By now, you've probably gotten all the advice from others that you can stand. Your family, friends, even total strangers have likely offered opinions on everything from toilet training to saving for college. Many probably have come up with names for your baby, especially if you've shared your child's gender with others. This is a common complaint for many pregnant women, and is, unfortunately, something to be weathered—it is nearly impossible to stop others from offering unsolicited advice. Remember that most people are coming from a place of kindness and desire to help.

BABY - WHAT'S HAPPENING:

Around this time, the loops and swirls that make your baby's toe and fingerprints unique should have finished developing. Also, your baby's body is developing a protective coating called vernix. This substance has the consistency of thin wax. It, coupled with lanugo, helps protect your baby's skin from long-term exposure to water in the amniotic sac.

TIPS AND ADVICE: Before you purchase big ticket items for your baby, such as a crib, stroller, bassinet, high chair, and car seat, do your homework. All products are not created equal, and there are several agencies and organizations that test and rate products based on safety, cost, and durability. Some websites to check out when you start researching are the U.S. Consumer Product Safety Commission (www.cpsc.gov) and Consumer Reports (www.consumerreports.org). It is a good idea to comparison shop and take your time before deciding on more expensive items.

DAILY JOURNAL

Mood:

Energy:

Cravings:

Symptoms:

Weight:

DAY 109: Date:___/___/___

MOM - WHAT'S HAPPENING:

You may have noticed an increase in strange or vivid dreams over the last few nights. The rush of hormones that accompanies pregnancy is partly responsible for this. Also, during sleep your brain processes some of the concerns you probably have: Will I be a good mother? Is my baby OK? The list of worries is almost endless. If you find your dreams disturb the amount of sleep you get, discuss them with your partner or keep a dream journal. Sometimes just talking or writing helps put them in perspective.

BABY - WHAT'S HAPPENING:

Your baby's lungs are continuing to develop and grow, and though they will not be completely mature until right before she is born, some big things are happening. Around this time, the tiny air sacs, called alveoli, are forming. Even though the baby is breathing nothing but amniotic fluid right now, the alveoli will be ready to process the flow of air as soon as she is born.

TIPS AND ADVICE: These days, you may find yourself on the receiving end of random belly-rubbers. These are people whom you barely know (or strangers) who act on the urge to touch your pregnant belly without asking you first. This will become more frequent as you get further along, so develop a strategy now for dealing with unwanted belly-rubbers. If you don't like it, verbalize that you would rather not be touched. Say something like, "I'd rather you didn't touch me," while taking a step back. It may be awkward, but you will be thankful later that you established boundaries now.

DAILY JOURNAL

Mood:

Energy:

Cravings:

Symptoms:

Weight:

DAY 110: Date:___/___/___

MOM - WHAT'S HAPPENING:

You may notice some numbness or "pins and needles" in your feet and legs today. This is the result of pressure exerted on your blood vessels by your growing uterus. You can relieve this condition by getting up and moving around or by changing position. If you notice these symptoms when on your back, try shifting to your left side. Simple stretching exercises or a brisk walk can often return circulation to your calves to a normal level, which should bring relief.

BABY - WHAT'S HAPPENING:

By this time, your baby's eyes are in their final, forward-facing position. The position of the eyes is important, since it allows for depth perception. The ability to judge how far away objects are will eventually enable your child to do things such as participate in sports, appreciate art, and drive a car. Also today, your little one weighs about 7 ounces and his tiny heart is increasing its muscle mass, and now pumps between 25 and 30 quarts of blood daily.

PREGNANCY FACT: Approximately 15 percent of pregnant women are plagued by a creepy, crawly, tingly, generally unsettled feeling in their legs and feet that cannot be controlled. In fact, it is almost as if the legs have a mind of their own. This is known as restless leg syndrome (RLS) and researchers are stumped by what causes it. Anecdotal evidence points to iron deficiency and/or food allergy, so it can help to keep a food journal and to make some dietary changes accordingly. However, most women who are affected by RLS find that there is no relief until they deliver their baby.

DAILY JOURNAL

Mood:

Energy:

Cravings:

Symptoms:

Weight:

DAY 111: Date:___/___/___

MOM - WHAT'S HAPPENING:

Since your lung capacity has increased by up to 40 percent since your baby was conceived, it is likely you are feeling short of breath today. At this point, shortness of breath occurs because you are breathing faster than you were before, which can feel scary at times. The best way to control your breathing is to pay attention to each breath, slow down, and focus on the rise and fall of your chest. It is important not to panic if you can't get a good, deep breath. Panic will only cause you to breathe shallower and could lead to hyperventilation.

BABY - WHAT'S HAPPENING:

As your baby's bones continue to ossify, or harden, you will need to keep up with his calcium demands, because remember: what he doesn't get from your diet, he takes from your bones. Interestingly, your baby's leg and inner-ear bones are among the very first to harden, which may be why you feel his kicks before his punches and why he responds to sounds so early in his development.

PREGNANCY FACT: If you have chosen to have a midwife monitor your pregnancy and help you during delivery, be sure she is certified by the American College of Nurse Midwives (ACNM) and/or the North American Registry of Midwives (NARM). Midwives are most often used by women who have low-risk pregnancies that want to have a natural birth at home or in a birthing center. A midwife offers direct emotional and physical support and care to the mother and helps to ensure that there is little to no medical intervention during delivery.

DAILY JOURNAL

Mood:

Energy:

Cravings:

Symptoms:

Weight:

DAY 112: Date:___/___/___

MOM - WHAT'S HAPPENING:

Your uterus is getting closer to your belly button, and today you should be able to feel the fundus just about 1 inch below it. It can be fun to keep track of the changes your body is going through. Since pregnancy brain is probably in full swing, you should keep track of these changes in this book for your family's posterity.

BABY - WHAT'S HAPPENING:

Your baby is now approximately 6 inches long and weighs just over 7 ounces. This means she will more than triple her length by the time she is born—the average length of most full-term babies is between 19 and 21 inches long. Also, by now your baby is sleeping and waking in a pattern that resembles that of a newborn. As mentioned earlier, she will likely be lulled to sleep by your movements during the day and become more active at night. Thus, don't panic if you don't notice your baby's flutters and kicks while you're at work or running errands.

TIPS AND ADVICE: A wonderful way to connect with new and veteran mothers is to attend a breast-feeding support group while you are still pregnant. Spending time with those who recently went through labor and delivery can be a great educational experience. New moms are eager to tell their stories and to help other moms learn from their experiences. Asking a few of the mothers to share their stories, and what they wished they had known or asked or done, can give you invaluable tools heading into your own baby's birth. This will also prepare you for the beauty and challenges of breast-feeding.

DAILY JOURNAL

Mood:

Energy:

Cravings:

Symptoms:

Weight:

Lunar Month

Five

PHOTO

Place a photo of you during your fifth month here

My Monthly Update

Waist Measurement: ____

Weight: ____

Mood: ____

Lunar Month five . . . .

PREGNANCY CHECKLIST

- ❑ Your baby should start kicking and moving — tell you doctor when you first feel it
- ❑ Get 8 hours of sleep or more each night. Take naps and breaks during the day if you're feeling tired
- ❑ Time to tell your employer and update yourself on your company's maternity leave policy
- ❑ Start researching your childcare options
- ❑ Decide if you want to find out your baby's sex, or if you want to keep it a surprise
- ❑ If you haven't had one lately, schedule a regular dental checkup
- ❑ Your sex drive may be back full force. Talk to your doctor about how to get comfortable with sex during pregnancy.
- ❑ Treat pregnancy heartburn, but don't take laxatives or antacids without consulting your health care provider
- ❑ Try prenatal yoga to relax and rejuvenate
- ❑ Continue talking to your partner about parenthood and your expectations
- ❑ Prepare for your group B strep test
- ❑ Minimize pregnancy brain by getting plenty of rest, writing yourself notes, eating well, and staying hydrated
- ❑ Register for your baby shower

MY PERSONAL CHECKLIST:

- ❑ ....
- ❑ ....

MY HOPES FOR THIS MONTH:

....

....

....

Lunar Month Five

Second Trimester

THIS MONTH SHOULD BE CALLED "REALITY CHECK" month, because you will find that you really connect the idea of pregnancy with the reality that there is a tiny human being growing inside your uterus. This is because if you haven't already felt your baby moving, you will by the end of this month. For many women, having a baby doesn't feel real until they feel their wee one moving around with some regularity. As you look forward to and depend on those movements for assurance that your baby is OK, you can expect to experience an increase in anxiety this month tied to how often you feel your baby's kicks and flutters.

Another reason your pregnancy may seem more real to you this month is that your belly will really start to round out. This is exciting, as the combination of fetal movement and your protruding navel are an internal and external affirmation that everything is progressing as it should.

WHAT TO EXPECT THIS MONTH

You can expect to see your health care provider for your monthly checkup. It will likely be similar to the appointments in previous months, though you may have an ultrasound around lunar week 18 (20 weeks LMP) that will be able to tell you whether you are having a boy or a girl (unless your baby is camera shy and facing the wrong way). During your appointment your doctor will also check the height of the fundus, listen to your baby's heartbeat, check your urine for sugar and protein, and field your questions and concerns regarding your symptoms.

An exciting development this month is your ability to feel your baby's kicks and other movements with some regularity. Keep in mind that your baby will sleep most of the day, so don't worry if you do not feel him while you're going about your day. Most women find that their babies are most active first thing in the morning and at night.

THINGS TO CONSIDER

Lunar month 5 places you at the midway point in your pregnancy. This means you should start planning for your baby's arrival. If you haven't already, register for items you hope to receive at your baby shower. It is also the time to take a look around your house to figure out whether you will be able to have a dedicated nursery or if another room—such as your bedroom or the office—will have to double as the nursery. It may not seem like much, but everything that you do now in preparation for bringing baby home will make things that much easier later on.

In addition, simply taking the time to evaluate what needs to be purchased, planned for, and done around the house is a huge step forward in the getting-ready-for-baby-process. So, don't put it off. At this point in your pregnancy, the chances of miscarriage are minute and thus it is not only safe but smart to start chipping away at the steps required to get set up for your newest family member.

TIPS FOR COPING

As you settle into the reality of your pregnancy and begin to make preparations for bringing your baby home, you may feel anxious, overwhelmed, and financially incapable of handling your new responsibility. Compounding these feelings is the calendar, which indicates that you are halfway to the day when you will meet your new baby, making it seem like you do not have enough time to pull it all together.

Very few mothers are able to do everything before baby comes home. To keep your sanity and avoid pushing your partner off the deep end, limit your list-making to necessities. Be true to the word "need" when you consider what needs to be done before baby comes home. If you follow this rule, you will find your list is short, manageable, and less expensive, which should cut down on your anxiety level and that of your partner.

WHAT TO EAT

This month is a time to focus on what not to eat. As you are in the midst of the honeymoon phase of your pregnancy and your appetite increases, you may be tempted to treat yourself to those foods that turned your stomach in the first trimester. Of course, a plate of nachos now and then is perfectly acceptable, and it can be helpful to your overall disposition to indulge yourself now and then. However, if you find that you're "treating" yourself to pints of ice cream and drive-through fast food several times a week, work hard to control your impulses and cravings. As you know, it is important not to put on excess weight during your pregnancy.

A good way to satisfy the urge to splurge is by substituting healthier options for your most indulgent cravings. So, instead of eating a quarter-pound cheeseburger with large fries and a milkshake, consider making a veggie burger at home with low-fat cheese. Enjoy it with a baked potato and low-fat sour cream and have a serving of frozen yogurt for dessert. This may not be as appealing as the fast-food, but you will be serving yourself and your baby much better than if you indulge those high-fat, low-nutrient cravings.

HOW MUCH WEIGHT TO GAIN

This month you should continue to gain between 1 and 2 pounds per week. As mentioned above, you may be tempted to eat fatty or sweet foods since your appetite is on the rise, but try to limit such indulgences. The guidelines that determine how much weight a women should gain are designed to keep you and your baby as healthy as possible. Also, consider that the weight you pack on now is the very same weight you will have to fight to lose after your baby is born. Excess weight gain can also cause complications at delivery, so be sure to choose your calories wisely.

EXERCISE TIPS AND ADVICE

Your exercise regimen should be similar to last months. However, because your center of balance has shifted a bit, you will be more prone to accidents. Also, your joints will continue to loosen due to the hormone relaxin. These changes can make activities like jogging or aerobics more precarious. So, consider changing your exercise routine to feature walking or swimming instead. Whatever your exercise of choice is, be sure to do something for at least 20 to 30 minutes each day. This will help with swelling, circulation, and weight control.

POTENTIAL SYMPTOMS AND HOW TO ALLEVIATE THEM

The usual suspects of symptoms continue to hang around this month. Some may intensify, such as round ligament pain. This is because your uterus is stretching and expanding constantly to make room for your growing babe. You may feel pain low in your groin. It may also appear all the way up your sides and into your hips and lower back. It will feel something like general achiness and will intensify if you get up too fast from a sitting position. For some women, this pain is like daggers in the abdomen and can have them doubled over, taking them up to a minute to recover. To avoid these attacks, get up slowly from lying and seated positions. Also, warm compresses, such as a heated wash cloth or even a warm bath, can offer relief as well.

Also causing trouble in the abdominal area this month are gas, heartburn, and bloating. The reasons for this are basically the same as last month—your digestion is slowed to allow your baby to absorb the maximum amount of nutrition from your diet. Also, your growing uterus is putting additional pressure on your lower intestines and stomach. The remedy for these remains the same—continue to eat several small meals daily and avoid high-fat or greasy foods. Also, be sure to drink lots of water. Staying properly hydrated can help you flush out excess fluid and calm stomach acids.

WAYS OTHERS CAN HELP

Since you're about halfway through your pregnancy, you may need some serious encouragement to keep going this month. Naturally, because you are the one carrying the child, the burden falls on you to make daily choices to keep your baby alive and healthy. However, your partner can offer support by engaging in the same decisions and sacrifices that you do. For instance, if you're watching your calories carefully, it will not help to see your husband eating a pepperoni pizza while you eat a salad. If he hasn't already done so, ask your partner to eat what you eat and to be sensitive to your cravings and aversions.

Your partner can also help make social events more pleasant for you by abstaining from alcohol while you are pregnant. Being the only one to have to turn down a glass of wine or a beer can be difficult. Ask your partner to team up with you in this area. Finally, it is definitely time for your partner to quit smoking, if he hasn't already. Having your partner make responsible life choices with you will help affirm your new lifestyle as a healthy family and take some of the pressure off you.

"A mother's joy begins when new life is stirring inside... when a tiny heartbeat is heard for the very first time, and a playful kick reminds her that she is never alone."
~ Author Unknown

Week 17

Starting Weight: _________

OVERVIEW

This week you can expect to feel an increase in round ligament pain as your uterus continues to expand upward and out. Also this week, you may feel leg cramps creep in at night. These can be so painful, they might even wake you from a sound sleep. Deep, twisting leg cramps are common during pregnancy. If you start to experience them now, odds are the will intensify in the third trimester. To prevent a muscle spasm in your calf from worsening, fight the urge to pull your heel up to your knee. Instead, force your toes up toward the ceiling. This can decrease tension and help to release the spasm. If leg cramps plague you often, soak in a warm bath, stretch before bed, and work on your relaxation techniques, as stress can make them worse.

Meanwhile, this is a big week for your baby. If you are having a girl, her uterus will start to develop. By week's end, her ovaries will contain approximately 6 million eggs. By the time she is born, however, she will lose most of those eggs and have around 1 to 2 million left. If you are having a boy, his genitals will be plain as day on the ultrasound. However, there is a small percentage of error that occurs when a technician reads an ultrasound, so it is slightly possible (though unlikely) that you will have a girl even if you've been told "it's a boy!"

DAY 113: Date:___/___/___

MOM - WHAT'S HAPPENING:

You've made it 113 days—just 153 days to go! At this point, there's relatively little that is likely to go wrong. However, on rare occasions, problems can crop up, and you should be watching for the following problem signs around this time. If you feel strong contractions that come at regular intervals, call your health care provider immediately: these could be a sign of premature labor. If caught in time, premature labor can usually be stopped with treatment. Your provider might prescribe bed rest or possibly have you admitted to the hospital.

BABY - WHAT'S HAPPENING:

Around now, your baby has grown buds for her permanent teeth. These will complement the buds she has already developed for her milk or "baby" teeth. Her permanent teeth buds are located behind the milk teeth buds. They will stay buried until all of her baby teeth fall out and her adult teeth start to work their way down through the gums.

TIPS AND ADVICE: After this many visits, you should feel confident in your OB-GYN. If for any reason you do not feel comfortable with your OB-GYN, switch doctors sooner rather than later. Assuming you are happy with your doctor, however, start talking with him or her about delivery day. Ask your doctor who will deliver your baby if he is not available. Your doctor will likely do his best to be there when you deliver, but there's always the chance that you will go into labor while he is on vacation. You can even ask to meet the back-up doctor, if it will help ease your mind.

DAILY JOURNAL

Mood:

Energy:

Cravings:

Symptoms:

Weight:

DAY 114: Date:___/___/___

MOM - WHAT'S HAPPENING:

Around now, you may notice that your navel feels sore and itchy—you may even start to see stretch marks. Though you can't prevent them, you can soothe the irritation with lotion—cocoa butter is particularly effective. While some itching is normal, severe itching is not. If you have severe itching that does not let up after applying lotion, let your doctor know right away. This can be the sign of a rare liver complication that needs treatment.

BABY - WHAT'S HAPPENING:

Your baby is continuing to produce vernix to coat and protect his skin. This wax-like substance also lubricates your baby's body, which helps him get through the birth canal. Also, your baby's brain is further specializing its functions. For instance, his senses are becoming more refined, and thus he will kick, wiggle, or turn when he encounters spicy foods, music, and bright lights aimed at your uterus.

FOR YOUR HEALTH: Give up sleeping on your stomach for the remainder of your pregnancy. Chances are you've already done so, as it can be quite uncomfortable to have added pressure on your uterus. Odds are, as your pregnancy progresses you will not even be capable of rolling onto your stomach, but to avoid unnecessary pressure on your lower abdomen, take precaution to prevent accidentally rolling onto your stomach while asleep. Consider building a pillow wall around you at night to prevent rolling over.

DAILY JOURNAL

Mood:

Energy:

Cravings:

Symptoms:

Weight:

DAY 115: Date:___/___/___

MOM - WHAT'S HAPPENING:

You may be getting the "spins" more often now. These can be very disconcerting. Feeling cooped up and stuffy can exacerbate dizzy spells, but taking precautions can help you be prepared to handle the spins when they strike. If you commute to work, get some fresh air by cracking your car window—even in winter. If you ride public transportation, make it known that you are pregnant, and someone is bound to give you a seat. Always keep water and a few snacks on hand, such as nuts and raisins for a quick blood-sugar-stabilizing pick-me-up.

BABY - WHAT'S HAPPENING:

Your baby weighs just about 8½ ounces by now, and is slightly longer than 6 inches from head to bum. If you could see her, you might catch her going through the motions of crying, though she makes no sound yet. Your baby may also look like she's having a conversation with herself, as her mouth opens and closes many times throughout the day.

PREGNANCY FACT: You may find yourself thinking, "Are my shoes getting smaller?" No, you're not crazy. Expectant women's feet both swell and spread over the course of their pregnancy. The swelling occurs due to excess blood and fluids pooling in your feet. This will go away about a week after you deliver your baby. Foot spread happens thanks to the loosening of the ligaments in your feet—this, unfortunately, is permanent. So, be prepared to go up one-half to a whole shoe size during the course of your pregnancy.

DAILY JOURNAL

Mood:

Energy:

Cravings:

Symptoms:

Weight:

DAY 116: Date:___/___/___

MOM - WHAT'S HAPPENING:

As you know, your doctor measures the height of your fundus at each appointment. Usually, this measurement matches up with the week you are in with a margin of error that is plus or minus 2 centimeters. If your doctor tells you that your fundal height measures large this week, don't panic. There are many reasons your fundal height may be more than it should. You might have loose abdominal muscles from a previous pregnancy. Or, your due date may have been miscalculated. Occasionally, a large measurement indicates a large baby, twins, gestational diabetes, or placenta previa.

BABY - WHAT'S HAPPENING:

Your baby's hair continues to grow along his scalp. Hair grows in a pattern established by the hair follicles. Over the next few weeks, your baby will finish developing the rest of his hair follicles. In fact, by week 20, your baby will have all of the hair follicles that he will need on his body—about 5 million!

PREGNANCY FACT: There is a pleasant and surprising side effect of eating healthy and having an expanded circulatory system: all these extra nutrients are flooding your skin cells. This is partly responsible for why you appear to have that pregnancy "glow." All this extra goodness is having an impact on your hair and nails as well. In fact, you should notice that both your hair and nails are growing longer and thicker than before you were pregnant. This is the perfect excuse to indulge in a manicure or take a trip to your favorite hair salon.

DAILY JOURNAL

Mood:

Energy:

Cravings:

Symptoms:

Weight:

DAY 117: Date:___/___/___

MOM - WHAT'S HAPPENING:

Around this time in your pregnancy, high levels of estrogen may cause you to develop small clusters of blood vessels near the surface of your skin. These clusters look like tiny red spots, and they'll probably vanish after your baby is born. They most often appear on your nose, cheeks, breasts, and belly. They are harmless, but if their appearance bothers you, a simple face powder should cover them up nicely.

BABY - WHAT'S HAPPENING:

If you are having a baby girl, her uterus has started to develop this week. She has made approximately 6 million immature egg cells in her ovaries. By the time she is born, she will have lost many of these egg cells and be left with between 1 and 2 million eggs. This is the maximum number of eggs a woman will ever have. As she menstruates and ages, she will continually lose them. In fact, out of the original 1 or 2 million, only around 400 will ever reach maturity.

FOR YOUR HEALTH: If your doctor tells you that your fundal height is smaller than expected, don't panic. Some women measure small in later appointments because the initial measurement was off. A small measurement could also be due to the fact that your due date was miscalculated. Finally, you might just be having a small baby! If your doctor suspects that your baby isn't on track with his growth, he will order an ultrasound to confirm his suspicions. Depending on what the ultrasound reveals, he will come up with a plan to get you and your baby on track.

DAILY JOURNAL

Mood:

Energy:

Cravings:

Symptoms:

Weight:

DAY 118: Date:___/___/___

MOM - WHAT'S HAPPENING:

You may never have thought it could happen so fast, but as you got dressed this morning, you may have noticed that your breasts have grown even larger than they were just last week. Your breasts continue to grow due to increased circulation and fluids. Also, your milk ducts are expanding with every week you are pregnant. These may also make the veins in your breast more prominent—they may even bulge in places.

BABY - WHAT'S HAPPENING:

Your baby's brain is making staggering progress. Around this time, her brain is creating millions of neurons that tell her muscles what the brain wants them to do. This connection between her movements with her brain are the early stages of her motor skills. She will begin to make conscious movements now, in addition to the involuntary ones. It will be hard to tell which is which on an ultrasound, but if you see that she's waving—assume it is on purpose!

FOR YOUR HEALTH: Diarrhea is one of the more uncomfortable and unpleasant side effects of pregnancy you may have encountered by now. However, if you experience diarrhea for more than 24 hours, tell your doctor. Diarrhea can be the result of a stomach flu, parasite, or food poisoning. Stay hydrated and avoid over-the-counter medications unless recommended by your doctor. Some intestinal ills are best beat by letting your body flush them out. If you are too sick to eat or drink for more than 24 hours, call your doctor or go to the emergency room.

DAILY JOURNAL

Mood:

Energy:

Cravings:

Symptoms:

Weight:

DAY 119: Date:___/___/___

MOM - WHAT'S HAPPENING:

By now you have probably experienced a variety of skin changes. The skin around your armpits may have darkened, and you may have seen the appearance of "skin tags," which are very small flaps of excess skin. You also might see darkening around your inner thighs and even the appearance of red splotches on the palms of your hands. All of this is normal and should go away after you have your baby.

BABY - WHAT'S HAPPENING:

The placenta continues to grow and pass nutrition on to your baby. It is also starting to move up and away from the cervical opening. Your baby continues to swallow amniotic fluid and his kidneys are making sterile urine that circulates back through the surrounding fluid. In fact, most of his organs are doing some version of what they are intended for at this point.

TIPS AND ADVICE: Ultrasounds are valuable diagnostic tools and come in many dimensions. At some point, your doctor might suggest that you have 3-D images taken of your baby in utero. This ultrasound technology is more advanced than normal 2-D ultrasounds. They must be read by a skilled technician. Thus, if you visit a retailer who offers 3-D ultrasounds, know that these are not medical professionals. They cannot diagnose problems and will not be able to tell you if things are progressing normally. In general, it is wise to avoid novelty ultrasounds not conducted by professionals.

DAILY JOURNAL

Mood:

Energy:

Cravings:

Symptoms:

Weight:

Week 18

Starting Weight: ________

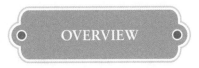

OVERVIEW

According to your last menstrual period (LMP), you are now at the halfway point in your pregnancy! Remember, though, that your baby is actually in his 18th week of development. Big things happen this week for both you and your baby. By the end of this week, your uterus will expand to the point that it is level with your belly button.

At this point, you should be used to being pregnant. You should be in tune with your body's limitations and with your baby's dietary needs. Because you are so well adjusted, now is a great time to start looking ahead. Feel free to book childbirth classes, because they can fill up pretty quickly. Taking this step is a big deal for many parents-to-be, as signing up for birth and delivery classes makes the arrival of their baby seem more real than ever.

While you are preparing for the birth of your baby, he is doing what he does best—growing and developing. By the end of this week, your baby will be the size of a banana. He will be approximately 10 inches long from the backs of his heels to the top of his head and weigh as much as 10½ ounces. His kicks might be hard enough that your partner can feel them if he places his hand in the right spot at the right time!

DAY 120: Date:___/___/___

MOM - WHAT'S HAPPENING:

You may notice the line that stretches from your pubic bone to your navel has darkened. This is called the linea nigra, and it is caused by the increased hormone levels in your body. For many women this—coupled with the pushing out of their belly button—is an exciting piece of pregnancy evidence. If you do not experience either of these side effects, don't be alarmed. Everyone's skin pigmentation and body shape are different, so not all women develop these signs of expecting.

BABY - WHAT'S HAPPENING:

Your baby's skin has started to become less transparent as it develops into three layers. Her skin thickens as it starts the process of creating the outermost layer, called the epidermis; the middle layer, the dermis; and the deepest, fatty layer of skin, the subcutis. Interestingly, 90 percent of skin is made up of the dermis. As your baby develops her fat stores, her skin will fill out, becoming less wrinkled and more opaque.

FOR YOUR HEALTH: If you were prone to uterine fibroids (nonmalignant growths) before you were pregnant, there is the chance that you will develop them while you are pregnant. Thus, it is important to let your doctor know about a previous history of fibroids, and also to let her know if you notice pain or pressure in your lower abdomen that is accompanied by a fever. This can be a sign that a fibroid has twisted or has become very large. In most cases, however, fibroids will not affect the health of your baby and should not interfere with delivery.

DAILY JOURNAL

Mood:

Energy:

Cravings:

Symptoms:

Weight:

DAY 121: Date:___/___/___

MOM - WHAT'S HAPPENING:

You may be tired of paying strict attention to your diet by now, and who could blame you? It is important to keep it up, however. Take time today to evaluate whether you are getting enough iron in your diet. Remember, good sources of iron are lean red meat, pork, dried beans, fortified cereals, oatmeal, dried fruits, and spinach. To make sure you are getting enough iron, plan your meals in advance to include these foods.

BABY - WHAT'S HAPPENING:

Since your baby swallows more frequently, she ingests more of the contents floating around in the amniotic fluid. Her first bowel movement, called meconium, accumulates in her bowels, however. It is possible that your baby will pass a little of this sticky green or black substance while she is in utero or during delivery. This should not be a problem unless she inhales it into her lungs, in which case she will need special attention at birth.

FOR YOUR HEALTH: At your first prenatal appointment, you had a blood test to determine your Rh factor. If you were Rh positive, you have nothing to worry about. But if you were Rh negative and your partner is Rh positive you will need an injection of Rho (D) immune globulin at 28 weeks, and again after you deliver. This injection prevents your immune system from attacking your baby as if it were a virus. It is likely that you are in the clear, however, since a negative Rh factor occurs in only 15 percent of the population, while 85 percent of people have a positive Rh factor.

DAILY JOURNAL

Mood:

Energy:

Cravings:

Symptoms:

Weight:

DAY 122: Date:___/___/___

MOM - WHAT'S HAPPENING:

Around today, you may notice your nasal congestion is back—particularly as a post-nasal drip. This may be constant and cause you to feel "flooded" when you first wake up in the morning. For relief, run a humidifier while you sleep and put blocks under the head of your bed to raise you up while you sleep (which makes it easier to breathe).

BABY - WHAT'S HAPPENING:

By now, your baby's entire body is covered in lanugo and vernix. This allows his skin to develop its layers while it is protected from the saturating effects of constant immersion in the amniotic fluid. In fact, his skin is becoming thicker and more opaque with each passing day. Brown fat is accumulating in various parts of his body. This particular kind of fat provides insulation and heat. While it will be with your baby when he is born, it will only exist in trace amounts by the time your child is an adult.

FOOD FOR THOUGHT: Start your mornings out right by including oatmeal in your diet at least a few times a week. Oatmeal has been shown to lower cholesterol and is a heart-friendly food. There is also evidence it may reduce the odds of developing certain types of cancers. It contains several essential minerals and vitamins, including iron, fiber, protein, and complex carbohydrates. Because oatmeal slows digestion, it will make you feel full longer and can help quell heartburn and nausea. Finally, oatmeal is a convenient snack, as it usually comes in transportable packets.

DAILY JOURNAL

Mood:

Energy:

Cravings:

Symptoms:

Weight:

DAY 123: Date:___/___/___

MOM - WHAT'S HAPPENING:

By now, you are looking quite pregnant, as your uterus has grown to the point that it is level with your belly button. You probably spend quite a bit of time admiring your belly bump in the mirror—from all angles. As you're inspecting yourself, keep in mind that each woman "shows" in her own way, depending on her size and shape before becoming pregnant. Also, you may have heard others claim all sorts of wisdom about your baby based on how high or low you carry. However, there is no scientific evidence that supports a correlation between the shape of your belly and the gender of your baby.

BABY - WHAT'S HAPPENING:

As your baby starts to stretch out her legs, you will likely be able to feel her kick and move around with some frequency. Up to this point, she has been curled up, thus her length has been measured from the top of her head to her bum. From this point on, however, she will be measured from head to heel.

PREGNANCY FACT: Approximately 25 percent of pregnant women develop a condition called rectus diastasis at some point in the second trimester. This occurs when the stomach muscles are pushed apart due to uterine growth and the hormone relaxin. It is sometimes called a "gap," but there is no actual gap between the muscles. Instead, the tissue that joins the stomach muscles gets stretched very thin as the muscles are pushed apart. The muscles should return to their normal position within a few months after delivery.

DAILY JOURNAL

Mood:

Energy:

Cravings:

Symptoms:

Weight:

DAY 124: Date:___/___/___

MOM - WHAT'S HAPPENING:

If you notice sharp pains that start in your lower back and extend to your buttocks and thighs, this is probably sciatica. This is a frequent complaint during the second trimester, but is likely to go away once the baby is born. Unfortunately, as your pregnancy progresses, sciatica flare-ups will occur more frequently (especially when sitting). If you experience numbness down one of your legs or in one of your feet, let your doctor know. There is little that can be done, however, other than resting, taking warm baths, and stretching.

BABY - WHAT'S HAPPENING:

If you are carrying a girl, her uterus is fully formed by now, and her vaginal canal is in the early stages of development. If you are housing a boy, his testicles are continuing their slow descent down to where his scrotum will be. Once the scrotum is developed, his testicles will drop and his external genitalia will be complete.

FOR YOUR HEALTH: Of the percentage of women who develop preeclampsia during pregnancy, 1 out of 10 will also develop a condition known as HELLP syndrome. H (hemolytic anemia) EL (elevated liver enzymes) LP (low platelet count) can become serious very quickly, causing severe complications for both you and your baby. Therefore, it is important to notify your doctor immediately if you experience the following: pain and/or tenderness in your upper right side, constant all-over itching, general lethargy, and nausea and vomiting.

DAILY JOURNAL

Mood:

Energy:

Cravings:

Symptoms:

Weight:

DAY 125: Date:___/___/___

MOM - WHAT'S HAPPENING:

In addition to other stomach ills, today you may start to experience mild to severe acid reflux. This can be quite uncomfortable and will literally leave a bad taste in your mouth. If you find you are regurgitating your food more often than you can stand, speak to your doctor about possible remedies that are safe for your baby.

BABY - WHAT'S HAPPENING:

It is possible at this point that your doctor (and you and your partner) will be able to hear your baby's heartbeat with a stethoscope instead of having to use the Doppler (though your doctor will continue to use the Doppler for accuracy). You may be thinking of buying a personal device that amplifies your baby's heartbeat and can be heard using headphones. These products range in price. If you do purchase one, keep in mind that these are often inaccurate. In addition, it can be difficult for you to locate your baby's heartbeat based on where she is resting in the womb.

TIPS AND ADVICE: Now is the time to start looking into childbirth education classes. If you are thinking of skipping them, think again. Childbirth education classes are often held in the hospital where you will give birth and end with a tour of the labor and delivery floor. This alone is worth the cost, as the tour helps demystify the environment in which you will have your baby. Also, these classes are full of important information. You will meet other expectant parents and be able to share your experiences with them. Check with your insurance company as many offer free or inexpensive classes.

DAILY JOURNAL

Mood:

Energy:

Cravings:

Symptoms:

Weight:

DAY 126: Date:___/___/___

MOM - WHAT'S HAPPENING:

Today you may be feeling generally achy in the abdomen. This is due to several factors that are all great for your baby, but painful for you. You know by now that as your uterus expands, the ligaments that anchor it are stretched, which causes pain from the front of your abdomen and into your sides. Also, your stomach muscles are being forced apart. This can cause the tissue that links them to stretch and become thin and painful. Add to all of this gas and bloating, and odds are you are pretty uncomfortable. Just remember to keep your eye on the prize and know that you are only about 20 weeks away from meeting your baby.

BABY - WHAT'S HAPPENING:

Your baby is giant today compared to his size at week 8. At your first ultrasound, he was about the size of a raspberry. Today he is more like a large banana! Most of his major development has occurred by now. The remaining time in utero will be spent improving his developed systems.

TIPS AND ADVICE: If your first baby was your pet pooch, consider registering for a Dogs and Babies class when you are signing up for other childbirth education classes. These classes offer valuable information on how to integrate your baby and dog into your family. Classes are often just one day and cover topics such as bringing baby home, training your dog to walk next to a stroller, and how long and why to keep your baby and dog separate. This class is a must for dog lovers.

DAILY JOURNAL

Mood:

Energy:

Cravings:

Symptoms:

Weight:

Week 19

Starting Weight: ________

OVERVIEW

This is a slow week for both you and your baby. Though baby continues to develop and put on weight, there are few major milestones. What is exciting, though, is that you have begun the first week in the second half of your pregnancy! This is a time to relish in the relative comfort and calm that settles in before some of the third trimester symptoms hit you. By now, you should be used to the aches and pains that the second trimester brings and, hopefully, you've learned how to make symptom management part of your daily routine.

Spend this week getting a head start on arrangements that need to be made before you bring your baby home. Start thinking about nursery ideas. Plan menus for cook-and-freeze meals you can pop into the microwave those first few days home from the hospital. Whatever planning you can do now will be a tremendous asset to you later when you are scrambling for time.

While you plan and make lists, your baby is getting bigger and stronger. This week those flutters and butterflies will start to feel like kicks and prods. Enjoy each and every one of them! You will miss that intimate feeling when he is on the "outside."

DAY 127: Date:___/___/___

MOM - WHAT'S HAPPENING:

This week is big for varicose veins, so be sure to keep an eye on your legs. If you notice that the veins in your calves or thighs are bulging, employ the maternity hose mentioned earlier. It will also help to be mindful of your position and when blood is most likely to pool in your legs, such as while sitting or sleeping. Remind yourself to change positions every 30 minutes or so while awake and sleep on your left side. Also, remember that if your mother had varicose veins, odds are that you will get them as well.

BABY - WHAT'S HAPPENING:

Your baby's white blood cells, which are a key component of the immune system, are forming now. White blood cells will fight off infections and are your baby's natural defense against bacteria, colds, and viruses. However, for some months after birth, he will mostly be dependant on antibodies he receives through your breastmilk.

FOOD FOR THOUGHT: Variety is the spice of life and, thus, garbanzo beans are a great addition to your pregnancy diet. Garbanzo beans, or chickpeas, are both versatile and healthy. They are featured in many yummy Middle Eastern dishes, which are flavorful and good for you. Garbanzo beans are loaded with folate, fiber, protein, and iron—all necessary for the healthy pregnancy diet. For your convenience, note that canned garbanzo beans have the same nutritional value as dried—therefore they make a convenient addition to nearly any recipe.

DAILY JOURNAL

Mood:

Energy:

Cravings:

Symptoms:

Weight:

DAY 128: Date:___/___/___

MOM - WHAT'S HAPPENING:

Today, your uterus is approximately a ½-inch above your belly button. Thus, you really look pregnant! Many women find it reassuring to watch their abdomen get bigger as pregnancy progresses, because it signifies that baby is growing and gaining good weight. It can be strange to watch your body change so dramatically. Just remember that you won't always look pregnant. It can be fun to have your partner take a picture of you each month so you can look back in awe at how much your has body changed.

BABY - WHAT'S HAPPENING:

Your baby's tongue, including her taste buds, is completely developed now. Your baby has begun swallowing several ounces of amniotic fluid each day. Your baby gets some of her nutrition from this practice, but mainly it functions as a drill for when she must digest breast milk or formula.

TIPS AND ADVICE: If your partner expresses feeling left out of your pregnancy, try to be as reassuring as possible. Often, it only takes a small gesture to bring him in and make him feel connected. Include him in childbirth classes, nursery plans, and of course, let him in on your fears as well. Men often feel one step removed from baby while their partner is pregnant. This can carry over into the first few days or weeks of baby's life when mom is still the sole source of nutrition. So, be sensitive to your partner's desire to participate and feel connected to your baby before she is born.

DAILY JOURNAL

Mood:

Energy:

Cravings:

Symptoms:

Weight:

DAY 129: Date:___/___/___

MOM - WHAT'S HAPPENING:

Your pregnant body has been like a chemistry lab with a mad scientist (your baby) at work on hormones required to sustain your pregnancy. Up to this point, your body produced a bit more progesterone than estrogen. Around now, however, these two hormones even out. This should result in a more emotionally stable you. However, as your pregnancy progresses, estrogen will become the dominant hormone, and your mood swings might return in the third trimester.

BABY - WHAT'S HAPPENING:

Though the placenta is still responsible for most of your baby's nutritional needs, your baby is able to digest some nutrients from the amniotic fluid that he swallows—particularly sugar. Therefore, it is important to control how much sugar you ingest. Whatever sugar your baby absorbs must be processed with insulin, and if you flood your system with sugar your baby will have to produce enough insulin to digest it.

FOR YOUR HEALTH: Approximately 1 in 100 pregnancies end in the second trimester due to an incompetent cervix. This occurs when the cervix prematurely opens due to pressure from the uterus and its contents. It happens in women who have a genetic disposition to the condition, were exposed to DES (diethylstilbestrol) while in utero, or have a previously damaged cervix. Tell your doctor if you are aware of any of these preexisting conditions so she may stitch your cervical opening closed. This procedure may not be 100 percent effective but is the only known treatment.

DAILY JOURNAL

Mood:

Energy:

Cravings:

Symptoms:

Weight:

DAY 130: Date:___/___/___

MOM - WHAT'S HAPPENING:

Your monthly goal for gaining weight should now be around 4 pounds. You can expect to gain between ½ to 1 pound per week, depending on your diet and exercise regimen. As long as you're eating a well-rounded, healthy diet, try not to obsess over your weight gain. Though you should have gained between 10 and 15 pounds by now, there are variables to consider with each individual pregnancy, and so there is no use getting stuck on these numbers.

BABY - WHAT'S HAPPENING:

If you are having a baby girl her vagina has fully formed by now (though external genitalia for either sex will continue to develop and mature until birth). Also, your baby's legs have reached a length where they are in proportion with the rest of his body. You can be sure he will be kicking and moving his legs (and every other body part) in your spacious uterus. As time goes on and your baby grows, he will eventually start to be crowded in utero.

PREGNANCY FACT: By now you should be feeling your baby move with some regularity. You have probably also noticed that your baby is most active at night when you are ready to settle down and rest. Now, imagine trying to get some shut-eye when you have two (or more) babies kicking their way around your uterus! Interestingly, if you are having twins they do kick each other with some frequency but are not in danger of hurting each other. This is because twins are separated by a thin, elastic membrane that protects them from each other's acrobatics.

DAILY JOURNAL

Mood:

Energy:

Cravings:

Symptoms:

Weight:

DAY 131: Date:___/___/___

MOM - WHAT'S HAPPENING:

By this time, your expanding uterus has probably had a telling effect on your abdominal and hip skin in the form of stretch marks. These red or purple lines probably cannot be completely prevented, though there is anecdotal evidence that drinking plenty of water can reduce the severity of stretch marks. Also, if you haven't been consuming enough calcium you may notice a slight gray tint to your teeth. In fact, some women have been known to lose a tooth with each pregnancy! Make an appointment to see your dentist at the earliest sign of dental trouble.

BABY - WHAT'S HAPPENING:

Your baby's sleeping and waking hours will become more consistent as she takes her cues from your schedule of eating, working, and sleeping. All babies are different, though. Some are lulled to sleep by daytime activities. Others respond to the motion and noise of daytime and sleep when mom sleeps.

TIPS AND ADVICE: Though many women find that their hair becomes shinier, thicker, and healthier thanks to great pregnancy nutrition, some women find their hair takes a nosedive. If you are depressed over lackluster locks, avoid the urge to get a perm or to use relaxers. These hair treatments are made up of very strong chemicals that get absorbed through your scalp and end up in your bloodstream. While there is no specific evidence linking these hair treatments to fetal distress or birth defects, the risk simply is not worth the benefits.

DAILY JOURNAL

Mood:

Energy:

Cravings:

Symptoms:

Weight:

DAY 132: Date:___/___/___

MOM - WHAT'S HAPPENING:

Today you might be marvelling at the size of your swollen ankles and feet. This is to be expected and can be eased by making the effort to move around during the day. Also, make an effort to put your feet up for at least 30 minutes each evening. Drink plenty of water and consider limiting foods that cause you to retain water, such as food with a high salt content or diuretics.

BABY - WHAT'S HAPPENING:

Your little one's heart is getting stronger by the day and, if you haven't already, you will be able to hear his heart beating through a stethoscope. Your baby is enjoying the whooshing sounds your blood makes as it rushes through your body. He is often lulled to sleep by the soothing sound of your heartbeat. If you were to be subjected to the noise of your body functions at the decibel level your baby hears, you would need ear plugs. Your baby, however, actually takes great comfort in these constant and noisy body sounds.

PREGNANCY FACT: Fetal heart development goes through many stages. In in each of these stages, your baby's heart will resemble that of a particular animal—from a fish to a snake and finally that of a human. Once your baby is born his heart will be roughly the same size as his fist. As he grows so will his heart—keeping pace with the size of his fist throughout his life. Heart size can often indicate heart health—for example, an enlarged heart often indicates cardiac distress and a small heart points to developmental issues.

DAILY JOURNAL

Mood:

Energy:

Cravings:

Symptoms:

Weight:

DAY 133: Date:___/___/___

MOM - WHAT'S HAPPENING:

Just think, in about 133 days your sweet baby will be crying her head off. She'll be nursing, pooping, and snuggling up against you as she sleeps. How does that make you feel? Now is a good time to check in with yourself and your emotions. If you are still ambivalent about your pregnancy, it is OK—don't be hard on yourself. Some women don't connect with their babies until they are actually born, and even then it can take a few days for the maternal instinct to kick in.

BABY - WHAT'S HAPPENING:

Your baby is 10½ inches long and weighs nearly 13 ounces. She continues to build fat stores under her thickening skin and, at this point, looks like a miniature newborn baby. Her eyelids are finished forming and are lined with lashes, though her eyelids are still fused shut. She's also got a set of impressive eyebrows and if her hair is coming in dark it is visible.

TIPS AND ADVICE: Be sure to make time for intimacy with your partner. Keep in mind it will be much more difficult to make time for just the two of you when there is a newborn to care for. So, each morning or evening, turn off the television, don't answer the phone, and cuddle up with your honey. The physical closeness will do wonders for both of your stress levels, and if it leads to sex, that's great! Unless you've been ordered by your doctor to avoid penetration or orgasm, sex is perfectly safe—and beneficial—for you and your partner.

DAILY JOURNAL

Mood:

Energy:

Cravings:

Symptoms:

Weight:

Week 20

Starting Weight: _________

OVERVIEW

This week, your uterus will rise about ¾ of an inch above your belly button. This means your navel will protrude quite a bit more than just a few weeks ago. Unfortunately, you may find that as your belly becomes larger, others act as if it has become public property. Everyone from family members to coworkers to complete strangers may find themselves mesmerized by your belly and will reach out to put their hands on you without asking. This is a strange but common phenomenon. The fact is that most people wouldn't dream of touching a woman's stomach if she wasn't pregnant, so what is it that compels people to do this when she is? While there is not just one answer, you might want to chalk it up to the magical allure of the pregnant belly. Develop a strategy that works for you for how to handle unwanted belly-touchers, either by asking them to respect your space, letting them touch once or twice, or by turning so they get the message that your body is not for public consumption.

Meanwhile, inside your belly is where the magic is happening. This week, your baby's senses are becoming more alert and she will be exploring her newly discovered sense of touch. She constantly moves her hands and fingers over her face, umbilical cord, and sucks her thumb or other fingers. This is just the beginning of a very long career in curiosity for your little one.

DAY 134: Date:___/___/___

MOM - WHAT'S HAPPENING:

Today you might be forgetting how big you have gotten! You may find that you bump your belly into countertops or against the stove or refrigerator. This is harmless to your baby but it may frustrate you. You may even get a little bruised if you bang your belly often. This is very common, especially for first-time moms. Though you may feel like a bull in a china shop, you are probably not as big as you think you are. Also, keep mind you are more likely to bump into things when you are rushing, so take your time and slow down.

BABY - WHAT'S HAPPENING:

As your baby continues to fill out, he looks more and more like a newborn baby, though he is far from the plump little boy with chubby knees that he will become in the months after he is born. Also contributing to his newborn appearance is soft tissue, or cartilage. Today this is forming in his nose, giving it more of a defined shape.

PREGNANCY FACT: Ancient Egyptians believed that children were a blessing and so many families had between 4 and 15 children. However, pregnancy was difficult then, and infant mortality was very high. The Egyptians used many salves and plant remedies to aid the mother in her delivery. The Ancient Egyptians believed that pregnancy lasted between 271 and 294 days. When it was time to give birth, the mother squatted, sat, or kneeled on a birthing seat. Often, a pot of hot water was placed below her, because it was thought that the steam would make her delivery easier.

DAILY JOURNAL

Mood:

Energy:

Cravings:

Symptoms:

Weight:

DAY 135: Date:___/___/___

MOM - WHAT'S HAPPENING:

Today, take a moment to think about your footwear. Interestingly, the shoes you wear while pregnant can exacerbate or reduce your level of back pain. Thus, if you're used to wearing heels, trade them in for a flatter shoe. Shoes that are too flat, however, such as flip-flops and sandals, may cause you grief as well, because they aren't supportive enough. Therefore, stick to low-heeled, supportive shoes—you will be shocked at how much your pain will improve.

BABY - WHAT'S HAPPENING:

As your baby's taste buds become more sensitive, she might react to the foods you eat. In fact, if your OB-GYN is having trouble hearing your baby's heartbeat because of his position or because you are very overweight, he may suggest that you drink orange juice or eat a cookie before you come in to see him. This is because many babies "wake up" and get moving when they get a taste of sweet foods.

TIPS AND ADVICE: Now is a great time to start kicking around baby names with your partner. This sounds like a lot of fun but it can turn ugly if either or both partners are insensitive when they reject each other's choices. A good way to deal with this is to write down five of your favorite names on a piece of paper. Then, trade lists with your partner. Mark off the names that you absolutely cannot live with and give the list back to your partner. If you find you have two or three names left between you, you are off to a great start!

DAILY JOURNAL

Mood:

Energy:

Cravings:

Symptoms:

Weight:

DAY 136: Date:___/___/___

MOM - WHAT'S HAPPENING:

The expansion of your uterus has reached the point that you may have trouble seeing your feet while standing up straight. Your blocked view, combined with a shifting center of gravity, means you should be extra cautious as you walk so as to avoid falls. This is particularly true while going down stairs, exercising, and while carrying older children.

BABY - WHAT'S HAPPENING:

Your baby's brain is busy linking up nerves and commands to body parts and functions. For instance, your baby's brain is developed enough that it is able to process what it feels like to touch. Thus, your baby is constantly touching something—his face, feet, belly, and the umbilical cord are all fair game. This early tactile exploration is just the beginning of your baby's initiation into the world of his own senses.

TIPS AND ADVICE: Vacationing at high altitudes—7,000 feet or above—can be dangerous to you and your baby. This is because it will take awhile for your already-taxed respiratory and circulatory system to adjust to the lower oxygen levels. In fact, you may not adjust fast enough to supply necessary oxygen to your baby, which can cause fetal distress. If you must go to a high-elevation destination, make sure to ascend no more than 2,000 feet per day. Also, attempt to book your accommodations below 6,500 feet so that you are sleeping in a more oxygen-rich environment.

DAILY JOURNAL

Mood:

Energy:

Cravings:

Symptoms:

Weight:

DAY 137: Date:___/___/___

MOM - WHAT'S HAPPENING:

You may be experiencing occasional bouts of wet underwear. Chances are this is caused by tiny amounts of urine leaking from your bladder when you laugh or cough. If you notice more than a small amount of leakage, though, see your doctor to make sure you are not leaking amniotic fluid. There will be a difference in how these two fluids smell, so one way to check whether it is urine is to scent-check your underwear. Urine will be yellowish and smell something like ammonia. Amniotic fluid may have no scent or a "clean" smell and can be clear, pink, brown, or green.

BABY - WHAT'S HAPPENING:

If you are having a boy, his testes have begun their descent from his pelvis into his scrotum. If you are having a girl, her vagina continues to become more mature in its formation. If you've opted to know your baby's gender, you likely know by now what you are having—this does not mean you have to share with anyone but your partner, however.

FOR YOUR HEALTH: There are some cases in which you should avoid intercourse while pregnant. These include bleeding that cannot be stopped or explained, after the amniotic sac has ruptured, and when mom has a history of miscarriage or premature labor. Other reasons to avoid intercourse during the second and third trimesters are when there is known placenta previa or if mom is carrying multiple babies. If you are unsure whether penetration is safe, be sure to ask your doctor. This is not the time to be shy!

DAILY JOURNAL

Mood:

Energy:

Cravings:

Symptoms:

Weight:

DAY 138: Date:___/___/___

MOM - WHAT'S HAPPENING:

You will remember that a hormone called relaxin has been circulating in your body for quite some time now. It has helped to loosen your joints in preparation for giving birth and now is causing your spine to curve, giving you a severely arched back. This can cause you to feel achy and like someone is pushing into your lower back. As your belly gets larger, so too will the arch in your back. A good way to balance this out is to bend your knees slightly and lean forward, placing your hands on your thighs. This gentle forward bend can be done anytime and will give your aching back a rest.

BABY - WHAT'S HAPPENING:

Your baby's skin still looks wrinkly because she hasn't yet accumulated enough fat to fill out her skin. Keep in mind that she will continue to look wrinkly for the first few days or even weeks of her life as she fills out and her skin gets used to her new environment.

FOR YOUR HEALTH: If you are seeking a way to relieve the aches and pains of pregnancy, give reflexology a try. Reflexology is a form of physical therapy given through pressure applied to various points on the feet, hands, and ears. This noninvasive technique is safe while pregnant. However, when choosing a reflexologist, be sure the practitioner has worked on expectant women before. This is important because putting pressure on specific areas can cause contractions. Thus, the reflexologist you select will have to know which points to completely avoid while you are pregnant.

DAILY JOURNAL

Mood:

Energy:

Cravings:

Symptoms:

Weight:

DAY 139: Date:___/___/___

MOM - WHAT'S HAPPENING:

Today, you may be suffering from an itchy rash on your chest, stomach, or elsewhere. This is most likely a heat rash and is fairly common during pregnancy. You can use baby powder or cornstarch to absorb perspiration, which will help ease the itching. You may also want to wear clothes made from breathable cotton. Try to avoid scratching because bacteria under your fingernails can enter your bloodstream and cause infection. You might also want to try soaking in a tepid oatmeal bath. Be sure to completely dry off before getting dressed.

BABY - WHAT'S HAPPENING:

Your baby's lips are becoming more defined around this time. Though they are thin, they are filling out to a kissable size as your baby fattens up. If you could peek into your uterus, you would see that your baby is rubbing his closed eyes and grabbing his nose. You would also catch him sucking his thumb—a behavior he will take with him after he is born.

TIPS AND ADVICE: Now is a great time to either start or continue with meditation. Studies show time and again that meditation lowers stress hormones and improves overall health. Meditation will also help you filter out all the "noise" that surrounds your pregnancy—adverse symptoms, offensive inquiries from well-meaning family members, and the ever-accumulating lists that keep you up at night. Meditation is most effective in a quiet, private room. You should carve out 20 to 30 minutes each day (twice a day is even better) to simply "be" and focus on your breathing.

DAILY JOURNAL

Mood:

Energy:

Cravings:

Symptoms:

Weight:

DAY 140: Date:___/___/___

MOM - WHAT'S HAPPENING:

Many women find themselves suffering from insomnia at this point in their pregnancy. This is due, in part, to having difficulty getting comfortable enough to sleep, but most moms admit that what keeps them pacing at night are their own racing thoughts. It is normal to worry about the health of your baby and how you will get everything ready in time, but you must get your rest. Think of how hard your body is working each day to support both of you! Give yourself a break and thoroughly decompress before you hit the sack.

BABY - WHAT'S HAPPENING:

Your baby now weighs approximately 1 full pound and is 11 inches long. He is long and skinny and is electric with the excitement of discovering his senses. At this point, the little guy can hear, taste, and touch. So that is what he spends his time doing—he listens to your voice and heartbeat, he tastes the foods you eat, and is constantly touching whatever he can get his hands on.

PREGNANCY FACT: Many women start to worry about preterm labor at this point in pregnancy. This is because second trimester symptoms, such as backaches, dull cramping, and discharge can also signify preterm labor has begun. If you are afraid you will experience preterm labor, there is a test your doctor can perform. This test looks for a protein called fetal fibronectin (fFN), which is only present in the amniotic sac before 22 weeks and after 38 weeks. The presence of fFN in vaginal secretions between 22 and 38 weeks is a red flag that you may, indeed, be at risk for preterm labor.

DAILY JOURNAL

Mood:

Energy:

Cravings:

Symptoms:

Weight:

Lunar Month

Six

PHOTO

Place a photo of you during your sixth month here

My Monthly Update

Waist Measurement: ______

Weight: ______

Mood: ______

PREGNANCY CHECKLIST

❑ Manage back pain by wearing low-heeled shoes or flats. Light exercise and not standing for long periods of time will help

❑ Alleviate constipation by drinking water or fruit juice and eating more fiber

❑ Help with heartburn by eating 4 or 5 smaller meals during the day

❑ Have your vision checked — changes in vision are common but can be a sign of complications

❑ Manage varicose veins by propping your legs up during bed rest

❑ Feel confident about your rapidly changing body by tossing your sweats and purchasing pretty maternity outfits

❑ Take time to pamper yourself with a warm bath or manicure

❑ Start creating your baby's nursery

❑ Try meditation to relieve stress

❑ Tend to pregnancy back aches. Talk to your doctor about the possibility of seeing a chiropractor

❑ Negotiate the details of your maternity leave

MY PERSONAL CHECKLIST:

❑ ....

❑ ....

❑ ....

MY HOPES FOR THIS MONTH:

....

....

....

....

....

Lunar Month

Six

Second Trimester

AT THIS POINT IN YOUR PREGNANCY you are probably starting to wonder if your baby will ever arrive. But rest assured, he will be born before you know it, and you will wonder where the time went. Indeed, pregnancy plays tricks on women—it simultaneously flies by and drags on endlessly. If you are among the unlucky percentage of women who suffer from nausea and vomiting throughout your pregnancy, it may seem like each minute lasts a hundred years. However, even for you, at some point you will look back on this time and think, "It went so fast."

Now that you are ready to savor the remaining months of your pregnancy, consider how to commemorate this truly special time in your life. One excellent way is to photograph your growing belly at the beginning of each new month. Another great idea is to keep a pregnancy journal that details the books you read, how you feel, names you're considering, when you first felt your baby kick, and what it felt like to hear his heartbeat for the first time. If you haven't already started doing these things, it is not too late to start. Pick up the camera and your journal, and get busy. Find a quiet spot to reflect on your pregnancy before it is over.

WHAT TO EXPECT THIS MONTH

This month you can expect to really start to show. As your uterus grows higher above your belly button and pushes your entire abdomen out, there will be no denying that you are pregnant. If you have been able to avoid maternity clothes up to this point, odds are by the end of this month most of your outfits will feature at least one piece of maternity wear.

As your belly grows up and out, your hormones will level off. Indeed, you should notice a change around week 22. The amount of progesterone and estrogen that your body produces will be even for a short time until estrogen levels surpass that of the progesterone. You can also expect to have low blood pressure until week 22 or 23 when it may return to what it was before you became pregnant. Also, by the middle of this month your body's production of red blood cells starts to match its production of plasma.

Something that is exciting for your baby this month is that his lungs are developed to the point that if he was born in this month he has a chance at survival. Of course, you want him to stay put until at least week 37 or 38 so that he puts on enough weight and is as healthy as possible.

THINGS TO CONSIDER

If you haven't done so, it is seriously the time to register for childbirth classes. There are several types of classes to choose from, and you should complete your classes by week 35 in case you go into early labor. Be sure to also register for a breast-feeding class. Though it may seem like it will come naturally, many women have trouble getting the hang of it at first. When the baby comes, you will be glad you were prepared.

Another great class to register for is infant CPR. Even if you are certified in adult CPR, take the infant class. It's a much different procedure and proper technique can be the difference between life and death. Make sure that your partner attends classes with you, and you may want to insist that whoever is going to take care of your child (babysitters, daycare, or grandma) attend infant CPR as well. Don't forget to check with your insurance carrier to find out if they offer classes at a discount or for free.

While you have the insurance company on the line, you should also inquire into their pregnancy benefits. Find out if you have a co-pay and how much it is, as well as what is covered under the co-pay. Be sure to ask about coverage in the event of necessary medical interventions, such as Cesarean or episiotomies.

TIPS FOR COPING

Honestly, at this point in your pregnancy, it is likely that your biggest issue to cope with is feeling as if you will be pregnant forever. This is a common feeling for pregnant women at this point in the process. Some women even start to feel trapped by bodily functions, diet, doctor visits, and general limitations, such as abstaining from alcohol. If you're sick of talking about pregnancy—take a break!

If you have time, consider joining a book club or taking a cooking class. Engaging in activities that have absolutely nothing to do with being pregnant is healthy and necessary for your mental health. So, accept your co-workers' invitations to happy hour and participate in the gossip and play pool while you sip virgin margaritas. Remember that you need to take care of your whole self and that means engaging the person you were before you were pregnant. She's still in there, after all!

WHAT TO EAT

There is no reason to change your diet if you've been eating a healthy mix of fruits, vegetables, complex carbohydrates, and protein. Of course, you must continue to consume enough folate, iron, and calcium. And you will want to limit your sugar and saturated fat intake. Though, you should certainly treat yourself now and then to cheese fries or a piece of carrot cake!

HOW MUCH WEIGHT TO GAIN

Assuming that you are not eating 3,000 calories a day, your weight gain should level off at about a pound per week. For some women, this fluctuates—they gain ½ pound one week and 2 pounds the next. The goal you should set for yourself is to gain 4 pounds total for the month. This way, if you gain more or less than a pound in a given week, you can pay more attention the next week. However, don't drive yourself crazy trying to stick to this formula. If you gain 6 pounds this month, it isn't the end of the world. And no matter how much weight you end up gaining this month, do not for one second consider dieting next month. Dieting will be harmful to both you and your baby right now, so save it for after your little one has arrived.

EXERCISE TIPS AND ADVICE

It's likely that you are becoming less graceful as your pregnancy progresses and that you have become more accident-prone. Don't worry—this clumsiness will not last! As you know by now, your body is flooded with the hormone relaxin, which is loosening up your joints and ligaments in preparation for the big day. This, coupled with your shifting center of gravity, can make exercise a precarious undertaking. For all these reasons, it is important to avoid activities that require precision or coordination. Instead, exercises like walking, swimming, and yoga are excellent ways to stay in shape and keep your weight under control.

POTENTIAL SYMPTOMS AND HOW TO ALLEVIATE THEM

You should still be feeling pretty good this month, though there are a few symptoms that will give you trouble. Your back is forced into a deep arch as your belly continues to grow out and pull your muscles forward. This will give you the feeling that your shoulders are constantly being pulled back as your stomach is being pushed forward. Your lower back ends up feeling taxed and achy almost constantly. In order to alleviate some of this stress, do gentle forward bends a few times a day, take warm baths, elevate your feet while sitting down, and sleep with a pillow between your knees.

Another symptom that will increase this month is edema, or swelling of your feet and ankles (and possibly your wrists as well). This is somewhat unavoidable, but you can control the level to which you swell by taking walks after sitting for awhile, elevating your feet and hands whenever you can, and drinking plenty of water. If your swelling seems extreme, let your doctor know, because it could be an early sign of preeclampsia (pregnancy-induced hypertension).

WAYS OTHERS CAN HELP

If you are feeling hemmed in by your pregnancy, let your partner know. Dads can be a great resource for coming up with ideas on how to spend your time together that has nothing to do with pregnancy. If you haven't already taken a weekend getaway, now is the time to plan one, dad! Another great way to make mom feel pretty and special is by arranging a spa day and then going out for a lovely dinner for two. Remember to take advantage of this "just the two of us" time because soon it will always be "and baby makes three."

"Loving a baby is a circular business, a kind of feedback loop. The more you give the more you get and the more you get the more you feel like giving."

~ Penelope Leach

Week 21

Starting Weight: _________

OVERVIEW

At this point in your pregnancy you have probably gained between 12 and 15 pounds. If you have gained more or less, it is OK as long as your doctor is comfortable with it. You can expect to gain 1 more pound this week, though if you are retaining a lot of fluid, you may gain more. To avoid this, drink plenty of water—this helps flush your system and makes sure your kidneys are doing their job. Avoid coffee, soda, and tea because they are diuretics and will cause you to retain more fluids. All this extra weight and fluid may have you feeling heavy and clumsy, but this is perfectly normal feeling. Continue to take care of yourself and remember—you are pregnant and are supposed to get bigger and heavier!

Your belly will be telling the world you are pregnant this week, as your uterus is now 1½ inches above your belly button. Your uterus is also sitting right on top of your bladder, which can cause you to experience a return to a frequent need to pee. It might even cause you to leak a little urine now and then from the pressure. You are probably already wearing panty liners and, aside from that, there really isn't much you can do about this inconvenience. It may help a little to completely empty your bladder with each trip to the bathroom.

DAY 141: Date:___/___/___

MOM - WHAT'S HAPPENING:

You may be having trouble with hemorrhoids today. You might even notice some blood on the tissue when you wipe following a bowel movement. Bleeding from hemorrhoids is not dangerous, but it is still smart to let your health care provider know about it. For relief, put a cold compress on them whenever is convenient. You may also use topical compresses that contain hazel, such as Tucks pads. Finally, warm baths can offer relief from stinging and itching.

BABY - WHAT'S HAPPENING:

Some days your baby is punching and kicking like crazy, and on other days she is very quiet. This is completely normal. Babies (even ones that haven't been born yet) have days when they're less energetic, just like the rest of us. If you don't feel your baby moving around at all for several hours in a row, though, give your doctor a call. She may want to bring you in for an ultrasound to make sure everything is all right.

PREGNANCY FACT: Many women experience the sensation of pins and needles in their arms, hands, legs, and feet. In pregnancy, these sensations do not indicate anything is wrong with your circulation. During pregnancy, fluids build up in all parts of the body, putting pressure on various nerves. When these nerves are pressed upon, it affects the feeling in your extremities. To avoid pins and needles, switch positions often. Experiment with elevating your feet and hands to move some of the fluid around and away from the nerves that are causing you trouble.

DAILY JOURNAL

Mood:

Energy:

Cravings:

Symptoms:

Weight:

DAY 142: Date:___/___/___

MOM - WHAT'S HAPPENING:

Around this time, many women experience a mild level of anemia. If you feel unusually tired or lack the energy for even low levels of exercise, mention it to your health care provider. Hopefully, anemia will not be a problem for you. If you've been getting an adequate amount of iron, your red blood cells should be caught up to your plasma production. If you feel exceptionally tired, do not self-diagnose anemia or take iron supplements. Instead, call your doctor and schedule an appointment.

BABY - WHAT'S HAPPENING:

Your baby's middle ear is continuing to form and the bones within it are hardening. This middle ear development gives your baby a sense of balance. It is how she will be able to tell whether she is upside down. It will help her experience the sensation of movement when you dance or walk. Your baby may even experiment with her own sense of balance by moving from side to side or doing somersaults.

PREGNANCY FACT: It is rare for babies to survive if they are born between weeks 20 and 24, but it has happened. Viability increases with each week of your pregnancy. About 33 percent of all premature babies born at 23 weeks survive. Fifty percent of babies born at 24 weeks will survive if they are cared for in the hospital's NICU. By week 28, the survival rate reaches 95 percent. In 2007, the world record for the youngest person ever born was broken by Amillia Taylor, who was born in Miami at just 21 weeks and 6 days.

DAILY JOURNAL

Mood:

Energy:

Cravings:

Symptoms:

Weight:

DAY 143: Date:___/___/___

MOM - WHAT'S HAPPENING:

Today you might find that your mood swings have returned as you settle into the reality of actual childbirth. If you've been reading about labor and vaginal and Cesarean deliveries, you may be feeling like you want to turn the clock back! Being afraid of birthing your child is a very common fear. To get a grip on your fear, connect with other moms in online chatrooms or live support group settings. Talk to your older relatives who have had children. Most of all, remember that giving birth is scary but doable—the human race wouldn't be here if it were impossible!

BABY - WHAT'S HAPPENING:

Your baby's pancreas continues to develop around this time, which is a very important stepping stone in his digestive health. The pancreas is responsible for producing insulin, which is necessary for your baby's body to process sugar. Interestingly, your baby's pancreas won't be fully developed until he is 2 years old.

TIPS AND ADVICE: A wonderful way to connect with new and veteran mothers is to attend a breast-feeding support group while you are still pregnant. Spending time with new mothers who recently went through labor and delivery can be a great educational experience. New moms are eager to tell their stories and to help other moms learn from their experiences. Asking a few of the mothers to share their stories, and what they wished they had known or asked or done, can give you invaluable tools heading into your own baby's birth. This will also prepare you for the challenges of breast-feeding.

DAILY JOURNAL

Mood:

Energy:

Cravings:

Symptoms:

Weight:

DAY 144: Date:___/___/___

MOM - WHAT'S HAPPENING:

Around now, you may start noticing some tensing and releasing in your lower abdomen. Yes, these are contractions. But they are short and come at irregular intervals, so don't panic. These are Braxton Hicks contractions, which do not signal the onset of labor. Braxton Hicks contractions will often appear during or after exercise, or after having an orgasm. If you notice contractions that seem regular or seem progressively closer together, call your doctor immediately.

BABY - WHAT'S HAPPENING:

Your baby's skin is still relatively thin and wrinkled. He is starting to take on a reddish color as more blood vessels form beneath his skin. Also, around this time the lanugo that covers his body will start to take on pigment. So, if your baby has inherited your dark hair, it will start to darken. Your tiny little baby is looking more and more like the newborn he will become with each passing day.

TIPS AND ADVICE: To deal with the forgetfulness typical of this stage of pregnancy, consider investing in a daily organizer. Or, better yet, hang a large dry-erase calendar on the inside of your front door so that you can see your daily task list as you leave the house. You may also want to phone your office or home and leave yourself messages so that if you forget something by the time you arrive, you will have a friendly reminder waiting for you. This may all seem very strange but pregnancy brain forces women to become quite resourceful to stay on top of everything.

DAILY JOURNAL

Mood:

Energy:

Cravings:

Symptoms:

Weight:

DAY 145: Date:___/___/___

MOM - WHAT'S HAPPENING:

The fear of labor and delivery may cause you to start having nightmares. These nightmares are your brain's way of exploring your worst fears in a safe way. Think of these as your mind playing out worst-case scenarios in order to make room for the best possible outcome on delivery day. If you find that your sleep is being affected more than one or two times a week by these nightmares, however, consider speaking to a therapist who can help you gain perspective.

BABY - WHAT'S HAPPENING:

Your baby's sense of hearing is becoming more fully developed and sounds that she hears in the womb on a regular basis will become so familiar that she will not flinch when she hears them after she is born. Studies indicate that baby is able to hear low-tone noises easier than high-frequency noises. This means dad's voice is getting programmed into baby's brain, so speak up and often, dad!

FOOD FOR THOUGHT: If you are pregnant around the holidays, you will be exposed to many meals with family members who will likely try and stuff you like a turkey. When faced with a buffet table of cheeses, sauces, cakes, and pies, you should, of course, allow yourself to indulge. However, a great rule to make for yourself is to taste a little of everything and to eat a lot of nothing. In other words, make yourself a plate that has a variety of foods, but not too much of any one of them.

DAILY JOURNAL

Mood:

Energy:

Cravings:

Symptoms:

Weight:

DAY 146: Date:___/___/___

MOM - WHAT'S HAPPENING:

Today, you might notice small lumps in one or both of your breasts. Chances are this is simply a clogged milk duct. It is hard to believe, but your breasts are already diligently preparing to feed your baby once he is born. As this construction is going on, there may occasionally be a glitch, such as a clogged duct. Applying a warm, damp washcloth over the lump can bring relief and allow the duct to clear itself. If the lump doesn't go away, or if it is accompanied by a fever, make sure to tell your doctor.

BABY - WHAT'S HAPPENING:

The blood vessels in your baby's lungs are starting to develop around now. These will prepare her to breathe once she is born. With every growing day, her body becomes more and more prepared to take that first breath—and the more anxious you become to meet her!

FOR YOUR HEALTH: If you are carrying multiple babies, you are at a higher risk for preterm labor. Therefore, it is very important that you know when to call your doctor. Some symptoms, such as Braxton Hicks contractions are normal, and not cause for concern. However if you experience any of the following, call your doctor right away: pelvic pressure or fullness, more than four contractions in an hour, cramping that does not go away, ruptured amniotic sac, discolored vaginal discharge or bleeding. If you experience more than one of these at the same time, head to the hospital.

DAILY JOURNAL

Mood:

Energy:

Cravings:

Symptoms:

Weight:

DAY 147: Date:___/___/___

MOM - WHAT'S HAPPENING:

Around this time you may notice small growths on your gums. Known as pyogenic granulomas or "pregnancy tumors," these are harmless and will go away shortly after your baby is born. Also, at this point you may actually be able to see your baby's acrobatics through your clothes! This is a sight that usually only very thin women are treated to, but women of all shapes and sizes will be able to feel their baby kick, punch, and roll around in their womb by now.

BABY - WHAT'S HAPPENING:

Your little baby is gradually becoming not-so-little. Weighing in at 1.1 pounds and stretching out to just over 11 inches, your babe is really able to throw his weight around now. Starting now and continuing throughout your pregnancy, your partner will be able to feel your baby's movements by placing a hand on the outside of your abdomen. You will also notice that at each prenatal checkup your baby's heartbeat sounds stronger and more persistent.

TIPS AND ADVICE: Now is a great time to purchase a few books about caring for a newborn. There are several reputable guides that will come in handy when it is 3 a.m. and you are wondering if your baby's poop should be that color. Starting your library now will cut down on last-minute runs to the bookstore will also help you to feel more prepared when you bring your bundle of joy home. If you are feeling too tired to go to the bookstore yourself, register for the books or order them online.

DAILY JOURNAL

Mood:

Energy:

Cravings:

Symptoms:

Weight:

Week 22

Starting Weight: ________

OVERVIEW

It is likely that sometime this week or next your doctor will order the glucose screening test, which is the first step in determining whether you have gestational diabetes. Between 2 and 5 percent of pregnant women develop gestational diabetes, and although most of those cases can be controlled through a special diet and exercise regimen. The reason the test is done around this time (weeks 24 to 28 LMP) is because your placenta floods your body with hormones that may inhibit insulin production. If your numbers are elevated, you will likely undergo a second screening, but if your numbers are very high, the doctor may skip the second test and get you started right away on controlling your gestational diabetes.

Also, this week you can expect an increase in itching as your skin continues to stretch across your abdomen and breasts. The stretched skin can become very dry and irritated, so be sure to use lotion to keep skin moist and supple. You may also experience an increase in heartburn, which can be relieved by sticking to smaller, more frequent meals, and avoiding eating late at night before lying down. If you find heartburn to be unbearable, speak to your doctor about taking over-the-counter liquid acid neutralizers, such as Mylanta.

DAY 148: Date:___/___/___

MOM - WHAT'S HAPPENING:

Today you may feel as if you are carrying around a heavy soccer ball. In fact, you'd be right: your uterus has expanded to around 2 inches above your belly button, and it is now the size of a soccer ball. This growth spurt will push up on everything above it, including your diaphragm and esophagus. This, plus the hormone relaxin, causes your stomach acids to squeeze upward, causing you discomfort.

BABY - WHAT'S HAPPENING:

Your baby is about to undergo a growth spurt this week. She will put on an impressive 6 ounces by the end of the week. Fat makes up much of her weight gain, as does bone and muscle mass. Her increase in size will make her kicks and punches feel as if you have a monkey in your womb. Enjoy these movements, share them with your partner and try to pay attention to when your baby is most active.

FOR YOUR HEALTH: From now until the end of pregnancy, heartburn will be your companion. Though it is safe to take Tums or Mylanta (with your doctor's approval) you may not want to rely on these. Instead, taking steps to prevent or avoid heartburn is your best course of action. Avoid spicy, fatty, or acidic foods. Wait at least two to three hours after eating before lying down, as this lets digestive acids flow up to your throat. If heartburn is particularly bad, try eating a small portion of plain oatmeal made with reduced-fat milk. This can be soothing and soak up some of those excess acids.

DAILY JOURNAL

Mood:

Energy:

Cravings:

Symptoms:

Weight:

DAY 149: Date:___/___/___

MOM - WHAT'S HAPPENING:

Around this time carpal tunnel syndrome (CTS) may make its first appearance or intensify if you've already started to experience it. This numbing, tingling sensation in your hands and fingers may have you dropping dishes and feeling weak in your wrists. If so, this is a great time to pass dish duty on to dad. And if you haven't already, invest in a good CTS brace, especially if you work on computers or tend to sleep on your hands.

BABY - WHAT'S HAPPENING:

Your baby's lungs are making an important advance—cells are beginning to form that will eventually produce a substance called surfactant. This is a key component in getting your baby's lungs ready to inflate when she takes a breath. Surfactant prevents the tiny air sacs in the lungs from collapsing under the pressure of inhalations. Babies born before surfactant is developed will have a difficult time breathing on their own and will require intensive care treatment until (at least) their official due date.

PREGNANCY FACT: Some women wake up one morning to find that most, or even all, of their symptoms have disappeared. This can be disconcerting and may or may not signal a problem. The best thing to do in this situation is to give your doctor a call and ask to come in for a Doppler. Hearing your baby's heartbeat can be the reassurance you need, or if there is a problem your doctor can advise the best course of action. Try not to panic, because is it likely that this is just brief respite and that your symptoms will return within a few days or weeks.

DAILY JOURNAL

Mood:

Energy:

Cravings:

Symptoms:

Weight:

DAY 150: Date:___/___/___

MOM - WHAT'S HAPPENING:

At this point in your pregnancy, your fundal height should correspond to the number of weeks from your last period. Thus, today you are 24 weeks from your last menstrual period (LMP), and so your fundal height should be just about 24 centimeters. If it is slightly more or less, don't worry. If your doctor is concerned about a due date mix-up, she will be able to determine the actual due date by other means.

BABY - WHAT'S HAPPENING:

Your baby's hands are developing creases and lines that make up his intricate and unique palms. Sometime in his early years of life, you will probably want to capture the preciousness of those little hands by commemorating your little one's hand print. His hands are becoming more coordinated and he is now able to suck his thumb or any fingers of his choosing when he feels the need to. He can also grasp at will and may be tugging on the umbilical cord as you read this.

FOR YOUR HEALTH: If your doctor orders bed rest for you at any time during your pregnancy, be sure to follow his instructions to the letter. It can be discouraging and difficult to have to lie down and stay there this early in your pregnancy, but keep in mind that your doctor has ordered this for a serious reason. Be sure to ask your doctor for specific instructions and to find out if you are on temporary bed rest (just a few weeks) or permanent (until your baby is born). Knowing why bed rest was ordered and for how long can go a long way in helping you feel prepared.

DAILY JOURNAL

Mood:

Energy:

Cravings:

Symptoms:

Weight:

DAY 151: Date:___/___/___

MOM - WHAT'S HAPPENING:

You may develop a new kind of lower back pain called posterior pelvic pain (PPP). This is different than lumbar lower back pain, upper back pain, or sciatica (with which PPP is often confused). Posterior pelvic pain is pain that originates at the back of your pelvis and radiates out to one or both of your buttocks. This can make it painful and difficult to sit for long stretches. Therefore movies or plays may no longer be as fun to sit through. It can help to sit on a pillow or to limit how long you are seated.

BABY - WHAT'S HAPPENING:

Your baby has started to develop sweat glands under her skin. There are four types of sweat glands—eccrine glands, which help regulate body temperature; apocrine glands, which do not function until puberty; ceruminous glands, which form in the ear and produce earwax; and mammary glands, which also do not function until after puberty.

FOR YOUR HEALTH: Sometimes women can develop a rash during pregnancy that signifies a serious problem. In fact, one out of every 500 to 1,000 pregnant women will develop this condition, known as intrahepatic cholestasis of pregnancy. A rash appears due to bile acids that build up in the liver, which also spills over into the bloodstream. One study conducted by the University of Birmingham found that this disorder may be the cause of up to 5 percent of stillbirths. Thus, if you develop a severe rash that doesn't go away in a day or two, call your doctor for an appointment.

DAILY JOURNAL

Mood:

Energy:

Cravings:

Symptoms:

Weight:

DAY 152: Date:___/___/___

MOM - WHAT'S HAPPENING:

You may be feeling like you're breathing fine today, as one symptom that should be on its way out is shortness of breath. You still may be breathing faster to accommodate your increased lung capacity, but shortness of breath will subside as your baby settles at the bottom of your pelvis. Also, your rib cage will start to expand to accommodate your growing uterus. In fact, by the time your baby is born, your rib cage will have expanded by 2 to 3 inches! It will return to its normal size shortly after you have your baby.

BABY - WHAT'S HAPPENING:

Your baby's brain is continuing its very intricate development of nerves and channels that will help him process information and perform bodily functions that are necessary for his survival, such as breathing, sleeping, suckling, and crying. If your baby was born this week, he would have about a 30 percent chance of survival, which will become greater as the days and weeks go by.

FOOD FOR THOUGHT: Trying to add a healthy, satisfying fat to your diet? Look no further than the avocado. This powerhouse fruit is loaded with vitamin K, potassium, folate, vitamin B6, and vitamin C. It is delicious mashed and spread over whole wheat toast, cubed and tossed with salads, or eaten by itself with a spoon. Avocados contain oleic acid, which has been linked to a reduction in bad cholesterol, and its high levels of potassium may aid in lowering high blood pressure. Avocados are also rich in vitamin E, which will keep your skin and hair healthy and shiny.

DAILY JOURNAL

Mood:

Energy:

Cravings:

Symptoms:

Weight:

DAY 153: Date:___/___/___

MOM - WHAT'S HAPPENING:

At this point in your pregnancy you may become troubled by your worsening memory. Though it is frustrating, "pregnancy brain"—increased forgetfulness and reduced attention span—is common. Be prepared to have your memory worsen and your attention span shorten until you have your baby. To stay on top of things, use organizational aids, such as calendars, day planners, personal digital assistants, and checklists.

BABY - WHAT'S HAPPENING:

By now your baby may be able to open and close her eyes! This means that she will become even more sensitive to light changes in her environment. You may also be able to notice that your baby frequently has the hiccups. This can be an adorable and very humanizing experience. As she hiccups, she may jostle her home around just enough for you to feel little flutters.

TIPS AND ADVICE: Now is the time to finalize your maternity leave plans with your human resources representative. You should have decided how long you plan to be gone and filing the paperwork will make the transition easier on you and your employer. You should also have the discussion with your partner about whether you will return to your job once your maternity leave runs out—and if you do plan to return to work, how you will arrange for childcare. Many facilities have wait lists, so it is best to put your name on them as soon as you know you will need their services.

DAILY JOURNAL

Mood:

Energy:

Cravings:

Symptoms:

Weight:

DAY 154: Date:___/___/___

MOM - WHAT'S HAPPENING:

As your 22nd week of pregnancy comes to a close, turn your attention to what needs doing before your baby's arrival—and focus on needs, not wants or wishes! Have a look at the lists you've been making and check things off as you complete them. Mounting anxiety over the future is normal, but you can feel more in control if you start taking action.

BABY - WHAT'S HAPPENING:

Your baby is a foot long by now. He weighs around 1.3 pounds. He is probably testing out his feet against your uterine wall and some women are even able to see their belly push out when the baby does this. Your doctor will ask you to count the number of times you feel your baby kick. Pay attention to when your baby is most active so that you are prepared for when you must start keeping track.

PREGNANCY FACT: If you are not feeling the number and intensity of kicks or movements that you were hoping to at this point, it doesn't necessarily mean there is anything wrong with your baby. The number of kicks a baby makes at this stage in its development varies from 50 to 1,000 per day. Most babies tend to kick 250 times daily, but you may not be able to feel their motions due to a number of factors. The placement of your placenta, for example, may be dulling the sensation of your baby's tiny blows.

DAILY JOURNAL

Mood:

Energy:

Cravings:

Symptoms:

Weight:

Week 23

Starting Weight: _________

OVERVIEW

This week you can expect to find that your hair is thicker than ever! This is because pregnancy hormones prevent you from shedding the amount of hair that you normally would. Enjoy your thicker hair now, because after you have your baby your hair will start to fall out. Don't worry—you won't be bald, but your hair will definitely thin out. Something else you may notice this week is that you are in an uphill battle with hemorrhoids. Keep in mind that constipation will exacerbate the occurrence of hemorrhoids, so consume enough fiber and drink lots of water. Also, walking every day helps keep circulation up, which prevents blood from pooling in the veins that cause hemorrhoids to appear. Managing hemorrhoids can be quite a miserable job but just keep reminding yourself that it is all going to be worth it once your baby is born.

Speaking of the little guy, this is a busy week for him! Over the next seven days, your baby's spine will make great strides in its development. A more developed spine will help him better control his movements and be more flexible as he cruises around inside your uterus. Your baby's facial features also continue to develop definition. He will also put on weight at a rate of approximately 6 ounces per week and will be about 13.6 inches long by the end of the week.

DAY 155: Date:___/___/___

MOM - WHAT'S HAPPENING:

Your expanding uterus is still about the size of a volleyball. It is incredible to think that your uterus started out at around the size of a pear! However, all of that stretching is bound to cause some discomfort, and you will likely feel generally achy in your lower abdomen. All of this front weight will likely cause your lower back to spasm occasionally if you do not stretch regularly. Consider purchasing a prenatal yoga DVD so that you can practice this very beneficial exercise in the convenience and comfort of your home.

BABY - WHAT'S HAPPENING:

Your baby is beginning to form all of the 33 rings, 150 joints, and 1,000 ligaments that make up the components of his spine. Once completely formed, a developed spine will help your baby stretch out and control her position inside your uterus. Your baby's bones also continue to ossify this week. As her bones harden, she will become stronger, and you will feel the results of this in the form of kicks.

FOOD FOR THOUGHT: Treat yourself to the healthy comfort of the good, old-fashioned potato. Potatoes are a fantastic source of vitamin B6, which the body needs to form new cells. Potatoes are also loaded with potassium, vitamin C, copper, manganese, and fiber. Potatoes are inexpensive and available all year round. Of course, it's how you eat your potato that makes the difference nutritionally. French fries and other greasy versions will not offer the health benefits of a simple but delicious baked potato. Try using low-fat yogurt for a topping instead of sour cream.

DAILY JOURNAL

Mood:

Energy:

Cravings:

Symptoms:

Weight:

DAY 156: Date:___/___/___

MOM - WHAT'S HAPPENING:

You may find that you have an increase in the number of times a day you get cramps in your calves. To minimize the occurrence of these painful spasms, avoid crossing your legs while standing or sitting. Stretch your legs often, and go for walks every day. Whenever you are sitting down, rotate your ankles and wiggle your toes. Make sure to stay hydrated, and try to get plenty of rest. And remember—if you awake to a leg cramp, do not curl your foot into the cramp but rather force your toes up toward your knee.

BABY - WHAT'S HAPPENING:

Your baby's hands are well-formed by now, and he is able to open and close his fist with ease. He is also able to close his hand around objects that rest in his palm, such as his other hand or the umbilical cord. But don't worry, the umbilical cord can withstand any tugging or twirling your baby may put it through.

FOOD FOR THOUGHT: You may be surprised to learn that you already have control over determining how your baby's tastes for food will develop. Studies have shown that babies are influenced by the flavors they taste while in utero. So, if you want to raise a child who will eat his veggies, be sure to ingest plenty of them while you are pregnant and also when you are nursing. Similarly, babies exposed to high doses of sugar while in utero or when breast-feeding may be slower to accept foods that are not sweet.

DAILY JOURNAL

Mood:

Energy:

Cravings:

Symptoms:

Weight:

DAY 157: Date:___/___/___

MOM - WHAT'S HAPPENING:

If you are still experiencing morning sickness, you are not alone! Though most pregnant women get relief from nausea during the second trimester, many do not. If you are still sick at this point, be sure to let your doctor know. This misery does not have to last—he can prescribe medication that will give you relief and is not harmful to your baby. If you are still vomiting and nauseous, it is likely that your nutrition is mediocre to poor, and it will be more beneficial for you and your baby if you are well enough to eat properly.

BABY - WHAT'S HAPPENING:

Your baby is like a little explorer who has discovered a new land. His sense of touch continues to develop and your baby will be constantly stimulating himself by grabbing everything he can get his tiny little hands on. If you are carrying twins, they will start to interact with each other through touch. This is thought to be the one of the earliest ways multiples bond.

TIPS AND ADVICE: It is not uncommon to wake up in the middle of the night feeling ravenous. If you do awake hungry after having nightmares, night sweats, or with a headache, there's a chance your blood sugar could have fallen during the night. To prevent this from happening, have a small snack that is high in protein before you go to bed. Good selections include a hardboiled egg, a string cheese stick, or peanut butter on a slice of whole wheat toast. These can keep your blood sugar even until morning.

DAILY JOURNAL

Mood:

Energy:

Cravings:

Symptoms:

Weight:

DAY 158: Date:___/___/___

MOM - WHAT'S HAPPENING:

It is a good time to get into the habit of breathing deeply and slowly several times a day. This helps to lower your heart rate and reduce anxiety. Deep breathing is also the very first step to any relaxation exercise, which you should be doing every night before bed. Practicing deep breathing now will make you comfortable with this very important tool that you will use when you go into labor. Making time for deep breathing exercises will also ease muscle tension and quiet your busy mind.

BABY - WHAT'S HAPPENING:

Today, your baby's lungs are continuing to produce blood vessels. These blood vessels will eventually be a very important part of the overall composition that gives her lungs a greater surface area on which to process oxygen into her blood while removing carbon dioxide. When she is born, she will have perfectly formed lungs that look something like tiny pink sponges.

FOOD FOR THOUGHT: When planning your meals, remember that your job is to supply the correct nutrition to support your baby's growth. During the first trimester, folic acid was the star ingredient for your baby's brain development. While folic acid is still important, in the second trimester new nutrients take center stage. At this point in your pregnancy, you need to consume at least 71 grams of protein, 27 milligrams of iron, and 1,000 milligrams of calcium each day. Don't forget about these important nutritional minimums as you plan your meals.

DAILY JOURNAL

Mood:

Energy:

Cravings:

Symptoms:

Weight:

DAY 159: Date:___/___/___

MOM - WHAT'S HAPPENING:

If you have opted to learn your baby's gender, you have known whether you are having a boy or a girl for a few weeks now. This knowledge can be very helpful as you decorate your nursery and start to purchase clothes. Indeed, getting a headstart on buying little dresses or khakis can be quite fun. But even if you and your partner have chosen to keep your baby's gender a secret until his or her birthday, you can still get a jump on the planning and decorating. Choose gender-neutral shades, such as green or yellow for your baby's nursery and wardrobe. And of course, most baby products, such as diapers, will fit either gender!

BABY - WHAT'S HAPPENING:

Your baby's face is becoming more distinguished as his nostrils begin to open and the nerves that surround his lips and chin become more sensitive. These nerves will help him develop the rooting reflex, which guides his mouth to your nipple when it is time to nurse.

PREGNANCY FACT: How many times a day do you eat? Hopefully, you've followed the advice in this book and you are eating five or six small meals daily. However, if you aren't, you are not alone. According to a poll conducted by Babycenter.com, just 23 percent of pregnant women eat six times a day or more. Thirty percent of pregnant women said they ate five times a day, 26 percent ate four times a day, 16 percent ate three times a day, and 5 percent ate just twice a day—which is not recommended. If you are eating just twice a day, you are likely starving yourself and your baby.

DAILY JOURNAL

Mood:

Energy:

Cravings:

Symptoms:

Weight:

DAY 160: Date:___/___/___

MOM - WHAT'S HAPPENING:

You are probably consumed by everything pregnancy-related: symptoms, diet and nutrition, your physique, environmental factors, nursery plans—all of which are worth thinking about. However, don't forget about your partner! Pregnancy is often the beginning of a major change in the dynamic between a couple, so taking steps now to stay bonded will help carry you through when tensions are running high. In fact, just letting him know you are aware that you've been completely obsessed with your pregnancy and may have neglected him can make him feel included in your experience.

BABY - WHAT'S HAPPENING:

Your baby's skin is still mostly translucent, but is thickening with each passing day. Eventually it will no longer be see-through. Capillaries beneath the skin are filling with blood, which increases her pink complexion. The opening of your baby's nostrils allow her to practice breathing through her nose as well as through her mouth.

PREGNANCY FACT: If you are the first among your group of friends to become pregnant, be prepared for some major changes in your friendships. Though you are all are well-meaning and want to try to keep things as they are, things will be different. Your needs and priorities will become different enough that you may find yourself seeing your friends much less than before you were pregnant. This can be a difficult transition, but your friends who are committed to your friendship will stick around and become a part of your baby's life.

DAILY JOURNAL

Mood:

Energy:

Cravings:

Symptoms:

Weight:

DAY 161: Date:___/___/___

MOM - WHAT'S HAPPENING:

Since you are likely feeling well these days, you and your partner are probably trying to get all your "ducks in a row." In addition to decorating the nursery, part of getting ready for baby's arrival may include discussing choosing a godparent for your child. Your baby's godparent will be a family member or deeply trusted friend who will care for and provide guidance for your child, should you and your partner pass away suddenly or otherwise be unable to care for your child. Although it might seem morbid to discuss, you will feel better knowing you have planned for your baby's care.

BABY - WHAT'S HAPPENING:

Your little one is becoming a heavyweight! She now weighs approximately 1½ pounds and is close to 13 inches long. Over the next few months your baby will gain between 6 and 7 pounds if she is of average birth weight. She is also busy perfecting her ability to swallow amniotic fluid.

TIPS AND ADVICE: If you do not already have a life insurance policy, start shopping around for one. You will need coverage for both you and your partner. You will first want to figure out what it costs to run your household annually. Be sure to include the added cost of having a new baby. It is advisable to purchase 6 to 10 times your yearly salary in coverage. Also, it is customary to have your partner be the recipient of the benefits, so that if something happens to one of you the other will have enough money to take care of the family.

DAILY JOURNAL

Mood:

Energy:

Cravings:

Symptoms:

Weight:

Week 24

Starting Weight: ________

OVERVIEW

Welcome to the last week of your second trimester! This week is another transitional week, during which old symptoms resurface as new ones are introduced. You can expect to gain another pound this week. Also, your belly will start to expand about ½ inch per week from now until the end of your pregnancy. At this point, you've probably gained between 16 and 22 pounds, but if you have gained a little more or less, don't panic. If you have gained less than 16 pounds, speak to your doctor about your symptoms and eating habits, because it is important to consume enough calories to support your baby's growth.

You will likely experience an increase in Braxton Hicks contractions this week, which is not cause for alarm. However, it becomes increasingly important that you familiarize yourself with the signs of preterm labor so that you can tell the difference between it and harmless "practice" contractions.

As your uterus becomes more active, so too, does your baby. You may feel like he's building a tree house in your uterus for all the banging around he's doing. You may even be able to interact with him by pressing on your belly and watching him push out back at you!

DAY 162: Date:___/___/___

MOM - WHAT'S HAPPENING:

Though you had a brief respite from feeling short of breath, you may find that it returns this week as your uterus expands. Your growing uterus crowds all the organs around it, including your lungs. It will even put pressure on your rib cage. This can be uncomfortable and will feel worse if you panic. Keep reminding yourself that even while short of breath, you are getting enough oxygen for both you and your baby.

BABY - WHAT'S HAPPENING:

This is an active week for your baby's lung development. Her lungs are now producing surfactant, which will enable her lungs to stay inflated once she starts to breathe air after she is born. Tiny air sacs called alveoli are also continuing to mature and develop. This is all great news for your baby's survival rate if you were to deliver early. If you could see your baby now she would look like she is breathing—though it is still just practice, as all she breathes is amniotic fluid.

PREGNANCY FACT: Baby showers in America are rooted in our nation's history. These parties got started after World War II, when women got together to celebrate a new child coming into their community. Families were often too poor to acquire everything they needed for the baby, so the community of women would gather and bring homemade clothing, food, and furniture for the new mom-to-be. Baby showers today are considerably different, but the heart of them still rests in helping a new family get started through gifts received at a celebration.

DAILY JOURNAL

Mood:

Energy:

Cravings:

Symptoms:

Weight:

DAY 163: Date:___/___/___

MOM - WHAT'S HAPPENING:

Another side effect of your uterus's expansion is the onset of aches and pains felt in your feet all the way up to your shoulders. This is because your uterus is actually pushing your bones out of the way to make room for its growth. This can hurt particularly in your ribs, pelvis, and hips. The best way to get relief is to change position frequently and take your time when getting in and out of your car or the bathtub, as these motions tend to cause the most discomfort.

BABY - WHAT'S HAPPENING:

Your baby may look like a little flirt on his next ultrasound. This is because as he open and closes his eyes, he looks a lot like he is winking or batting his eyelashes. This, added to all the other facial development, has your baby looking quite like he will after he is born. Your baby's eye color still hasn't developed, though pigmentation has begun in his irises.

FOOD FOR THOUGHT: A great way to have a healthy and easy home-cooked meal is to make a cream of vegetable soup. Sauté one small yellow onion and a clove of diced garlic in a tablespoon of olive oil. Add your nutrient-rich pregnancy vegetable of choice—broccoli, asparagus, or potato are great selections—then sauté until coated with the garlic/onion mixture. Add one carton of chicken or vegetable broth, bring to a boil then let simmer until vegetables are soft. Finally, puree the mixture in a blender and return to the pot. Add ½ cup of low-fat milk, stir, and serve!

DAILY JOURNAL

Mood:

Energy:

Cravings:

Symptoms:

Weight:

DAY 164: Date:___/___/___

MOM - WHAT'S HAPPENING:

That feeling of food sitting like a brick in your stomach is probably surfacing again. This is because progesterone has caused your digestion to slow down, making food stay longer in your stomach before being digested. As mentioned already, the only cure for this sensation is to eat smaller meals more often. Eating seven, even eight tiny meals a day may be your best option.

BABY - WHAT'S HAPPENING:

Now that your baby's retina are developed and her eyes can open and close, she is able to focus on images that are up close. This means she is able to see her hands, the placenta, and the umbilical cord. Interestingly, some light does get through into your womb, so she is also becoming aware of light and dark.

FOR YOUR HEALTH: Your doctor will order a glucose screening test sometime this week to screen for gestational diabetes. You will drink several ounces of glucose then wait an hour. Your blood will be drawn and tested. If the results are concerning your doctor may order a follow-up test called a glucose tolerance test. This test requires that you fast overnight and then drink more glucose solution. Your blood will be drawn several times over three hours and then your doctor will be able to determine if you have gestational diabetes.

DAILY JOURNAL

Mood:

Energy:

Cravings:

Symptoms:

Weight:

DAY 165: Date:___/___/___

MOM - WHAT'S HAPPENING:

If it hasn't already happened, there is an excellent chance that your belly button will pop out around this time. You will notice that it sticks out through your clothes and seems to be a magnet for other people's eyes. For those women whose belly buttons stay put—don't worry, this is also completely normal. Some women have a little too much padding between the back of their belly buttons the outer part for it to pop.

BABY - WHAT'S HAPPENING:

Your baby's brain waves are starting to fire up at this point, which means that his senses are becoming even more refined. Thus, if you haven't already done so, start to play with your baby using sound and movement. For example, you may notice that he stops moving if you dance around the room, and that the minute you stop, he starts moving again. He will also startle if a loud noise occurs near him, though you may or may not feel him "jump."

FOOD FOR THOUGHT: A delicious addition to nearly any meal is the California artichoke. There are several ways to prepare this yummy vegetable, and it is great for you. Artichokes are loaded with potassium, vitamin C, folate, and magnesium. One large artichoke has just 25 calories, zero fat, and lots of fiber. You can steam whole artichokes and peel off the leaves to eat the meat as well as the "heart." Artichokes are also available pre-cooked in a can and are a great topping for pizzas or salads. Just be sure to keep this vegetable healthy by avoiding dipping it in heavy sauces and butter.

DAILY JOURNAL

Mood:

Energy:

Cravings:

Symptoms:

Weight:

DAY 166: Date:___/___/___

MOM - WHAT'S HAPPENING:

You may be tired of thinking about what to eat for your next meal since food is on your mind so much these days. If you are a carnivore, be sure to incorporate fish into your diet. Good fish choices are bass, cod, flounder, and salmon. Eat only fresh fish and be sure that it is cooked thoroughly before eating. You can even get creative with spices and see how your baby reacts to Cajun seasoning!

BABY - WHAT'S HAPPENING:

Your baby's sweat glands are mostly formed by now and may have even started to function—though there is little need for them in the perfect temperature of the amniotic sac. Your baby continues to accumulate fat and his skin is becoming less transparent, though you can still see his veins. Also, at this point, he still has plenty of room to somersault and turn around, but fairly soon he will grow large enough to become cramped. This is when you will really be able to see his movements through your skin.

TIPS AND ADVICE: If you and your partner have life insurance policies, IRAs, and/or a 401(k), be sure to revisit them this week or next. At the time you opened these accounts you may have selected a beneficiary for your benefits that is no longer whom you want. If you have listed your partner, then you are in good shape. However, if you want one or all of these benefits to go into a trust for your child, now is a great time to make changes. The individual policy directives on these accounts will supersede your will, so it is important to make sure that all these documents are in order.

DAILY JOURNAL

Mood:

Energy:

Cravings:

Symptoms:

Weight:

DAY 167: Date:___/___/___

MOM - WHAT'S HAPPENING:

You have probably found by now that it is nearly impossible to find a comfortable sleeping position. There are many products that may help you get more comfortable. A foam wedge made specifically for pregnant women may help. You slide these under your belly for support. Similarly, body pillows and other gadgets designed to keep you supported and/or from rolling over onto your back are available in most stores or from websites that cater to pregnant women. You can also ask other pregnant women what they are using or check pregnancy-product message boards online.

BABY - WHAT'S HAPPENING:

Your baby's eyelashes, eyebrows, finger and toenails have all finished forming, though they will continue to grow longer and thicker. All of these attributes give your baby her unique appearance. The physical characteristics she develops in utero will mature after she is born, but the basic foundation for how she will look is already well underway.

FOR YOUR HEALTH: If you have a toddler at home, make use of all of your friends and relatives who said, "Let me know if there's anything I can do to help!" when you told them that you were pregnant. Ask someone to take your little one to the park on the weekend. It will make him feel special and give you a chance to rest while your partner takes care of household chores. Getting just an hour or two break to nap and rest can mean the difference between feeling a little stressed and having a complete meltdown. If none of your friends are available, hire a babysitter to come over during the day.

DAILY JOURNAL

Mood:

Energy:

Cravings:

Symptoms:

Weight:

DAY 168: Date:___/___/___

MOM - WHAT'S HAPPENING:

Welcome to the last day of your second trimester! This milestone likely has you feeling both excited and anxious. As you look ahead to the third trimester, you will probably become focused on how and when you will deliver your baby. You may even start having bizarre dreams in which you give birth to a litter of puppies or that you are drowning in a large body of water. Both of these themes are common to pregnant women and represent their anxiety over the impending responsibility they are about to face.

BABY - WHAT'S HAPPENING:

Your baby is far from the tiny raspberry he was at 8 weeks! By now he is just about 2 pounds and may be as long as 14 inches—about the size of a medium butternut squash. This may not surprise you considering how big you feel, but this is a huge step in your baby's viability should you go into preterm labor.

FOR YOUR HEALTH: Approximately 1 out of 200 pregnant women suffer a serious complication known as placental abruption. This occurs when the placenta separates from your uterus before you give birth. It is unclear why this happens, but some segments of the pregnancy population are more at risk. These include women who have had this condition during previous pregnancies, those pregnant with multiples, women with preeclampsia, and those with blood-clotting problems. If you experience a sudden and significant amount of vaginal bleeding, call your doctor immediately.

DAILY JOURNAL

Mood:

Energy:

Cravings:

Symptoms:

Weight:

Lunar Month

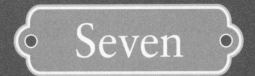

Seven

PHOTO

Place a photo of you during your seventh month here

My Monthly Update

Waist Measurement: ______

Weight: ______

Mood: ______

Lunar Month seven

PREGNANCY CHECKLIST

- ❑ Soak your feet in warm water or lie down with your feet raised to prevent ankle and foot swelling.
- ❑ If your hands and face swell suddenly, call your health care provider.
- ❑ Stretch marks may appear on the abdomen and breasts — use a stretch-mark eraser cream or cocoa butter
- ❑ Make sure you know the signs of premature labor
- ❑ Call your health care provider if you have more than 5 contractions in 1 hour
- ❑ Be aware that you will have a hard time with your balance, now that your belly is growing so much!
- ❑ After the 28th week, visit your health care provider every 2 weeks for prenatal care
- ❑ Get plenty of rest — your body is working hard
- ❑ Care for painful pregnancy hemorrhoids
- ❑ Start or continue childbirth education classes
- ❑ Have a blood test for gestational diabetes
- ❑ Consider hiring a doula
- ❑ Create your birth plan
- ❑ Decide who will be in the delivery room with you
- ❑ Understand your feeding options — breast or bottle?
- ❑ Know your cord blood banking options
- ❑ Buy your baby's crib and mattress
- ❑ Buy a stroller
- ❑ Have baby clothes and necessities, like bottles, ready

MY PERSONAL CHECKLIST:

❑ ....

MY HOPES FOR THIS MONTH:

....

....

Lunar Month Seven

Third Trimester

WELCOME TO YOUR THIRD and final trimester! It may seem as if your pregnancy has completely taken over your life, just imagine what life will be like once you bring home your tiny infant. In fact, preparing for life after pregnancy is how you should spend the majority of your third trimester. Hopefully, you will feel well enough for the majority of these last few months to be able to get your living space—and yourself—ready for bringing home baby.

Since there is so much to do to prepare for your baby's arrival, you and your partner may start to notice that your anxiety and stress levels increase. This is normal, of course, and is not indicative of you not being mature enough to handle having a baby. People panic when their baby's arrival is near, because it is overwhelming to know that in just 14 weeks or so you will be caring for a tiny human being who completely depends on you for all of her needs. Rest assured that no parent before you ever had a handbook—they all figured it out, and you will too. Also, once your baby is out, family, friends, and coworkers will be beating down the door to meet her—so try to enjoy these last few months of having the baby all to yourself.

WHAT TO EXPECT THIS MONTH

By the end of this month you can expect that your uterus will expand to approximately 4½ inches above your belly button. This will give you a pregnancy "shelf" just under your breasts. As your uterus moves up under your rib cage, you may feel uncomfortable in any position for too long. To give the various affected organs, muscles, and bones a break make sure to change positions frequently.

This month will also bring with it the excitement of being able to more frequently share your baby's movements with your partner and friends. This is because she is rapidly putting on weight—she will weigh close to 3 pounds by the end of the month, and may be as long as 16 inches. Indeed, her growth spurt will result in more definitive kicks, punches, and hiccups for you and your partner to enjoy on a regular basis.

THINGS TO CONSIDER

If you have not registered for childbirth classes, put this book down and do it right now! You want to try and complete all classes by week 35, which gives you just 10 weeks from enrollment until completion. You may not think you need classes after having read this book but classes are helpful, practical, and educational—especially if this is your first baby.

If this not your first baby, this month is a good time to have the first in a series of discussions with your older child about the fact that he or she is about to have a little brother or sister. There are several children's books that deal with this topic. They illustrate what is happening to mommy's body, as well as what it means to be an older sibling. If your child is very young, he or she may not fully comprehend what you are saying, but will get the idea eventually. Now is also an excellent time to come up with a plan for who will care for your older child when you go into labor and delivery. It is important to note that completely excluding your older child from the birth can be confusing and hurtful. So, if possible, have him or her present for early labor—before you are in too much pain (so the child is not scared). Also, be sure to arrange to have someone bring your child to your room after the baby is born so that your he or she can immediately participate in family bonding.

TIPS FOR COPING

For help coping with new and old symptoms this month, try identifying what your feelings are about the various components of the remainder of your pregnancy. Get in touch with your feelings regarding the birth of your baby and bringing baby home. Most women at this stage tend to become (understandably) fixated on labor and delivery. In fact, a good percentage of women would love to hear that there is an alternative means through which to have their baby. You are, of course, limited to either a vaginal or Cesarean delivery, so given these options—what are your fears? What are you curious about? What are you excited for? Indeed, identifying your fears, concerns, excitements, and curiosities, and sharing them with your partner is the best way to cope with last-trimester anxiety.

WHAT TO EAT

Beginning this month you should consume an additional 300 to 350 calories each day to keep up with your baby's nutritional demands. Make sure that these are high-quality calories and keep in mind it is possible to get these calories (and then some!) from a single cupcake or from just a few bites of a fast-food cheeseburger.

Therefore, these additional calories should be spent wisely. Of course, if you've been eating healthily all along this will not be difficult.

Getting creative with your snacks is the best way to add calories and prevent overeating. Never sit down to a plate of food with a goal of eating 350 additional calories. This mindset is likely to cause you to eat many more than 350 calories and feel bloated and uncomfortable for hours after. So, instead, add calories to your diet by eating healthy snacks in between meals, such as a sliced apple with 2 tablespoons of peanut butter—this nutritious snack equals just 310 calories.

HOW MUCH WEIGHT TO GAIN

Keep in mind that at the end of last month, your baby weighed just about 2 pounds—this means in the next three months she will gain between 5 and 7 pounds. This weight comes from those additional 350 calories you are eating. Indeed, much of the weight you gain from now until the end of your pregnancy will be diverted to your baby, the placenta, and to the amniotic fluid. You will still gain approximately 4 pounds per month, and if you are hitting that mark then you are on track with exercise and diet. If you are gaining much more than 4 pounds per month, examine your diet and make healthier choices—without dieting. Refer to the helpful nutritional information in the back of this book. This section makes it simple and convenient to plan healthy meals and be sure you are getting the proper nutrients from your pregnancy diet.

EXERCISE TIPS AND ADVICE

Unless your doctor has restricted your activity level, keep moving this month. Walking, swimming, prenatal yoga, and Kegel exercises are all beneficial to you. You may also want to add some gentle stretches to keep your shoulders loose and to relax your lower and upper back. In fact, now is an excellent time to introduce a yoga ball into your daily routine. It is great for gently moving while watching TV and will reduce tailbone pain caused by sitting.

POTENTIAL SYMPTOMS AND HOW TO ALLEVIATE THEM

There exists the potential for many symptoms to surface and resurface this month. Any symptoms that you have experienced before will be best relieved by doing what you already know works. This holds true for the following that will likely appear or increase this month: whitish vaginal discharge, sensitive and bleeding gums, congestion and nosebleeds, cramping in your calves, heartburn, constipation, hemorrhoids, varicose veins, headaches, insomnia, and backaches.

Also, at this point you should learn what preterm labor will look and feel like so that if it strikes, you can get to the hospital right away for intervention. As a reminder, preterm labor can include any or all of the following: abdominal cramps with or without bleeding, sudden and severe nausea, pelvic pressure, rupture of the amniotic sac, and contractions (not Braxton Hicks). If you ever suspect that you are in premature labor, call your doctor. If you cannot get ahold of him, head to the hospital—don't wait to hear back from him!

WAYS OTHERS CAN HELP

This is a good month for your partner to double as a forklift—you will probably need some help getting up off the couch or out of the bathtub. Let your partner help you, since the added strain of these motions on your abdomen, hips, and lower back can add to your overall achiness. Also, allow your to partner take on all heavy-lifting duties, including carrying groceries and laundry. Carrying these will not harm you or your baby, but relief from these duties will give your back a much-needed break.

> **"The most important thing she'd learned over the years was that there was no way to be a perfect mother and a million ways to be a good one."**
> **~ Jill Churchill**

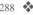

Week 25

Starting Weight: ________

OVERVIEW

This week marks the first week of your third trimester, which means you have entered the home stretch of your pregnancy. Your uterus is so large that the top rests in your rib cage, which prevents your lungs from completely inflating. This can cause you to feel short of breath. Though uncomfortable, it is not dangerous. Your respiratory system has become extremely efficient at processing oxygen to get the required amounts to both you and your baby. It is hard to say whether this symptom will stay with you, because some women find that they are short of breath until they deliver the baby. Others, however, experience relief once their baby drops down into the pelvis.

Meanwhile, your baby's lungs continue to grow and mature. Also, he will continue to practice breathing amniotic fluid. This exercise helps to develop his respiratory system, preparing him for that monumental first breath of air after he is born. Your baby's brain is also growing and refining its capabilities by practicing all of the various tricks it can do. So, if you are scheduled for an ultrasound this week, you may catch your baby waving, sucking his thumb, doing somersaults, and even blinking! Another exciting milestone occurs this week as your baby's retinas are developed enough that he will notice movements within the uterus and may even follow them by turning his head.

DAY 169: Date:___/___/___

MOM - WHAT'S HAPPENING:

Starting today, add between 300 and 350 calories per day to your diet until you deliver your baby. Do not mistake this directive for an all-access pass to consume treats and snacks: it is important to make these calories count by eating whole and nutritious foods. Keep in mind that adding 300 to 350 calories to your daily diet is not really very much at all—a small serving of low-fat yogurt, fruit, and granola will more than do the trick. When deciding where to add these extra calories, be smart—good sources to pull from are those high in calcium, fiber, protein, and iron.

BABY - WHAT'S HAPPENING:

Since your baby's retinas are nearly completely formed, she is able to distinguish between light and dark. She will be able to watch her hand as it moves through the amniotic fluid and up to her face. Her eyes stay open for longer stretches now and her waking and sleeping patterns have become semi-regular—as they will be after she is born.

FOR YOUR HEALTH: Approximately 1 in 7 women experience migraines for the first time during pregnancy. Though this usually occurs during the first trimester, it is possible they appear in the second or third. Unfortunately, the medications used to treat migraines are not advised for pregnant women. However, you may take acetaminophen or lie in a dark room with a cool compress on your head. Call your doctor if you suddenly develop migraines and have never had them before. At this point in your pregnancy it can be a sign of preeclampsia.

DAILY JOURNAL

Mood:
Energy:
Cravings:
Symptoms:
Weight:

DAY 170: Date:___/___/___

MOM - WHAT'S HAPPENING:

There is a good chance your blood pressure will start to go up early this week. It is probable it will even return to the level at which it was before you became pregnant. Also, around today you may start to have the sensation that your heart has skipped or added a beat. This is common during the third trimester and is usually is not cause for concern. However, it is a good idea to mention this to your doctor just to be on the safe side.

BABY - WHAT'S HAPPENING:

Your baby's lungs have produced enough surfactant and have enough air sacs that he is capable of breathing air. This means if you were to go into early labor, your little one has an improved chance of survival—more than 50 percent, in fact. Also, your baby's brain is undergoing rapid development as it creates billions of neurons necessary to process information and link up brain waves to body functions.

TIPS AND ADVICE: Include the following four simple activities into your daily routine, as they can help to prepare your body for labor: 1) Do Kegel exercises often. They will strengthen your pelvic floor and help control urinary incontinence now and after delivery. 2) Practice squatting. This strengthens your leg muscles and stretches your pelvic area. 3) Get down on all fours and stretch up like a cat. This pose stretches your back muscles and increases your abdominal strength. 4) Sit cross-legged on the floor. This will loosen up inner-thigh muscles and ease lower-back pain.

DAILY JOURNAL

Mood:

Energy:

Cravings:

Symptoms:

Weight:

DAY 171: Date:___/___/___

MOM - WHAT'S HAPPENING:

Unfortunately, progesterone continues to cause your digestion to be very slow so that your baby is able to pull every drop of nutrition out of the food that you eat. This means you are going to continue to experience heartburn and possibly see the return of constipation. Be sure to follow the tips throughout this book for managing heartburn and constipation. Finally, drink more water. This can help both heartburn and constipation and will keep you well-hydrated.

BABY - WHAT'S HAPPENING:

Although your baby is perfectly capable of stretching out, it is likely that he is spending much of his time curled up in the fetal position. As he gets bigger, he will be forced into the fetal position until he is born as he rapidly runs out of room. You will find even infants who are put to bed on their backs will wake up in the fetal position—this position helps to retain heat and is a familiar one that kept them safe and sound while inside the womb.

FOOD FOR THOUGHT: In addition to adding an assortment of vegetables to your pasta dishes, such as spinach, zucchini, and artichokes, consider switching to whole wheat pasta. It is more nutritious and higher in protein than white pastas. In fact, typical whole wheat pasta has between 8 and 9 grams of protein as well as 5 or 6 grams of fiber. Most white pastas, on the other hand, have around 5 grams of protein and just 2 grams of fiber. Thus, switching to whole wheat is an easy way to increase both your protein and fiber intake and still eat a satisfying comfort food.

DAILY JOURNAL

Mood:

Energy:

Cravings:

Symptoms:

Weight:

DAY 172: Date:___/___/___

MOM - WHAT'S HAPPENING:

Around this time you will probably experience an increase in leg cramps. This is because the extra weight you are carrying puts more pressure on the veins that circulate blood in the lower half of your body. When your muscles are deprived of blood they will cramp up—this is especially true when you are lying down. As mentioned earlier, stretching your calves before bedtime can help prevent cramps that come on while you are asleep (the most common time for pregnant women to experience them). This motion improves circulation, which can help alleviate and prevent cramping.

BABY - WHAT'S HAPPENING:

Your baby's hearing continues to improve as the nerves and connectors between his ears and brain become more fully developed. Though sounds are muffled by the amniotic fluid, your baby is able to hear noises on the "outside." So, don't be shy! Sing and talk out loud to your baby while doing chores or showering.

FOOD FOR THOUGHT: Pumpkin seeds are a delicious and nutritious addition to almost any dish. These gourds-to-be are jam-packed with manganese, magnesium, phosphorus, copper, iron, vitamin K, zinc, and protein. Pumpkin seeds can be eaten as a snack, added to salads and cereals, stir-fried with vegetables, or baked into cookies. They are best when dry-roasted so as to preserve their healthy oil content. One quarter of a cup of pumpkin seeds contains approximately 186 calories, and is a excellent way to meet the additional 300 to 350 third trimester calorie boost.

DAILY JOURNAL

Mood:

Energy:

Cravings:

Symptoms:

Weight:

DAY 173: Date:___/___/___

MOM - WHAT'S HAPPENING:

It is probably hard to imagine, but by now your uterus is about the size of a basketball. Though it seems impossible, you will continue to grow beyond this size. Today, you might be noticing the fluid retention in your extremities (particularly in your hands and ankles). Now is a good time to remove your rings and store them in a safe place until after delivery. Soon, your hands will become too swollen to take them off at all, which will be uncomfortable and possibly unsafe.

BABY - WHAT'S HAPPENING:

If you could see your baby, you would see she is making movements that she will take with her after she is born. In fact, some women are lucky enough to see a gesture on an ultrasound that they will see their baby perform again weeks or months after birth, such as sucking two fingers or a thumb.

FOR YOUR HEALTH: Usually, light or spotting bleeding during the third trimester is not cause for concern. It can usually be attributed to slight injury to the sensitive cervix as a result of intercourse or medical examination. However, you should always alert your doctor if you experience any bleeding this late in your pregnancy. Sometimes it indicates something very serious is going on, such as the result of a low-lying placenta, separation of the placenta, a tear in the uterine lining, premature labor, or in some rare cases—late miscarriage.

DAILY JOURNAL

Mood:

Energy:

Cravings:

Symptoms:

Weight:

DAY 174: Date:___/___/___

MOM - WHAT'S HAPPENING:

Today you might be experiencing the excitement of regularly feeling your baby's movements. In fact, you may even be able to see a foot extending out or notice when your baby's head is pushing out to one side. This will make it easier for your partner to feel your baby's acrobatics. You will notice that your baby is more active during certain times of the day. This is a great time to "tune in" to your baby and connect with her through movement and the sound of your voice.

BABY - WHAT'S HAPPENING:

Some of your baby's movements are likely caused by hiccups. Your baby is swallowing and "breathing" amniotic fluid regularly now, which can result in hiccups. These are harmless, and your baby is probably having fun with them. You may even be able to detect hiccups after eating a particularly spicy meal. It is interesting to experiment with food, sound, and motion to see how your baby responds to different stimuli.

TIPS AND ADVICE: It is likely that both you and your partner are having mood swings. It may even feel like your good moods rarely line up. Most often, dad's moods are in response to mom's, so if you find your crankiness can trigger arguments between you, try to steer clear of your partner until your mood improves. Though you are carrying the physical burdens (and joys) of pregnancy, remember that your partner is also stressed out, concerned about the health of you and the baby, and is probably losing sleep over upcoming familial and financial responsibilities.

DAILY JOURNAL

Mood:

Energy:

Cravings:

Symptoms:

Weight:

DAY 175: Date:___/___/___

MOM - WHAT'S HAPPENING:

Around this time you will find that your once slender ankles have become trunk-like and undefined. Edema, or swelling, is normal, but if you suspect your swelling to be excessive, let your doctor know. Severe swelling is one sign of preeclampsia, pregnancy-related hypertensia disorder. Even if you are unusually swollen, though, it does not mean you have developed preeclampsia—your doctor will test for protein in your urine and check your blood pressure. If these are fine, you have nothing to worry about except elevating your legs whenever possible.

BABY - WHAT'S HAPPENING:

Your baby is approximately 14½ inches long and weighs just about 2 pounds. This means that she will need to gain between 5 and 6 pounds over the next 11 weeks in order to be of average birth weight. If your baby was born now, she would have a more than 50 percent chance of survival—though she would require intensive medical care.

FOR YOUR HEALTH: There are some causes of premature labor that you can control. One cause completely under your controllable is your exposure to first and secondhand smoke. Alcohol and drugs (including over the counter and herbal), standing for many hours in a row, regularly lifting heavy loads, infection of the gums, and being either severely under or overweight can similarly increase your risk of going into early labor. Hopefully, you have given up many of these behaviors a long time ago, and now is more critical than ever to do so.

DAILY JOURNAL

Mood:

Energy:

Cravings:

Symptoms:

Weight:

Week 26

Starting Weight: ________

OVERVIEW

From here on out, you will probably see your doctor once every two weeks instead of once a month. For many women, this change seems to accelerate the passing of time, so be sure to take a look at your to-do list and take care of any items still lingering. Make sure you are keeping track of your symptoms in this journal so you may discuss them with your doctor. As you enter the final stage of pregnancy it is critical to be aware of potential late-term complications, such as preeclampsia and preterm labor. In general, keep in contact with your doctor about any new, strange, or intensifying symptoms.

This week, action may be taken on tests you took early on in your pregnancy. For example, if you had a high-glucose reading early on, your doctor will give you the follow-up glucose tolerance test. Also, if it was discovered that you are Rh negative, you will be given an Rh immunoglobulin injection (and another one after the birth of your baby).

By the end of this week, your baby's brain will have made great strides. Studies show that brain-wave activity in fetuses this age indicates evidence of different sleep cycles—even REM sleep. This means your baby may be dreaming. It is hard to say of what since she has no exposure to images, but it is interesting to think about.

DAY 176: Date:___/___/___

MOM - WHAT'S HAPPENING:

There is a good chance you will see the return of many first trimester symptoms this week, including nausea. This is unfortunate, but temporary. Remember, you have just 10 weeks left with your little one all to yourself, so try to keep perspective if you find yourself with your head in the toilet once again. Many women are lucky enough to avoid nausea until labor and delivery—if you are among this special group, relish it and continue to eat well. Nearly all of the weight you gain from here on out will be diverted to your baby, so remember to make those calories count.

BABY - WHAT'S HAPPENING:

Your little sweet pea is now made up of approximately 2 to 3 percent body fat. She has a long way to go, though, before she is of average birth weight. With each passing day fat stores will accumulate beneath her skin. This helps give her some bulk and will also make her skin less translucent.

PREGNANCY FACT: There are many causes of preterm labor you have no control over. Those who suffer from a hormonal imbalance, incompetent cervix, premature cervical effacement, placenta previa, or an irritable uterus are all at higher risk for going into preterm labor. Unfortunately, these conditions or physical reactions cannot be known until you are actually pregnant, so do not blame yourself for developing them. The best thing you can do for you and baby is to educate yourself about premature labor. Know the signs so if you enter it, you can act.

DAILY JOURNAL

Mood:

Energy:

Cravings:

Symptoms:

Weight:

DAY 177: Date:___/___/___

MOM - WHAT'S HAPPENING:

Today you might be dragging your feet. Indeed, fatigue tends to redescend at this point in pregnancy. The reason fatigue returns in the third trimester is your body is working extra hard to carry around your excess weight. Plus, your baby is in his final stage of fetal growth and development, so most of your energy is diverted to him. Sleep troubles also contribute to overall fatigue. You probably have difficult sleeping due to midnight bathroom visits and difficulty getting comfortable. The best way to ease the effects of fatigue is to rest when you can—catch a nap during your lunch break or as soon as you get home from work.

BABY - WHAT'S HAPPENING:

Your baby has already developed her olfactory neurons, and she would actually able to detect smells if she was outside of the womb. This is all a part of the remarkable brain development underway in the third trimester.

TIPS AND ADVICE: Though you should be thinking about whether you will return to work after your baby is born, put off making your final decision until you are at home with your newborn for a few weeks. Many mothers who prematurely decided they would not return to work find they do not enjoy the confines of staying at home with baby. Still other women find they have no interest in returning to their job once they get a chance to be a mom. Maternity leave protects your employment, so it is better to see what it is like to be home with your baby before making this critical life choice.

DAILY JOURNAL

Mood:

Energy:

Cravings:

Symptoms:

Weight:

DAY 178: Date:___/___/___

MOM - WHAT'S HAPPENING:

Your blood pressure is scheduled to rise this week, bringing with it a fluttery feeling in your chest. Occasional flutters and heart skips are a result of your blood pressure re-regulating itself. These sensations are nothing to fear if they last for just a minute or two. However, should you find you are having a spell of flutters, or if they come on very often, tell your doctor.

BABY - WHAT'S HAPPENING:

If you could look into your sweet baby's eyes, you might finally be able to see some color. However, this may not be his permanent eye color. Babies with blue-tinted eye color may not have their final shade set until they are 6 months old. Also, at this point your baby is sleeping for 20- to 30-minute stretches. When not sleeping, he is becoming increasingly active. You will probably find you are most able to feel your baby's movements while lying on your left side.

PREGNANCY FACT: At this point in your pregnancy your basal metabolic rate (amount of energy expended at rest) is 20 percent higher than before you were pregnant. This will cause you to feel hot most of the time. You may even perspire constantly, especially if you are pregnant in the summer. Many women experience sweaty feet, hands, and cheeks throughout their third trimester. While feeling hot is mostly uncomfortable, it is important to stay in tune with your body temperature to prevent overheating—particularly when exercising.

DAILY JOURNAL

Mood:

Energy:

Cravings:

Symptoms:

Weight:

DAY 179: Date:___/___/___

MOM - WHAT'S HAPPENING:

Your back might be screaming in pain today. As your weight and girth increase, so too will the frequency of backaches. Sometimes the uterus is placed in such a way that it puts tremendous pressure on the sciatic nerve. This can be quite painful, and there is little you can do to completely eradicate this symptom. Avoid standing except for very short periods of time. If you must stand for long stretches, put one foot on a step or a box and switch sides often to relieve some of the pressure.

BABY - WHAT'S HAPPENING:

Your baby has developed some very useful habits. Now that she is able to open and close her eyes, she blinks often. She is also able to move her head around to "look" at her surroundings. She has also started to cough and her sucking reflex has gotten a bit stronger. These are all impressive advances, considering she exists in darkness and is unable to observe these behaviors in others.

PREGNANCY FACT: It is usually fine to continue to make love with your partner well into the third trimester (unless your doctor advises you not to). Some women find that their baby either becomes more or less active after orgasm. Some babies are lulled to sleep by the rocking motion of sex and the vibrations of orgasm. Others are stimulated by these sensations and will kick back and bob around inside the womb. It is also normal to have Braxton Hicks contractions for a few minutes after orgasm—however, if they continue and intensify, call your doctor.

DAILY JOURNAL

Mood:

Energy:

Cravings:

Symptoms:

Weight:

DAY 180: Date:___/___/___

MOM - WHAT'S HAPPENING:

Your basketball-sized uterus is not only crowding your stomach but has actually pushed it out of its normal position. This can intensify heartburn, as stomach acids are squished upward toward your slackened esophagus. There is little you can do about your crushed anatomy, so control heartburn through what you consume. Drink plenty of water and avoid foods that kick up stomach acids, such as citrus and spicy peppers. You may also take relief in antacids such as Tums.

BABY - WHAT'S HAPPENING:

Though baby still has a lot of growing to do, her lungs have developed to the point where her chance of survival would be very good if she was born today. She has become a better breather, though she is just practicing with the amniotic fluid. The important thing is that she has the motion of breathing down now, which is necessary to her survival.

TIPS AND ADVICE: Now that your prenatal visits are scheduled every two weeks, you are hopefully becoming close to your doctor's staff. Making sure the nurses and front desk people remember you and your medical story will make visits more pleasant and productive. Their memory of you can lead to increased attention, such as call backs over small concerns. Maintaining good relationships with your doctor's staff, and treating them with respect and patience, makes it more likely that they will return your call sooner.

DAILY JOURNAL

Mood:

Energy:

Cravings:

Symptoms:

Weight:

DAY 181: Date:___/___/___

MOM - WHAT'S HAPPENING:

Today you might be noticing tiny blue or red webs of veins on your cheeks, chest, arms, and neck. Indeed, the third trimester brings with it additional weight and pressure on veins that cause them to become more pronounced. These are harmless and will likely disappear shortly after you deliver your baby. Varicose veins in the form of hemorrhoids are also likely to become prominent. As mentioned earlier in this book, relief can be found in warm baths and frequent walks to increase circulation. A "sitz bath" can help, too. This is a bath in which only your hips and buttocks are soaked in water or saline solution.

BABY - WHAT'S HAPPENING:

Your baby's eyelashes and eyebrows are filled in and ready to melt your heart. Also, her hair continues to grow in utero. If she has very dark hair, it may be quite thick when she is born. These features enhance your baby's human appearance. In fact, at this point, she looks like a shorter, skinnier version of herself at birth.

FOR YOUR HEALTH: It may seem preposterous to imagine you would ever fall and land on your belly, but it happens to at least 1 out of every 7 pregnant women. This is due to relaxin-induced clumsiness as the ligaments and joints loosen. If you should ever find yourself in this position, rest assured that your pride is more injured than your baby. He is protected by layers of fat, muscle, and amniotic fluid. Still, if you are concerned, ask your doctor if you can come in for a checkup just to be on the safe side.

DAILY JOURNAL

Mood:

Energy:

Cravings:

Symptoms:

Weight:

DAY 182: Date:___/___/___

MOM - WHAT'S HAPPENING:

At this point, your breasts have gained between 1 and 3 pounds. As a result, your back is probably killing you and you may find it impossible to maintain good posture. You may also start to leak colostrums. You should not worry about "running out" before your baby is born. That will not happen. If you are leaking, purchase nursing pads to wear inside your bra. These will absorb the additional moisture. If you buy the disposable kind, discard them after a few hours of use and replace with new ones.

BABY - WHAT'S HAPPENING:

By now your little babe is between 15½ and 16 inches long and weighs just about 2½ pounds. He is tiny, thin, and wrinkled, but looking very close to how he will when he is born. His sole job over the next 10 weeks is to put on weight. All of his major organ development is complete, except for some fine-tuning. As a result, he is technically viable, or able to survive outside of the womb, with medical assistance.

FOR YOUR HEALTH: As you've learned over the course of your pregnancy, never hold in urine when you feel the urge to go. The consequences become more serious in the third trimester. Not only does holding in urine increase the likelihood of developing a urinary tract infection, but it could cause your bladder to become inflamed, which can irritate your uterus. An irritated uterus can cause contractions, which may lead to preterm labor. Thus, even if it is your 14th time in the restroom for the day, go. The risks far outweigh the inconvenience of repeated trips to the bathroom.

DAILY JOURNAL

Mood:

Energy:

Cravings:

Symptoms:

Weight:

Week 27

Starting Weight: _________

OVERVIEW

This week you can expect to feel more of the same unpleasant side effects that you experience last week. Some, such as anxiety, heartburn, and constipation, may even intensify. It is possible to ease these symptoms through diet and exercise, but most women find these symptoms are just facts of life until the baby is born. If you are losing patience with not feeling well, know that you are in the home stretch. You have just 11 weeks left to be pregnant—just think of how quickly your first 11 weeks went! Relish these last few weeks, because they will go by in a flash. Use them to reflect on your pregnancy, enjoy the feeling of the baby being inside of you, and to take care of remaining tasks that are better done before your newborn is home.

This week is big for your baby's bone development. In fact, your baby's bones will be absorbing around 250 milligrams of calcium each day. If your baby doesn't get the calcium he needs from your diet, he'll take it from your bones and teeth. Thus, you must be diligent about consuming enough calcium over the next several weeks. This means eating lots of calcium-rich foods, such as yogurt, cheese, milk, and soy products. Other nutrients to focus on for the duration of your pregnancy are folic acid, vitamin C, iron, and protein. These are all crucial for your baby's brain and skeletal development.

DAY 183: Date:___/___/___

MOM - WHAT'S HAPPENING:

Unfortunately, you might be experiencing constipation again today. This will cause you a variety of abdominal discomforts, such as difficulty passing stools; passing hard, painful stools; gas; bloating; or not being able to defecate at all. For relief, drink between 80 and 96 ounces of water every day. Eat high-fiber foods, such as whole grain breads, products with bran, prunes, and other fresh fruits and vegetables. Finally, exercise for at least 20 to 30 minutes every day. If these suggestions don't work for you, speak to your doctor about taking stool softeners such as Colace or Metamucil.

BABY - WHAT'S HAPPENING:

Your baby's head is growing bigger in order to accommodate her enlarging brain. Brain development this week includes your baby's growing ability to regulate her own temperature. Her brain has not completely mastered this skill, however. Because the climate in which she resides is perfectly temperate at all times, there has not been a real challenge to her body temperature yet.

PREGNANCY FACT: Scottish doctor James Young Simpson was the first person to use anesthesia on a woman during labor on January 19, 1847. His method was simple—he poured ether on a cloth and covered the woman's nose until she fell asleep. This was highly controversial. People considered medicating laboring women an act against God, as women were supposed to suffer through childbirth to atone for the sins of Eve. Dr. Simpson kept at it, though, and switched from ether to chloroform, which was used by Queen Victoria when she had her son, Leopold in 1853.

DAILY JOURNAL

Mood:

Energy:

Cravings:

Symptoms:

Weight:

DAY 184: Date:___/___/___

MOM - WHAT'S HAPPENING:

Your growing baby, squished organs, gas, bloating, constipation, and your overall weight gain can make you feel, on some days, less like a woman and more like an elephant. Indeed, many women have trouble adjusting to their new size and underestimate how big they are when maneuvering through crowds, turnstiles, and other tight spaces. Don't be embarrassed if you get stuck in a turnstile or knock an item off a shelf with your belly—laughing it off will prevent you from feeling badly about yourself.

BABY - WHAT'S HAPPENING:

At this point, your baby's own bone marrow has taken over red blood cell production. This is a very important step in his development, because red blood cells are responsible for circulating oxygen throughout his body and for removing carbon monoxide from his blood. When your baby is a grown up, his bone marrow will produce 2 million red blood cells every second!

TIPS AND ADVICE: Now is the perfect time to think about your labor and delivery preferences. Discuss what you absolutely will not allow—such as your obnoxious brother-in-law recording the birth—and what you must have—an epidural or other pain medication. These and other preferences are your birth plan and should be written down. Make a copy for your doctor, the hospital, and put one in your hospital bag. Of course, this is just an outline for how you want things to go. It is entirely possible you will change your mind about the epidural on delivery day, so it is important to be flexible.

DAILY JOURNAL

Mood:

Energy:

Cravings:

Symptoms:

Weight:

DAY 185: Date:___/___/___

MOM - WHAT'S HAPPENING:

Today you may have more trouble than ever with urinary incontinence. This is due to pressure on your bladder from the baby and your oversized uterus. Incontinence affects most pregnant women, and the best two ways to handle this unfortunate side effect is to wear panty liners and practice your Kegel exercises. These can strengthen your bladder and will facilitate its return to normal functioning after you give birth.

BABY - WHAT'S HAPPENING:

Your baby's increasing size makes her living space smaller than it used to be. As a result, you will notice her movements have changed. Up to now her movements have felt big and sweeping. Now, however, she is running out of room. Her motions may consequently feel like little jabs and pokes. These are from elbows, hands, and feet. You may even catch her pushing outward on your belly; some women are able to see the outline of their baby's hand.

PREGNANCY FACT: In the 1950s and 1960s, it became popular for women to refuse pain medication during delivery. In those days, women were completely unconscious for the birth of their baby and missed out on the experience of bringing their child into the world. This also caused babies to be born drugged and unable to breathe immediately on their own. Thus, the natural childbirth movement became a popular alternative to the medicated birth. In the 21st century, however, epidurals have increased in popularity since women can actively participate in labor and delivery without feeling pain.

DAILY JOURNAL

Mood:

Energy:

Cravings:

Symptoms:

Weight:

DAY 186: Date:___/___/___

MOM - WHAT'S HAPPENING:

Your expanding belly is probably starting to feel tight and itchy. This is because as your skin stretches, it dries out. This has likely been an ongoing problem for you if you were very thin when you became pregnant. If you were heavier, this may be the first week you are experiencing this. Either way, avoid scratching. Instead, soothe your skin with aloe or lotions with cocoa butter or oatmeal. Take lukewarm baths and use a humidifier when you sleep. Hydrate your skin from the inside by consuming foods rich in vitamin E, such as avocados.

BABY - WHAT'S HAPPENING:

Your baby's head should be in proportion to his body at this point, though soon it will grow larger and appear to dwarf his body. In fact, it will take several months after your baby is born for him to develop the necessary neck-muscle strength to be able to hold his head up on his own.

FOOD FOR THOUGHT: One way to eat a healthy diet is to eat seasonally, meaning to eat foods that are in season in your region. Seasonal foods are fresh and on your table with little time to lose their nutritional value. They need not be preserved for travel, either. Winter squash is an excellent seasonal staple for women who are pregnant from August through March. It is packed with vitamin A, vitamin C, potassium, fiber, as well as folate and omega-3 fatty acids. Winter squash is versatile and can be added to soups, pastas, or baked and stuffed with couscous and raisins.

DAILY JOURNAL

Mood:

Energy:

Cravings:

Symptoms:

Weight:

DAY 187: Date:___/___/___

MOM - WHAT'S HAPPENING:

Today it might not be your back but rather your muscles giving you trouble. This is another side effect imposed by all the extra weight you are carrying. Also, your muscles must shift around with the rest of your body as your hips and rib cage expand. This pulls and stretches them, causing them to feel sore and weak. The best thing you can do for aching muscles is to stretch regularly and rest when you are feeling particularly exhausted.

BABY - WHAT'S HAPPENING:

Your baby's senses are becoming more refined, and she is able to detect light that filters in through your womb and react to it. She may look toward or away from it, but she definitely notices it. Also, her brain has gotten a handle on her breathing and if she was born today, she would have an excellent chance at survival—though she would certainly require several weeks of neonatal intensive care.

FOR YOUR HEALTH: Though you should always check with your doctor or midwife, there are a few herbs that are considered "likely safe" by the FDA. One is red raspberry leaf, which is rich in iron and found in most pregnancy teas. Peppermint leaf and ginger root are useful for relieving nausea and can also be ingested as a tea or added to your meals. Slippery elm bark has been shown to relieve heartburn when added to food and can also reduce nausea. Finally, calcium-rich oat straw is linked to calming restlessness and anxiety.

DAILY JOURNAL

Mood:

Energy:

Cravings:

Symptoms:

Weight:

DAY 188: Date:___/___/___

MOM - WHAT'S HAPPENING:

Your fundus is just about 3 inches above your navel. You may think you can't possible get any bigger—but you can, and you will. Remember, most of the weight that you gain from now until delivery is diverted to the placenta and to your baby. You may notice a slight drop in your appetite as nausea returns and heartburn increases. Keep your calorie intake up, because your baby is doing major growing and is counting on you to provide the necessary fat stores she needs to be strong and healthy for her birthday.

BABY - WHAT'S HAPPENING:

Your baby is accumulating white fat now, which is necessary for providing him with the energy he needs to kick, elbow, and push his way around inside your uterus. This is different from the brown fat he developed previously. Brown fat's job is to help your baby regulate his body temperature. The white fat that your baby is currently developing is the same kind of fat that you have beneath your skin.

FOR YOUR HEALTH: If you are carrying twins, triplets, or other sets of multiples, the American College of Obstetricians and Gynecologists (ACOG) recommends that you avoid aerobic exercises and any activity that requires you to lie flat on your back. This does not mean you have to be couch-bound, unless you are on bed rest. Walking, swimming, and other non-weight-bearing exercises are considered safe for women carrying multiples. However, call your doctor if you experience contractions, pelvic pressure, vaginal bleeding, or sudden and excessive swelling.

DAILY JOURNAL

Mood:

Energy:

Cravings:

Symptoms:

Weight:

DAY 189: Date:___/___/___

MOM - WHAT'S HAPPENING:

Today is a good day to start doing kick counts if you haven't already. Kick counts are when you keep track of the number of movements you feel your baby make per hour. You should notice at least 10 movements each hour, but will likely feel many more. These include kicks, nudges, flutters, tugs, and pushes. If you ever don't feel your baby moving at all, call your doctor so he can bring you in for the Doppler and an ultrasound. Sometimes, baby is simply napping and your doctor can ease your mind with a quick examination.

BABY - WHAT'S HAPPENING:

At the end of this week your baby should be between 16 and 17 inches long and weighs close to 3 pounds. He probably won't get too much taller—after all, the average length of babies born in the United States is between 19 and 20 inches. Thus, from now until he is born, your baby's main growth will be in weight. He will double or maybe even triple his weight over the next 9 weeks or so.

PREGNANCY FACT: The rate of teen pregnancy in the United States is higher than that of any other Western country. In fact, though pregnancy among underage girls is on the decline, every year 1 million U.S. teenage girls get pregnant and most are younger than 17 years old. Of those girls who become pregnant, approximately one-third will have abortions. Another third of the pregnancies will end in miscarriage. There are many theories for why teen girls have such a high miscarriage rate, which include poor nutrition and the intense stress of their situation.

DAILY JOURNAL

Mood:

Energy:

Cravings:

Symptoms:

Weight:

Week 28

Starting Weight: ________

OVERVIEW

With 10 weeks left to go you might be craving a good night's sleep, which probably eludes you more and more. This is mostly due to an inability to get comfortable in bed. If you haven't already picked one up, purchase a body pillow. They give your belly a ledge on which to rest and are long enough to be inserted between your knees. Both of these can help with lower back strain, allowing you to drift comfortably off to sleep. Another reason many women have difficulty sleeping at this point in pregnancy is because of intense heartburn and indigestion. To prevent digestive issues from interrupting your sleep, wait at least an hour after eating before you lie down. Also, sleeping in a recliner chair can be more comfortable than bed, since you are not entirely lying down (which helps stomach acids from flowing upward). Give it a shot the next time your heartburn is on the rise.

Meanwhile, your baby is starting to shed the lanugo that kept him warm all these months. Now that he has accumulated enough fat and his brain has taken over his thermostat, there is no need for his fuzzy covering. Many babies will still have some of this fine, downy hair when they are born, as not all of it is shed in utero.

DAY 190: Date:___/___/___

MOM - WHAT'S HAPPENING:

Today you may be experiencing mood swings similar to those you had during the first trimester. This is one of the many ways in which the first and third trimesters are alike for mom. Exercise helps temper your mood, so even when you don't feel like it, be sure to get in at least 30 minutes of walking in each day. When you start out you may feel like snapping at everyone you see, but by the end of the walk you'll feel better and will likely be in a more reasonable state for dealing with others.

BABY - WHAT'S HAPPENING:

Around now, your baby's permanent teeth have developed inside his gums behind the milk teeth. They will be ready to sprout once he starts losing his baby teeth. In addition, your baby continues to develop features that make him look more like he will when he is born. For example, today, his skin is in the process of smoothing out, as increased fat causes it to stretch and tighten.

PREGNANCY FACT: Epidurals are the most popular childbirth pain reliever used for both vaginal and Cesarean births. The popularity stems from an epidural's ability to keep mom awake during delivery, since the epidural causes only localized numbness. This means that mom is numb from her chest through her feet and does not feel any pain associated with the delivery of her baby. There is some risk for a drop in blood pressure but doctors are prepared to handle it. If you choose to have an epidural, be prepared for some side effects as it wears off, such as itching and shivering.

DAILY JOURNAL

Mood:

Energy:

Cravings:

Symptoms:

Weight:

DAY 191: Date:___/___/___

MOM - WHAT'S HAPPENING:

This is a good time to start investigating pain-relief options for when you deliver your baby. Unless an emergency develops while you are in labor, you should be able to select in advance whether you want childbirth medication and which kind is most agreeable to you. The most common pain relievers used by doctors include the epidural block, analgesics, and some narcotics. You will learn more about each option in the material yet to come in this book.

BABY - WHAT'S HAPPENING:

Approximately 9 out of 10 babies who are born at this point will survive with medical assistance. So, though you want to keep your little one on the inside for as long as possible, it is not the end of the world if you go into labor now. At this point your baby's head is approximately 3½ inches around and will continue to grow to around 10 centimeters in diameter—possible slightly larger—which may cause a vaginal delivery to be difficult.

FOR YOUR HEALTH: If you have complications with your pregnancy, or have certain preexisting medical conditions, your doctor may order a non-stress test at each of your appointments. This test is easy and painless. You will sit in a recliner while hooked up to an external device that monitors the baby's heartbeat. Your doctor then checks to make sure that your baby's heart rate increases with activity (when he kicks or moves) and goes down when he is less active. You may be asked to drink a glass of orange juice just before the test, because the sugar will make your baby more active.

DAILY JOURNAL

Mood:

Energy:

Cravings:

Symptoms:

Weight:

DAY 192: Date:___/___/___

MOM - WHAT'S HAPPENING:

You may find you have become even more of a klutz than in previous weeks as your center of gravity continues to shift. To compensate for this sensation, many women perfect the "pregnancy waddle." This is when you walk with your feet facing out in opposite directions. This can help steady you as you maneuver through your daily routine. Also, be sure to wear supportive shoes at this point. As you become clumsier, it is definitely to your benefit to sacrifice style for safety.

BABY - WHAT'S HAPPENING:

The umbilical cord has become thick, tough, and very efficient at doing its job. It is literally your baby's lifeline as it connects him to the placenta. All of his nourishment travels through the umbilical cord after being filtered through the placenta. Your baby is starting to store up calcium for his hardening bones, iron for his red blood cell production, and phosphorous, which is essential for all living cells, including your baby's teeth.

PREGNANCY FACT: A common analgesic given during labor is Demerol. This strong pain reliever can be administered through an IV or given as a single shot in a woman's rear. It can be given every two to four hours, with the last dose given two to three hours before delivery. Demerol can help with anxiety and also to regulate contractions. However, it may cause mom to feel sick, depressed, and lower her blood pressure. Demerol can also cause baby to be born drowsy and unable to suck if given too close to delivery.

DAILY JOURNAL

Mood:

Energy:

Cravings:

Symptoms:

Weight:

DAY 193: Date:___/___/___

MOM - WHAT'S HAPPENING:

As you get closer to delivery, your breasts may once again be tender to the touch. This is because the milk ducts are expanding and filling with milk so your body is ready to feed your baby immediately upon delivery. This feeling of fullness will increase during the first week after your baby is born, so get used to the sensation now. You can buy nursing bras now, as they will be more comfortable than your regular bras. Keep in mind that you will go up another bra size (maybe two!) once your milk comes in, so you may want to wait or only buy one for now.

BABY - WHAT'S HAPPENING:

Your baby's smooth brain is starting to wrinkle with grooves and indentations. These hills and valleys allow for more area of brain tissue to develop beneath your little one's skull. There are two areas in your baby's skull that will remain soft after he is born. These are called the fontanels and allow for continued brain growth after he is born.

PREGNANCY FACT: In some cases your doctor will recommend you have a spinal block if you are having a Cesarean birth. The spinal block is administered while mom lies on her side. A needle is inserted into the spinal fluid just before surgery. Many women experience nausea and even vomiting but anti-nausea medication can be given for relief. Similar to with the epidural, there is a risk for a drop in blood pressure, though you will be closely monitored. With the spinal block, mom will be required to lie flat on her back for about eight hours after delivery.

DAILY JOURNAL

Mood:

Energy:

Cravings:

Symptoms:

Weight:

DAY 194: Date:___/___/___

MOM - WHAT'S HAPPENING:

At this point in your pregnancy, your difficulty sleeping may turn into full-fledged insomnia. If you consistently have trouble falling asleep, wake up frequently, and feel exhausted all day long, then you may be suffering from insomnia. Try a variety of sleeping positions, since pregnancy-related insomnia is usually due to comfort issues. If this doesn't work, don't force yourself to stay in bed. Watch TV or read a book for half an hour, then try again. If anxiety is what is keeping you up at night, consider seeing a therapist and get in a good dose of exercise each day. If none of these help, speak to your doctor. He may be able to prescribe a mild sedative.

BABY - WHAT'S HAPPENING:

Your baby is doing more gaining today. She will gain about ½ pound each week until she is born. This number varies based on genetics and your diet, but this is the average rate at which fetuses gain weight during the third trimester.

FOR YOUR HEALTH: In some cases if mom's anxiety is through the roof during labor, the doctor will suggest using a tranquilizer, such as Vistaril or Phenergan. These are often used in conjunction with Demerol, as tranquilizers can enhance the effectiveness of analgesics. Like analgesics, tranquilizers are given once the doctor is sure that mom is well into her labor, but not too close to delivery. Doses vary, but small doses can take the edge off of severe anxiety without causing other impairments.

DAILY JOURNAL

Mood:

Energy:

Cravings:

Symptoms:

Weight:

DAY 195: Date:___/___/___

MOM - WHAT'S HAPPENING:

Your heart is pumping 20 percent faster than before you became pregnant, because your circulatory system has expanded to make room for extra blood. Most of this has already occurred by the second trimester but some continued circulatory system growth occurs during the third, adding to your fatigue today. This extra blood flow may also cause you to wake up to a swollen face and eyelids, because fluid pools in your face while you sleep. You can reduce swelling by using cold compresses and staying hydrated.

BABY - WHAT'S HAPPENING:

Today there are approximately 1½ pints of amniotic fluid around your baby. This amount will decrease as he takes up more space inside your uterus. At this point, he is urinating frequently and is capable of producing tears—though he probably will not cry while in utero. His vision is such that he can only see objects very close to his eyes. This will remain true after he is born.

FOR YOUR HEALTH: During emergencies when the mother's life or the life of the baby is at risk, the doctor will opt to use general anesthesia during a Cesarean delivery. General anesthesia will put mom completely out. As such, it is used only in extreme cases where there is no time to utilize other pain relief options for surgical delivery. Doctors will not choose this option unless absolutely necessary, because the fetus will also be sedated, which can cause respiratory troubles and depress the baby's urge to suck and feed after birth.

DAILY JOURNAL

Mood:

Energy:

Cravings:

Symptoms:

Weight:

DAY 196: Date:___/___/___

MOM - WHAT'S HAPPENING:

Your diaphragm is likely on the move today. In fact, by the time you are ready to deliver your baby, your diaphragm will have moved about 1½ inches from its normal position. The pressure on your diaphragm can make it hard to breathe. Though this is scary, rest assured that you are, in fact, getting enough oxygen for both you and your baby. The pregnancy hormone progesterone tells your brain to make your lungs breathe more deeply, which means that you are taking in more air per breath now than before you were pregnant.

BABY - WHAT'S HAPPENING:

Your baby's finger and toenails are growing, though they will remain thin and soft for the first few months after she is born. You will find her nails are surprisingly sharp for how thin they are, and you will need to trim them frequently after she is born to prevent her from scratching herself.

PREGNANCY FACT: Some women choose to forego drug interventions during labor and delivery and opt, instead, for alternative methods of pain relief. Such options include hypnosis, which causes you to become extremely relaxed, but focused. Hypnosis guides your mind, giving it control over pain. Another popular method for pain control is acupuncture. Needles are placed in key areas on the skin by a professional. Both methods are more readily available in birthing centers than in hospitals—though it is possible to bring a practitioner in with you with clearance from your doctor.

DAILY JOURNAL

Mood:

Energy:

Cravings:

Symptoms:

Weight:

Lunar Month

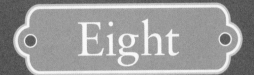

Eight

PHOTO

Place a photo of you during your eighth month here

My Monthly Update

Waist Measurement: ____________________

Weight: ____________________

Mood: ____________________

PREGNANCY CHECKLIST

- ❑ You may have trouble sleeping, so find ways to get more comfortable. Try putting several pillows under your head.
- ❑ Take it slow — you may have shortness of breath as the baby crowds your lungs
- ❑ Eat 5 or 6 smaller meals during the day to relieve pressure from the baby crowding your stomach
- ❑ Visit your health care provider every 2 weeks for prenatal care checkups
- ❑ Expecting a boy? Study up on circumcision and make sure you and your partner are on the same page
- ❑ Pack your hospital bag and keep it handy
- ❑ Arrange your ride to the hospital
- ❑ Buy your diaper bag, and stock up on diapering essentials
- ❑ Buy a high chair
- ❑ Attend your childbirth class
- ❑ Have your partner check to see if he's eligible for paternity leave
- ❑ Put together a family first aid kit
- ❑ Buy a nursing bra
- ❑ Shop for and learn how to install a car seat
- ❑ Attend your baby shower and write thank you notes now — you won't have time or energy later!
- ❑ Determine how you will share the news of the birth of your baby — by email or phone tree

MY PERSONAL CHECKLIST:

- ❑ ....
- ❑ ....

MY HOPES FOR THIS MONTH:

....

Lunar Month Eight

Third Trimester

WELCOME TO THE EIGHTH GESTATIONAL MONTH of your pregnancy! If you have been miserable for most of your pregnancy, take comfort in the idea that you can see the light at the end of the tunnel. On the other hand, if you have loved being pregnant, be sure to savor the remaining moments of your pregnancy, as they will go quickly. Or, with just nine weeks to go, you may find that your emotions are all over the map. You may feel elated one minute and crippled by anxiety the next. The important thing to remember is that you are not alone! According to the U.S. Census Bureau, one baby is born in the United States every eight seconds. That means you have lots of pregnant comrades out there going through exactly the same changes, worries, fears, and joys that you are.

WHAT TO EXPECT THIS MONTH

This month you can expect to experience many physical changes. Most of these changes are more of the same of what has already been happening, but they will intensify as you and your baby get bigger. In fact, by the end of this month your uterus will be about the size of a watermelon! Your baby will take up most of that space, and the tight squeeze will change the quality of his movements. Your baby will make movements that feel like pushes or nudges, though he may surprise you now and then with a kick or punch that you can actually see from the outside. You may even be able to feel where your baby's head and buttocks are if you press the right areas. If you are especially curious, ask your doctor to explain your baby's position, because she will be able to tell by either ultrasound or physical exam.

THINGS TO CONSIDER

You should start and finish your childbirth classes this month. Encourage your partner to attend the classes with you. Make a list of questions you want to ask the childbirth educator. In addition to questions, you will also want to take snacks, water, two pillows, a blanket, a notebook and a pen to each class. Consider opening up to the group if you are having a difficult pregnancy—you will be surprised at how many other women in your class can identify with you. Hopefully, your partner will be able to talk to some of the other dads as well. This type of camaraderie is important for parents-to-be, because it is very easy to become insular and isolated in this experience. Bonding with other expectant couples is a great way to make connections with others and to feel less alone. Who knows—maybe you will hit it off with another couple and your babies will be in a play group together! At the very least, you are likely to run into some of these people at the hospital when you have your baby and be able to compare stories.

TIPS FOR COPING

First trimester symptoms tend to return with a vengeance in the third trimester. If you were lucky enough to experience the honeymoon period at any time during the second trimester, this may be a particularly rough letdown. However, if you have been feeling awful throughout your pregnancy, then third trimester woes will simply be more of the same. Many women reach a point where they can't wait until pregnancy is over. This is mostly due to the discomfort of such excessive weight gain. To be clear—the weight you've gained is not excessive for pregnancy but for your frame and what you are used to it can feel like an awful burden after awhile.

The following suggestions will help get you through these next nine weeks. They all have something to do with keeping focused on what it is all been for—your baby. When you feel defeated by your symptoms, take a deep breath and do one of the following: Start a pregnancy scrapbook where you chronicle your feelings, keep track of symptoms, paste newspaper clippings of current events, and write notes to your baby. Buy some baby clothes. Spend time in the nursery and imagine sitting with your sleeping baby in your arms. All of these help you maintain perspective and cherish these last quiet weeks where you have your baby all to yourself.

WHAT TO EAT

If you have been eating a healthy and well-balanced diet—keep it up! You should be consuming an additional 300 to 350 calories a day. These calories should include vitamin C, folic acid, and healthy fats. In addition, there are specific nutrients you should focus on during the third trimester. Your baby is in the midst of a major growth spurt and must absorb 200 milligrams of calcium daily. He needs this for skeletal development. To support both you and your baby's needs, consume 1,000 milligrams of calcium from a variety of foods, such as milk, cheese, yogurt, tofu, and fortified orange juice.

Iron is another very important nutrient this month for the placenta as well as for your baby's bone marrow, which has completely taken over the production of his red blood cells. You will recall from your own body changes that iron is necessary for red blood cell production. So, be sure to ingest the necessary 27 milligrams each day by eating iron-rich foods, such as pumpkin seeds, fortified cereals, liver, beans, lentils, and potatoes with the skin. You must also make sure your protein intake reaches 71 grams daily. Many of the foods already mentioned will meet this need—lean meats, beans, tofu, and low-fat dairy products are all good sources of protein, as are nuts and eggs.

HOW MUCH WEIGHT TO GAIN

By now, you have probably gained between 21 and 27 pounds. You will continue to gain between ½ and 1 pound per week until you deliver your baby. This rate will keep you on track for normal weight gain. If you are gaining more or less, this could be attributed to your unique metabolism, exercise level, and diet. Notify your doctor immediately if you have a sudden jump in weight gain. This could indicate you are retaining excessive amounts of fluid due to pregnancy-induced hypertension or preeclampsia, which need immediate evaluation and intervention.

EXERCISE TIPS AND ADVICE

When it comes to exercise, the best advice is to listen to your own body. Your ligaments, joints, and muscles are loosening in preparation for the birth, and your center of gravity is not what it used to be. You have also put on a considerable amount of weight in a relatively short amount of time. Take all of these facts into consideration when you evaluate the best exercise routine for yourself. Some forms of exercise are safe bets throughout pregnancy, such as walking, swimming, and prenatal yoga. However, some women find they are able to continue to jog or do aerobics if they were extremely physically active before becoming pregnant. Whatever exercise you choose, be sure to do something active for at least 30 minutes each day and stop immediately if you experience painful contractions, bleeding, or become overheated and light-headed.

POTENTIAL SYMPTOMS AND HOW TO ALLEVIATE THEM

As mentioned earlier, the third trimester mimics the first in many ways when it comes to potential symptoms. The standards include heartburn, constipation, nausea, sleeplessness, back pain (lower and upper), breast tenderness with potential leakage, mood swings, vaginal secretions, hemorrhoids, and edema. There is little to be done to eliminate any of these symptoms, but you can manage them the same way you have been over the past eight months as they've come and gone. If any of these is unmanageable, however, be sure to let your doctor know. In extreme cases of nausea or heartburn, medical intervention may become your only option for relief.

WAYS OTHERS CAN HELP

This is the time for partners to really dig in and get involved in the pregnancy. Dad, be sure to go to as many doctors appointments with mom as possible. Try and schedule these appointments during lunch breaks or days off so dad is available to go. Also, partners should attend childbirth classes. This is where you will learn how to be a coach and what to expect during labor. For example, some women want to be massaged, while others cannot stand to be touched. This is something you want to learn about your partner now. This month is also when you want to make arrangements with family or friends to take care of older children and pets while you are in the hospital. You may also want to have a cooking party where you invite friends over to cook dishes that freeze well so you don't have to worry about what to eat once you bring baby home.

"There is only one pretty child in the world, and every mother has it."
~ Chinese Proverb

Week 29

Starting Weight: _________

OVERVIEW

This week you can expect an increase in Braxton Hicks contractions. These do not hurt and last between 30 and 60 seconds. They should come at irregular intervals and be relatively infrequent. Of course, if you have regular, painful contractions that stretch out longer and get closer together, call your doctor, as this can indicate you've gone into preterm labor. Even if you are only experiencing Braxton Hicks, you should let your doctor know. You are probably seeing your doctor every 2 weeks at this point. If this happens to be the week for your prenatal appointment, you can expect to have the usual checkup, which includes having your weight and blood pressure checked. Your doctor will also perform an external examination where she feels for the position of the baby. Your doctor will also measure the height of your fundus and ask you to do kick counts daily until you go into labor.

Your baby's length-wise growth will slow down this week, but he will continue to put on weight relatively rapidly. Accumulating white fat cells will make your baby's reddish color tone down to a healthy pink. This is because fat helps prevent a baby's skin from being translucent, thus you can no longer clearly see his blood cells. This is also another major week for your baby's brain development—his brain will create billions of new cells and he will become more aware of the sights, sounds, and flavors that surround him.

DAY 197: Date:___/___/___

MOM - WHAT'S HAPPENING:

Today, your uterus is approximately 4½ inches above your belly button. This means your uterus is really stretching out, which can cause your abdomen to be achy most of the time. As you recall, this round ligament pain occurs as the ligaments that connect to the uterus stretch to accommodate its growth. Though you cannot do much about the achy feeling, you can avoid the stabbing pain that accompanies rising too quickly from a seated or lying down position by being mindful of your movements.

BABY - WHAT'S HAPPENING:

Your baby's reproductive system is still developing. If you are having a girl her clitoris is clearly visible, though her labia are not yet large enough to cover it. If you are having a boy his testicles are continuing their descent into his scrotum. All major organs are formed, and the last to mature are the lungs. Your baby continues to practice breathing amniotic fluid.

FOOD FOR THOUGHT: Many pregnant women wonder if their cravings or aversions are the body's way of making sure they get the nutrition they need. In some cases, this seems to make sense—aversions to coffee, alcohol, and cigarettes, for example, certainly keep your pregnant body protected. Most of the time, however, it is simply a case of preference. For example, our taste buds can only detect four flavors: salty, sweet, sour, and bitter. Thus, if you are craving ice cream it is not because your body has detected low blood sugar, but rather you are in the mood for something sweet.

DAILY JOURNAL

Mood:

Energy:

Cravings:

Symptoms:

Weight:

DAY 198: Date:___/___/___

MOM - WHAT'S HAPPENING:

Now is an excellent time to choose your pediatrician. You have enough time to ask around, set up appointments, and meet a few of the doctors before you deliver your baby. If this is your first baby, you may feel like a fish out of water, but pediatricians are used to expectant parents interviewing them before making a decision. Know that the doctor you select may not be the doctor who tends to your baby in the hospital. This is typical, and you will be able to see the pediatrician you selected a few days after you are discharged.

BABY - WHAT'S HAPPENING:

The nerve cells in your baby's brain are starting to fire up and become active. In fact, this week, she is developing billions more nerve cells in her brain and all five of her senses are developed and ready to taste, touch, smell, see, and hear the world outside. In utero, she is able to practice four out of her five senses, with smell being impossible without air, of course.

TIPS AND ADVICE: At this point you may want to turn a deaf ear to those who want to share birth experiences with you. For some unknown reason, people gravitate toward sharing horror stories, and this is the last thing you need right now. Make sure to surround yourself with only positive people who want to say encouraging things. Hearing how your friend's cousin labored for 25 hours and ended up with a Cesarean anyway is not beneficial to you. Surround yourself with people who can share positive birth stories, or seek them out in online communities.

DAILY JOURNAL

Mood:

Energy:

Cravings:

Symptoms:

Weight:

DAY 199: Date:___/___/___

MOM - WHAT'S HAPPENING:

Many women experience urinary incontinence around this time, while others have been dealing with it for months now. If this bothersome side effect is just starting for you it is because your expanding uterus is putting pressure on your bladder. Therefore, when you laugh, sneeze, or cough, you are unable to contain fluid that has collected in your bladder. Also, hormones cause your ureters to relax, This slows the flow of urine, putting you at risk for developing a urinary tract infection (UTI). If it burns when you urinate or if you develop a fever that is accompanied by lower abdominal pain, tell your doctor. Left untreated, UTIs can lead to preterm labor.

BABY - WHAT'S HAPPENING:

It is possible that you will notice your baby jump when there is a loud noise near you. You may also find that your baby is most active when you are listening to music. She may even become receptive to a particular genre!

FOR YOUR HEALTH: The condition known as pruritic urticarial papules and plaques of pregnancy (PUPP) affects approximately 1 out of every 150 pregnant women. PUPP is evident when itching on the abdomen becomes severe and is accompanied by a raised, red rash. There doesn't seem to be one particular cause of PUPP, but it starts on the abdomen and spreads to the hips, buttocks, and upper thighs. It is important to see your doctor if you develop an itchy rash, because there can be several causes, including PUPP, and all must be treated with prescribed medication.

DAILY JOURNAL

Mood:

Energy:

Cravings:

Symptoms:

Weight:

DAY 200: Date:___/___/___

MOM - WHAT'S HAPPENING:

It may seem like your job in the third trimester is to watch for problems and manage symptoms. Though this is true for the most part, there are many pleasant aspects as well. As mentioned earlier, it is likely that your hair and nails have never looked thicker or better. It is also likely that by now you are not breaking out as often and consistently shine with pregnancy glow. When you have sex, it is a much more intense experience, because all of your nerve endings are filled with extra blood and, therefore, much more sensitive. You have also been without PMS or menstrual cramps for eight months! These are all things to celebrate.

BABY - WHAT'S HAPPENING:

Your baby's irises have matured to the point where they will dilate and contract in response to light that filters into your uterus. It may seem impossible to imagine that light makes it in there, but some does, especially through your lower abdomen.

FOR YOUR HEALTH: If any of the following occur, call your doctor immediately as something may be seriously wrong: vaginal bleeding, frequent and painful contractions, severe headache that is accompanied by vomiting and vision problems, severe abdominal pain, leg cramps that are accompanied by redness and excessive swelling, vomiting with fever, fever of more than 102 degrees, broken water, and fainting. Also, if you are in pain of any kind that cannot easily be explained, or if you have not felt your baby move for awhile, you should also call your doctor immediately.

DAILY JOURNAL

Mood:

Energy:

Cravings:

Symptoms:

Weight:

DAY 201: Date:___/___/___

MOM - WHAT'S HAPPENING:

You have been pregnant for 201 days! Take a moment to consider that you have just 65 days left in your pregnancy if you carry your baby full-term. You've come a long way, and are now a regular pro at managing symptoms and taking the good with the bad. However, if you are depressed, let your doctor know. Depression can cause problems for you during labor and delivery, and may indicate that you are a candidate for postpartum depression, which requires close monitoring.

BABY - WHAT'S HAPPENING:

By now it is possible that your baby's fingernails have grown long enough that they reach the end of his nail beds. Earlier it was mentioned that a baby would not be able to scratch himself while in utero because the fluid would keep his nails very soft. However, though it is not particularly common, it can happen if your baby's nails are uncommonly long or sharp.

TIPS AND ADVICE: You may experience pain in your ribs at this point. This is because your rib cage has to expand outward to make room for your extra lung capacity, enlarging uterus, and shifting organs. Compounding this is the fact that your baby is running out of room, and so his legs and feet are jammed up inside your rib cage. To get your baby to shift positions, try getting on all fours and doing the cat/cow stretch where you raise your head and drop your middle. This can encourage your baby to shift and find less painful stomping grounds.

DAILY JOURNAL

Mood:

Energy:

Cravings:

Symptoms:

Weight:

DAY 202: Date:___/___/___

MOM - WHAT'S HAPPENING:

It is normal at this point to notice an increase in sinus-related problems. Allergies, post-nasal drip, and a constantly running nose are all par for the course. You will remember that this occurs because pregnancy hormones cause your mucus membranes to swell, which causes irritation in your sinuses. Even though post-nasal drip may be contributing to your nausea and have you feeling miserable, ask your doctor before taking any allergy medications.

BABY - WHAT'S HAPPENING:

Your baby is behaving as he will when he is born. He has sleeping and waking patterns and makes faces and movements in response to stimuli. He can often be caught sucking his thumb, which is great practice for nursing or bottle feeding. In fact, some babies are born with tiny calluses on their thumb or fingers from such constant sucking. The fingers that baby sucks in utero are the very same he will choose to pacify himself with in the weeks after he is born.

FOR YOUR HEALTH: Rectal bleeding can be a relatively common problem during the third trimester. It is usually caused by hemorrhoids, but in some cases it happens as a result of anal fissures (tearing). Anal fissures are tiny cracks or tears in the anus that can cause bleeding. Anal fissures are usually caused by constipation. You can prevent this painful and messy pregnancy symptom by eating a high-fiber diet, drinking plenty of water, and exercising.

DAILY JOURNAL

Mood:

Energy:

Cravings:

Symptoms:

Weight:

DAY 203: Date:___/___/___

MOM - WHAT'S HAPPENING:

As your 29th lunar week of pregnancy comes to a close, your head is likely swimming with images of what it will be like to hold your baby for the first time. Just as that lovely image sets in, you suffer a twinge in your back that pulls you out of your warm, fuzzy fantasy. Unfortunately, back pain is the number one complaint of pregnant women in the third trimester. This is because it only gets worse, not better. Therefore it is very important that you rest whenever possible, put your feet up often, and spend some quality time with a heating pad. You may even want to schedule weekly prenatal massages or ask your partner to give you a good rub down each night. You deserve it, so don't hesitate to ask.

BABY - WHAT'S HAPPENING:

Your baby weighs between 3½ and 4 pounds by now, and still hovering just around 17 inches long. This means your baby is forced into the fetal position and is unable to stretch out.

PREGNANCY FACT: A developing fetus's calcium needs are greatest during the final 12 weeks of pregnancy. This is when the baby's bones ossify, or harden, into the skeletal frame he will be born with. A human baby has 350 bones that make up his skeleton. This is interesting to note, because the human adult has just 206 bones—more than half of which are in the hands and feet. How can this be? Well, as babies bodies grow and mature, many of their bones fuse together, which reduces the number of separate bones.

DAILY JOURNAL

Mood:

Energy:

Cravings:

Symptoms:

Weight:

Week 30

Starting Weight: ________

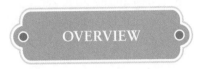

OVERVIEW

You can expect to feel a Braxton Hicks contraction almost every day this week. Though they are painless and infrequent, they can be surprising and uncomfortable. Look for tips in the forthcoming entries on how to safely deal with them, and keep in mind that these early contractions are your body's way of practicing for the real thing. Of course, it is necessary for both your safety and that of your baby that you are able to tell the difference between Braxton Hicks contractions and real labor. The key difference is that contractions that signify the start of labor will be painful and come at increasingly frequent intervals. Braxton Hicks contractions, on the other hand, are irregular and have no pattern or increased frequency. You should also pay attention to the amount and quality of your vaginal discharge. Some women may start to leak amniotic fluid as they get closer to laboring. Your doctor is able to measure the amount of fluid that surrounds your baby by guided ultrasound.

While you've got your antennae raised for preterm labor, your baby is just as comfortable as can be, doing what he should be doing—growing. Your baby's growth is mainly focused on putting on weight, at a rate of about ½ ounce per day. Of course, some babies will gain a bit more or less, but this is the average rate at which fetuses gain weight during the last 12 weeks of gestational development.

DAY 204: Date:___/___/___

MOM - WHAT'S HAPPENING:

Around this time the height of your fundus is just about 5 inches above your belly button, making the total length of your uterus about 32 centimeters. Interestingly, the size of your uterus usually corresponds with the number of weeks pregnant you are based on your last menstrual period (LMP) due date calculation. Thus, this week you are 32 weeks pregnant according to the LMP schedule, so your uterus should measure just about 32 centimeters from the top of your pubic bone to the height of the fundus.

BABY - WHAT'S HAPPENING:

Your baby's hearing is becoming more refined as time passes, and she is probably able to hear more clearly the sounds that pass through your womb. She may even respond to familiar, distinct noises by kicking or even by getting quiet, perhaps to concentrate on what she is hearing or to be lulled to sleep by your voice.

PREGNANCY FACT: Only 1 in 10 women have their water break before contractions start. You should be aware of what this sensation feels like in case it happens to you. Once your water breaks, you must get to the hospital immediately. So, have a bag packed and call your doctor en route if you experience an intense need to void your bladder followed by a gush of sweet-smelling, clear fluid, or a constant trickle of fluid that does not smell like urine. If either of these happens to you, get to the hospital right away, because you are in labor.

DAILY JOURNAL

Mood:

Energy:

Cravings:

Symptoms:

Weight:

DAY 205: Date:___/___/___

MOM - WHAT'S HAPPENING:

Today is a good day to start preparing for your baby shower. It is likely that your friends and family will have plans for one by now. Find out what they have planned and dress accordingly. Even if you are not feeling up to it, make an effort to look like your prettiest, pregnant self. Make decisions about whether you will allow other children to attend your shower, and if you don't mind if your guests drink mimosas or other alcoholic drinks.

BABY - WHAT'S HAPPENING:

You should be able to count at least 10 movements each hour, despite the fact that your baby spends 95 percent of his day sleeping. This is a lot more shut-eye than he will get after being born, of course. It is true that during the first week of life babies sleep most of the day but as they become more aware of their surroundings their waking patterns will become longer and more frequent. So, enjoy this peace and quiet while you still can.

PREGNANCY FACT: The University of California, Irvine, conducted a study in the 1990s that found that college students who listened to Mozart sonatas while they studied had improved spacial reasoning and concentration. Though there is little evidence that proves playing classical music for your fetus will increase her intelligence, there is anecdotal evidence that babies are able to recognize sounds they heard in utero after they are born. So, put a set of headphones on your belly and play a variety of classical pieces while you still have a say in the music your child listens to.

DAILY JOURNAL

Mood:

Energy:

Cravings:

Symptoms:

Weight:

DAY 206: Date:___/___/___

MOM - WHAT'S HAPPENING:

Now is a good time to start weighing the benefits of breast-feeding versus bottle feeding your baby. It is important to at least know how you want to start out feeding your baby. Your instructions for this will be included in your birth plan, which will be available to the nurses who tend to your family. In the event there is an emergency during delivery or if you have a Cesarean section, the staff will know how and when you want to nurse your baby.

BABY - WHAT'S HAPPENING:

Your baby's skin is getting thicker, pinker, and less wrinkled as the days go by. His face has smoothed out considerably compared to just 4 weeks ago. Most babies have lost much of the lanugo that covered them by now. This soft fuzz will be digested by your baby as he swallows amniotic fluid. It will be one of just a few components that make up your baby's first stool, or meconium.

FOR YOUR HEALTH: Your doctor may mention the possibility of inducing your labor for several reasons. You may have developed preeclampsia and both you and your baby's health are at risk by letting your pregnancy go on too long. Or, you may have entered your pregnancy as a diabetic or developed gestational diabetes while pregnant, and your doctor is concerned about the size and health of the baby. Another reason could be that a non-stress test indicates that the placenta is not functioning properly. Finally, your amniotic sac may have ruptured and labor is not starting on its own.

DAILY JOURNAL

Mood:

Energy:

Cravings:

Symptoms:

Weight:

DAY 207: Date:___/___/___

MOM - WHAT'S HAPPENING:

At this point, your body is producing between 40 and 50 percent more blood since before you were pregnant. This increase in blood volume is necessary for both you and your baby, but it also serves as a buffer for blood loss during childbirth. Indeed, it is normal to lose some blood when you give birth. It is usually a minimal amount and not cause for concern. In case you were considering banking your own blood before birth, think again—it is not safe to donate blood while you are pregnant. In fact, The American Red Cross and other organizations will turn you away.

BABY - WHAT'S HAPPENING:

By now your baby's arms, legs, and head are in proportion to each other and she looks just like a smaller version of how she will look on her birthday. Your little one has also got an impressive head of hair by now, especially if you and your partner have dark skin and hair.

FOR YOUR HEALTH: It is not considered safe to take Echinacea while pregnant. This is especially true during the third trimester, because Echinacea can stimulate your uterus enough to cause contractions strong enough to induce preterm labor. Another reason to avoid Echinacea is because your immune system makes adjustments to support your pregnancy, and this herb can negatively interfere with those changes. If you are coming down with a cold, just stick to orange juice and get lots of rest—let the Echinacea sit on the shelf until the next flu season.

DAILY JOURNAL

Mood:

Energy:

Cravings:

Symptoms:

Weight:

DAY 208: Date:___/___/___

MOM - WHAT'S HAPPENING:

The hormone relaxin is hard at work preparing your body for labor and delivery. This hormone is helping your hips spread wider apart and encouraging the bones in your pelvis to shift to make room for when your baby drops. Though it may cause you to be clumsy and achy now, you will be grateful that this bone shifting is happening gradually before you give birth.

BABY - WHAT'S HAPPENING:

By now, your baby's head measures approximately 4 inches around. It can be stimulating for your baby to expose him to all kinds of sounds and flavors. So, try stepping outside of your everyday routine. Visit a record store and play different types of music through the sample headphones. Try food from an Afghan restaurant. Your baby may get a kick out of hearing different sounds and tasting different spices.

TIPS AND ADVICE: Studies show that babies born to women who work where noise levels are so high that protective headphones must be worn are more likely to be born with some hearing loss. In fact, it has been shown that low-decibel noises are amplified by amniotic fluid, while high decibel noises (like mom's voice) are buffered by it. Thus, if you work in a venue where live music is played every night, such as in a club or bar, you may want to take a leave of absence until after your baby is born to avoid risking hearing loss.

DAILY JOURNAL

Mood:

Energy:

Cravings:

Symptoms:

Weight:

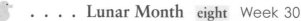

DAY 209: Date:___/___/___

MOM - WHAT'S HAPPENING:

Some women experience a condition known as diastasis during the third trimester (and sometimes as early as the second trimester). Diastasis is the separation of abdominal muscles. These muscles meet along the line of the belly button. When they separate from your uterus, a small bulge may appear. This condition ranges from painless to painful, and there is nothing to do be done except delivering your baby and allowing your body to return to normal.

BABY - WHAT'S HAPPENING:

The placenta has another very important job besides feeding your baby and filtering out toxins. Its many layers also prevent your blood from mixing with your baby's blood—a potentially fatal occurrence if your blood types are different or if you are Rh negative. This is one reason why prenatal visits are so important—doctors can check the condition of the placenta by ultrasound and intervene if there is a problem.

PREGNANCY FACT: Most babies produce at least four detectable movements per hour. These can include kicks, punches, hiccups, and other movements that are discernible to you. If you are carrying a baby who is not very active in the womb, she will still be healthy at birth. However, if you feel like baby is too still, have a small glass of juice or water and lie on your left side for 30 to 60 minutes. If two hours have passed and you haven't felt at least 10 movements, give your doctor a call so that you can get an immediate checkup.

DAILY JOURNAL

Mood:

Energy:

Cravings:

Symptoms:

Weight:

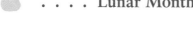

DAY 210: Date:___/___/___

MOM - WHAT'S HAPPENING:

With just 8 weeks left in your pregnancy, your head is probably spinning with questions, fears, and anticipation. It is recommended that you do your best to get as much rest as possible from now until you have your baby. Chronically fatigued pregnant women tend to have higher rates of depression and anxiety, as well as more intense back pain. If you know you are in danger of chronic fatigue, consider taking an early leave from work so that you can adequately rest before the baby comes.

BABY - WHAT'S HAPPENING:

At this point your baby is 17 inches long and weighs 4 pounds. You have probably noticed that your baby's height has not increased much over the last couple of weeks, but that is to be expected. Your baby's priority is to put on weight and that is exactly what he is doing. In fact, half of the weight you gain from now until you deliver your baby will be diverted to him.

FOR YOUR HEALTH: Sometime before you go into labor you may pass what is called "bloody show." It can appear in the toilet or in your underwear. This happens when the mucus plug that blocks the cervical opening falls out as a result of your body preparing for labor. Your cervix will start to thin out, which will loosen the plug enough for it to become dislodged. This does not necessarily mean that you are going into labor—bloody show can happen up to two weeks before labor starts. It is still a good idea to let your doctor know, however.

DAILY JOURNAL

Mood:

Energy:

Cravings:

Symptoms:

Weight:

Week 31

Starting Weight: _________

OVERVIEW

This week you can expect to feel heavier and perhaps more bloated. Pregnancy hormones cause you to retain water, and you may find your lower legs look more like elephant trunks than ankles by the end of the day. Swelling is uncomfortable, especially if you work with your hands. In fact, some women develop a pretty nasty case of swelling-related carpal tunnel syndrome at this point. As you may recall, carpal tunnel happens when all of that extra fluid puts pressure on the nerves in your wrists. You may even experience periodic numbness and tingling in your fingers—particularly upon first waking up. Despite the swelling, refrain from cutting back on your liquid consumption. Drinking water and staying hydrated actually promote kidney function, which facilitates the flushing of excess fluids.

Though this week may be rough for you in the symptom department, your baby is doing just fine. She continues to accumulate fat stores beneath her skin and her soft skeleton is getting harder by the day. As she gets longer and more plump her skin continues to stretch out and become less wrinkled, giving her a distinctly human baby appearance. By the end of this week your baby will be longer than 17 inches and weigh nearly 4½ pounds.

DAY 211: Date:___/___/___

MOM - WHAT'S HAPPENING:

At this point in pregnancy, 75 percent of women experience moderate to severe bouts of insomnia. This is due to frequent trips to the bathroom during the night, inability to get comfortable, vivid dreams, and anxiety. When dealing with insomnia, it is important to address the causes instead of trying to force the result (sleep). Do not eat too close to bed time, take a warm bath, and limit your fluid intake a couple of hours before you go to lie down.

BABY - WHAT'S HAPPENING:

The amount of amniotic fluid in your womb has reached its maximum level around now. Your baby is much larger than he was just two weeks ago and, as a result has less fluid between him and the outside world. This means that he can hear more clearly and can also tell the difference between day and night as more light filters in through your thinning uterine walls.

PREGNANCY FACT: There are several ways to distinguish between false and true labor. False labor causes irregular, inconsistent contractions; true labor produces contractions at regular intervals that come closer together. False labor contractions are weak, painless, and do not intensify; true labor contractions, on the other hand, last for at least 30 seconds at first, then longer, and get stronger with each set. Finally, contractions from false labor go away, but contractions from true labor do not and may intensify with activity.

DAILY JOURNAL

Mood:

Energy:

Cravings:

Symptoms:

Weight:

DAY 212: Date:___/___/___

MOM - WHAT'S HAPPENING:

By today, you have probably gained between 22 and 28 pounds. The height of your fundus is about 5 inches above your belly button. A few women will start to see a decrease in appetite at this point in their pregnancy. This is mostly due to pressure on the stomach from the uterus, as well as from the return of nausea—and even vomiting. If you cannot eat as many calories as you need to, try drinking a nutritious smoothie infused with protein, calcium, and vitamin C. These can be tasty, easy to digest, and give you a healthy calorie boost.

BABY - WHAT'S HAPPENING:

At this point your baby is swallowing about a pint of amniotic fluid per day. He is also still producing sterile urine that is recycled through the amniotic fluid only to be swallowed again. Fluid levels will decline slightly as you get closer to your delivery date. Some of the contents are digested and stored by your baby in the form of fat and meconium.

PREGNANCY FACT: Since your heart is pumping up to 50 percent more blood than it was before you became pregnant, there is a chance you may develop a heart murmur during your pregnancy. A murmur is a sound your heart makes when the valves open and close as blood passes through them. It can be normal or it can signify an underlying problem. Your doctor listens for this at each of your checkups. If a murmur is detected he will be able to tell whether it is normal and pregnancy-related or something more serious.

DAILY JOURNAL

Mood:

Energy:

Cravings:

Symptoms:

Weight:

DAY 213: Date:___/___/___

MOM - WHAT'S HAPPENING:

Your body is in overdrive, preparing for the birth of your baby. This is particularly evident in your breasts. Stimulated by the hormone oxytocin, the glands that produce milk have expanded further and are filling up with colostrum and perhaps even some milk. Your breasts may start to feel slightly lumpy, and you may have even gone up another half size in bras.

BABY - WHAT'S HAPPENING:

Thanks to the extra calcium you are consuming, your baby's skeleton continues to harden. Your baby's skull, however, will remain soft to make it possible for her head to fit through the birth canal. This amazing feat of nature allows the baby's head to compress into an almost cone shape while squeezing through your pelvis. Babies born vaginally will keep their conehead shape for a while after they are born. Babies born via Cesarean section do not develop this shape, of course, because they are surgically removed from the womb.

TIPS AND ADVICE: Start deciding whether you will want to circumcise your son. Circumcision is the cutting away of the foreskin around the head of the penis. This procedure is done either at the hospital or in your pediatrician's office within the first week of life. In Judaism, parents circumcise their baby on the 8th day after his birth in a ceremony called a bris. However, circumcision is elected by Americans of all faiths. There is evidence both supporting and contradicting the necessity of circumcision, which is why you should do your research before being faced with the decision.

DAILY JOURNAL

Mood:

Energy:

Cravings:

Symptoms:

Weight:

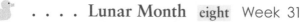

DAY 214: Date:___/___/___

MOM - WHAT'S HAPPENING:

Now is a good time to evaluate whether your exercise routine is too strenuous. As your body prepares for labor and delivery the tendons, ligaments, and soft tissue in your pelvic region are loosening to the point where you may feel as though your legs are a separate entity. This can decrease your coordination and make you more accident-prone. This is not to say you should sit on the couch until you deliver, but it may be time to switch to an activity that puts very little stress on your joints, such as swimming.

BABY - WHAT'S HAPPENING:

An important development has occurred—your baby's immune system has matured and is able to fight off mild infections on its own. This was made possible by antibodies passed on from you as well as increased white blood cell production by your baby's bone marrow, spleen, and thymus. He will be born with a natural immunity to some viruses and will acquire others from you if you breast-feed him.

FOOD FOR THOUGHT: A great number of pregnant women are lactose intolerant and thus may find it difficult to get enough calcium in their diets. If you did not know this about yourself before you were pregnant, it may be hard to decipher these symptoms from normal pregnancy-related issues. However, if you are painfully bloated after drinking a glass of milk or end up with diarrhea every time you eat pizza, there is a good chance that you are lactose intolerant. If so, eat lots of other calcium-rich foods, such as tofu, broccoli, spinach, sardines, and fortified juices and cereals.

DAILY JOURNAL

Mood:

Energy:

Cravings:

Symptoms:

Weight:

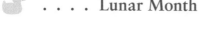

DAY 215: Date:___/___/___

MOM - WHAT'S HAPPENING:

Getting comfortable any time of day is becoming more of a challenge. This may mean that long, romantic dinners with your partner may need to change locations from your favorite restaurant to the couch. Sitting for any length of time on a hard chair is not ideal for you at this point. In fact, feel free to skip events where you know you will be uncomfortable. You will be able to go back to socializing normally after your baby is born—though you will probably be too exhausted!

BABY - WHAT'S HAPPENING:

Can you tell where your baby's head is? Some mothers swear they are rubbing their baby's sweet head at the top of their fundus, when, in fact, they are actually rubbing baby's bum! To the untrained hand baby's head and bum can feel quite alike. It is fun to guess but hard to know just exactly which way baby is facing at this point without asking your doctor.

FOR YOUR HEALTH: The synthetic form of oxytocin, called Pitocin, is what most doctors use to induce labor when there are health problems for mom or baby. Pitocin is also used to initiate labor in an overdue mother, or to expedite a particularly long labor that is not progressing. Pitocin-induced contractions are usually more intense than those generated naturally by the body. They can cause labor to progress very quickly through each stage, which poses some risk to mom and baby. Thus, both mom and baby will be very closely monitored should Pitocin be used.

DAILY JOURNAL

Mood:

Energy:

Cravings:

Symptoms:

Weight:

DAY 216: Date:___/___/___

MOM - WHAT'S HAPPENING:

Some women start to experience pain in their vagina around now. This is part of your body getting ready to deliver your baby. All of the bones below your belly button are spreading apart to make room for baby's grand entrance and this can affect your pubic bone and the muscles in your vagina. Continue to do Kegel exercises to strengthen these muscles. A warm bath can also help ease vaginal muscle pain. If it is troubling or too intense, tell your doctor. He will probably advise you to take a couple of Tylenol for pain relief.

BABY - WHAT'S HAPPENING:

Your baby continues to practice breathing. This exercise will encourage his lungs to produce more surfactant, which is necessary to keep his lungs inflated. Though his lungs are not finished developing yet, they are at the point where if he was born he would be able to survive and have an excellent chance of being healthy newborn—though he would have to spend time in the neonatal intensive care unit (NICU).

PREGNANCY FACT: The neonatal intensive care unit (NICU) is an isolated section of the maternity ward where babies born with special medical needs reside until they are healthy enough to go home with their parents. Pediatricians developed the NICU in the 1950s to provide babies with protection from infections in a temperature-controlled incubator where they receive respiratory support from specialized machines. Babies in the NICU are allowed few visitors and even parents are required to wear protective gear when spending time with their baby.

DAILY JOURNAL

Mood:

Energy:

Cravings:

Symptoms:

Weight:

DAY 217: Date:___/___/___

MOM - WHAT'S HAPPENING:

There are just 49 days left in your pregnancy if you carry baby to full term. You can expect to gain approximately 7 more pounds between now and when you deliver your baby. Of course, this number can fluctuate up or down based on diet and body type. Nerves may cause your appetite to plummet, but stay on track with your healthy diet. Never reduce caloric intake when you are pregnant—especially not at this stage when your baby is counting on you for the final push in his development.

BABY - WHAT'S HAPPENING:

As this week comes to an end, your baby has grown to be an impressive 17½ inches long and weighs 4½ pounds. Also, in the past week, your baby's head circumference has increased by 3/8 of an inch as his brain remains in a stage of rapid growth and development. Your baby will continue to put on about ½ pound per week until he is born—which is coming up very quickly!

FOR YOUR HEALTH: An episiotomy is a small incision made in your perineum during delivery. It is usually done when your baby's head is too large to fit through your vagina and it has become a medical emergency. The majority of women will tear during vaginal delivery—the tear can range from tiny to relatively large. Both natural tears and episiotomies make for a painful recovery, but the choice is yours (barring medical emergency), so be sure to educate yourself and let your doctor know your preference—and remember to include it in your birth plan.

DAILY JOURNAL

Mood:

Energy:

Cravings:

Symptoms:

Weight:

Week 32

Starting Weight: ________

OVERVIEW

This week you can expect to alternate between feeling fatigued and overcome with energy. These energetic bouts may be the nesting instinct kicking in. This is not a myth! Women really do experience a push to clean, organize, and get everything ready for when baby comes home. Sometimes this can supersede your exhaustion and keep you up at night scrubbing floors or folding baby clothes. Try to contain your need to clean to normal waking hours and reserve night time for whatever sleep you are able to get. Also, consider using natural and organic cleansers instead of chemical-based ones. It is dangerous for you to inhale toxic fumes from cleansers at this point. Include your husband in these projects so you don't run yourself ragged—plus, this is an excellent way for your partner to participate in a pregnancy-induced symptom.

While mom and dad are racing the clock trying to prepare for the big day, baby is looking and acting more like a newborn. If your baby was born this week he would have a 99 percent chance of survival without long-term major medical issues. By the end of this week your baby will be 18 inches long and weigh close to 5½ pounds. Also, your baby's immune system continues to improve as you provide him with antibodies that help fight a variety of infections. And finally, though your baby is far from having cute dimples and rolls that chubby babies are famous for, his arms, legs, and face are plumping up as fat continues to accumulate.

DAY 218: Date:___/___/___

MOM - WHAT'S HAPPENING:

If you are carrying twins, you have just entered the prime time for going into labor. Indeed, 50 percent of women who are pregnant with multiples will go into labor between 32 and 35 lunar weeks. Even if you are not pregnant with multiples, you are probably experiencing an increase in the intensity of Braxton Hicks contractions. They should still be painless and irregular, however. If you haven't already, pack your hospital bag—just in case.

BABY - WHAT'S HAPPENING:

Vernix, the white, waxy coating on your baby's skin, will start to thicken slightly at this point. Remember that its job is to facilitate your baby's passage through the birth canal and protect his skin. As you get closer to delivery, the vernix will become thinner, but he will still be nice and slippery for his grand journey into the world. There will be remnants of this substance in the folds of your baby's skin after he is born, though much of it will be cleaned off shortly after delivery.

PREGNANCY FACT: If you are expecting triplets, you may be extra nervous about how your band of babies will enter the world. Though it is true that most women who are pregnant with triplets end up delivering at least one baby through Cesarean section, it is possible to experience vaginal delivery with at least one of the babies. This, of course, requires that mom and babies are in good health and stay that way through labor. But if the baby who is closest to the birth canal is head down, odds are good that this baby, at least, will be delivered vaginally.

DAILY JOURNAL

Mood:

Energy:

Cravings:

Symptoms:

Weight:

DAY 219: Date:___/___/___

MOM - WHAT'S HAPPENING:

If your vision is blurrier than it used to be, you are probably suffering from moderate to severe edema. Indeed, the same fluid that builds up in your ankles and wrists puts pressure behind your eyes, which changes their shape. This is a temporary condition that will go away once you deliver your baby. Contacts may be uncomfortable, so stick to wearing your glasses until your eyes return to their normal shape. You may also be experiencing very dry eyes, so keep a bottle of eye lubricant on hand to alleviate this discomfort.

BABY - WHAT'S HAPPENING:

If you are having a boy, his testicles are close to their final position in his scrotum. However, between 3 and 4 percent of boy babies' testicles do not descend until after they are born. Also, your baby's central nervous system is maturing, which means he will be more in control of his movements—including sucking and swallowing, which is necessary for him to feed after he is born.

PREGNANCY FACT: There are three stages of labor you will pass through before you are able to rest and snuggle up with your baby. The first stage of labor covers the onset of contractions through active labor and transition from labor to pushing—this is the longest and often most painful stage. The second stage is from when pushing starts until your baby is actually delivered—the amount of time it takes to push baby out varies. The third and final stage of labor is delivery of the placenta. This usually occurs within one hour of delivering your baby.

DAILY JOURNAL

Mood:

Energy:

Cravings:

Symptoms:

Weight:

DAY 220: Date:___/___/___

MOM - WHAT'S HAPPENING:

Your belly button might be extremely sensitive right about now. If your belly button is an outie, your clothes may feel particularly uncomfortable against the skin. Some easy fixes are to wear light, cotton fabrics, and low waistbands. Some women like to put a band-aid over the belly button to decrease irritation. You should also ask your partner to avoid touching that area when he is spending "hands-on-time" with you and baby, as touching your sensitive belly button can send shivers through your entire body.

BABY - WHAT'S HAPPENING:

Your baby's eyes are open for longer stretches now and closed tight when he is sleeping. This is because he is becoming aware of the difference between night and day as light filters into your womb. This is impressive, but won't last. Many babies have day and night confusion for the first couple months after birth. This can make for an exhausted family but, with time, your baby will settle into a routine.

TIPS AND ADVICE: If you and your partner have life insurance policies, IRAs, and/or a 401k), be sure to revisit them this week or next. At the time you opened these accounts you may have selected a beneficiary for your benefits that is no longer whom you want. If you have listed your partner, then you are in good shape. However, if you want one or all of these benefits to go into a trust for your child, now is a great time to make changes. The individual policy directives on these accounts will supersede your will, so it is important to make sure that all these documents are in order.

DAILY JOURNAL

Mood:

Energy:

Cravings:

Symptoms:

Weight:

DAY 221: Date:___/___/___

MOM - WHAT'S HAPPENING:

Today is a good time to familiarize yourself with terms related to birth and delivery. This way, when you are in the hospital or birthing center, you are able to understand what the medical staff is talking about. One term you will hear often over the next few weeks is effacement, which describes the thinning of your cervix. Effacement is measured in percentages, and when you are 100 percent effaced you will be ready to start pushing your baby out into the world.

BABY - WHAT'S HAPPENING:

Your baby has developed an impressive grip at this point. In fact, he is probably grabbing anything he can get a hold of, including the umbilical cord, other fingers, his toes, ankles—whatever is within reach. Since his nails are now at the edge of his fingertips, don't be surprised if he is born with a few scratches here and there. Indeed, clipping his nails may be one of the earliest parental acts you will get to perform for your baby.

PREGNANCY FACT: In 1952, anesthesiologist Virginia Apgar developed a set of tests (called APGAR) to determine a newborn's health. The APGAR test is still used today. It assigns a number between 0 and 2 for each of the following: baby's heart rate, color, breathing, muscle tone, and reflexes. Babies are tested again at 5 minutes after birth. A total score of 7 to 10 indicates baby is doing well and will not require any special measures. Scores below 7 indicate baby will need special care, and scores below 4 require serious medical intervention.

DAILY JOURNAL

Mood:

Energy:

Cravings:

Symptoms:

Weight:

DAY 222: Date:___/___/___

MOM - WHAT'S HAPPENING:

Today you likely have the best proof of how much you have changed physically over the past 222 days. When you stand up, you can no longer see your feet. In fact, tying your shoes at this point is a chore better left until after your feet don't seem like a distant planet. Store any lace-up shoes in your closet and stick to supportive, slip-on shoes. Sandals with a low heel are your best bet and are usually pretty inexpensive as well as versatile.

BABY - WHAT'S HAPPENING:

At this point your baby has almost completely shed all of the lanugo that covered his body. As fat stores under his skin he ceases to need lanugo to help regulate his body temperature. In fact, his brain and the fat he's accumulating will work together to get baby's body temperature in line. Still, parents of babies born with residual traces of lanugo find the fuzz makes their baby all the more adorable.

FOR YOUR HEALTH: Complications during childbirth have been reduced to extremely low rates in the United States. Occasionally, however, complications do occur during labor and delivery that require medical intervention with forceps. Your doctor will only use forceps after your baby's head is already very low in your pelvis and it is clear that baby is stuck or that you are unable to push him out on your own. What looks like two large spoons will be inserted into your vagina and placed around your baby's head. As you push, your doctor will pull, helping to ease baby out of the birth canal.

DAILY JOURNAL

Mood:

Energy:

Cravings:

Symptoms:

Weight:

DAY 223: Date:___/___/___

MOM - WHAT'S HAPPENING:

Today it is probably that fluids—including blood—are pooling at the lowest point in your body. Getting up too fast doesn't give your body enough time to circulate blood back up to your head. This will cause you to feel light-headed, dizzy, and even to faint. Thus, it is important to get up in stages. If you've been lying down, sit up for a few minutes before standing and hold on to a piece of furniture as you rise. Remember to steady yourself before stepping away from your support.

BABY - WHAT'S HAPPENING:

Your baby is able to blink, which can give him a flirtatious ultrasound appearance. Blinking is a function for your baby to perfect, because it will help protect his eyes once he is born. Blinking helps keep an overabundance of airborne particles from entering the eyes—it also cleanses the eyes and lubricates them with three different layers of moisture necessary for optical health.

FOR YOUR HEALTH: In cases that require an assisted birth, your doctor may choose to use a vacuum extractor rather than forceps. When the vacuum extractor is used, the doctor places a plastic cup on baby's head and activates a pump that creates suction, which will aid mom in pushing. Of course, like with forceps, baby must be far enough down into the pelvic area. The vacuum extractor is less invasive to the mother than the use of forceps, but does pose some risk to baby. Sometimes neither forceps nor vacuum extraction does the trick, in which case the baby will be delivered by Cesarean.

DAILY JOURNAL

Mood:

Energy:

Cravings:

Symptoms:

Weight:

DAY 224: Date:___/___/___

MOM - WHAT'S HAPPENING:

By now, the height of your fundus is around 5½ inches above your belly button. The total length of your uterus from your pubic bone to the top of the fundus is approximately 34 centimeters. You have gained another pound, half of which has gone directly to your baby. You may feel like the other half pound is in your head. It is normal to be forgetful and to feel like you are operating from within a haze. Fatigue, anxiety, raging hormones, fluid retention, carrying around extra weight, and other physiological changes are taking their toll on your mind. Don't worry—your brain will return to its normal level of functioning after you have your baby.

BABY - WHAT'S HAPPENING:

At the end of this week your baby is about 18 inches long and weighs 5½ pounds. She is looking remarkably like a newborn baby, and her in utero behaviors are similar to how she will act after she is born—sleeping, waking, sucking, swallowing, yawning, blinking, and looking around.

PREGNANCY FACT: If either parent has a congenital heart defect, your OB/GYN may recommend that you see a specialist who can perform a fetal echocardiogram. This is performed the same way as the ultrasound, but is catered especially to zoom in on your baby's heart. It is read by a pediatric cardiologist. Fetal echocardiograms are good for detecting glaring problems in utero, which can help everyone be prepared when baby is born. If a defect is detected your doctor will request that a pediatric cardiologist be present at the birth to assess your baby immediately.

DAILY JOURNAL

Mood:

Energy:

Cravings:

Symptoms:

Weight:

Lunar Month

Nine

P H O T O

Place a photo of you during
your ninth month here

My Monthly Update

Waist Measurement: ______________________

Weight: ______________________

Mood: ______________________

Lunar Month nine

PREGNANCY CHECKLIST

- ❑ After the 36th week, visit your health care provider once a week for prenatal care checkups
- ❑ Decide if you are going to breast-feed or formula-feed
- ❑ Read up on newborn vaccines and find out what's best for your baby
- ❑ Talk to your doctor about your baby's position and how it may impact childbirth
- ❑ Finalize your baby name selections
- ❑ Pick out your baby announcements
- ❑ Know your contractions. Recognize the differences between Braxton-Hicks contractions and true labor
- ❑ Time your contractions to determine when you go into labor
- ❑ Buy a baby sling or baby carrier
- ❑ Prepare yourself mentally for labor and delivery. Talk to your doctor about any fears or concerns you may have.
- ❑ Learn the pros and cons of inducing labor and decide how you feel about it
- ❑ Wash and put away your baby's new clothes
- ❑ Prepare for the weeks after you give birth. Ask friends and family members for help around the house and with the baby
- ❑ Enjoy the last few days of your pregnancy and get plenty of rest

MY PERSONAL CHECKLIST:

- ❑ ....
- ❑ ....
- ❑ ....

MY HOPES FOR THIS MONTH:

....

....

....

Lunar Month Nine

Third Trimester

CONGRATULATIONS! You are truly about to enter the final leg of your pregnancy. You have been through a lot, mom: body changes, emotional upheaval, mood swings, not to mention the mounting expectation of who this tiny person you've carried inside you for so long will turn out to be. In the upcoming month you will finish your childbirth classes, which will help feel prepared and less anxious about labor and delivery. You will also make the final push to get your house and nursery ready for when baby comes home. Aside from taking care of the basics for your little one, you should spend as much time resting as possible. Sleep, more than anything else, is going to help you be ready for your baby's birthday.

WHAT TO EXPECT THIS MONTH

You can expect your doctor to increase your prenatal visits from once every two weeks to once a week. Most of these exams will be similar to those you have already experienced, but now your doctor will start to do vaginal exams to track the thickness of your cervix (effacement) as well as to monitor when it starts to dilate (open). Many women find that once they start seeing the doctor once a week time really begins to fly. This thought may cause you to feel like you will never accomplish all you wanted to before baby's arrival—and that is fine! Your priorities at this point should be to prepare to go on leave from work and to rest. In fact, if you have any complications, including gestational diabetes, preeclampsia, or any issues with placental placement, your doctor may urge you to stop working earlier than you planned. If he does, don't fight it. Your health and your baby's health could be at stake if you fail to follow doctor's orders.

THINGS TO CONSIDER

The nesting instinct is going to kick into high gear this month. This will have you running ragged trying to get the house ready but try to contain your urge to bleach all the surfaces in your home. At this point, heavy-duty cleansers can be harmful to both you and baby. Leave that kind of work to your partner. Instead, focus on making sure you are mentally, physically, and situationally prepared to care for your child. Be sure you have enough newborn-sized clothing that is seasonally appropriate. Install and practice using a car seat. Review your registry and pick up last-minute items. Stock up on diapers (either cloth or disposable). Finally, make a decision about your sleeping situation once baby comes home and set up the crib and/or bassinet. You may also want to purchase either a rocking chair or glider in which to feed and rock your baby.

TIPS FOR COPING

You are probably feeling overwhelmed, exhausted, and manic all at once. This is to be expected, but to avoid system overload, it is important that you make time to take care of you. The very best way to do this is to continue to eat well, walk for as long as you are comfortable each day, and rest as much as you can. Another way to deal with the stress is to make time to connect with your partner. Unless you've been ordered not to, have sex. Spend time exploring your pregnant body together, because you will be back to your old self in just a few months. Try to savor these last few weeks together without baby. Do special things together that you can both think back on later when there is little time for such intimacy.

WHAT TO EAT

At the beginning of this month you will probably have little appetite as your baby continues to encroach upon the space in which your stomach and other organs reside. Your stomach is so squished, you may even lose some weight this month. Not to worry, though, because this is normal. Just stay hydrated and continue to eat small, healthy meals until your appetite returns.

Sometime in the middle or end of this month your baby will drop down into your pelvic region to prepare for birth. Once she does this you will find that the pressure is off your stomach, esophagus, and diaphragm, and your appetite will return. This, plus the fact that you are busy finishing up with work and getting the house ready, may tempt you to eat fast-food regularly. Avoid this temptation! Your baby needs you to stick to a healthy diet.

HOW MUCH WEIGHT TO GAIN

At this point, you have probably gained between 24 and 29 pounds. You can expect to gain another 2 to 4 pounds between now and the end of your pregnancy. You have been gaining approximately 4 pounds per month thus far, but this month may be lighter than others since you are likely starting out with very little appetite. This is fine, so don't feel like you have to make up the difference when your appetite does return by eating donuts three times a day.

EXERCISE TIPS AND ADVICE

More than in previous months, you will have to evaluate what your limits are when it comes to exercise. Certain activities are inappropriate at this point because of the risk of injury. These include running, hiking, high-impact aerobics, and other exercises that require precision or serious coordination. You should still be able to go for moderately paced walks for 20 to 30 minutes each day, and you should also still be able to do prenatal yoga. Swimming is also an excellent, no-impact way to work your whole body.

Of course, if you are having any complications, do exactly as your doctor advises. If he says you are not to exercise at all—listen to him. There are activities that even women on bed rest can do, such as arm curls with 2- or 3-pound weights and, of course, Kegels.

POTENTIAL SYMPTOMS AND HOW TO ALLEVIATE THEM

At the beginning of this month you will still be battling shortness of breath, heartburn, constipation, fatigue, and back pain. These are the pregnancy staples, and by now you know what you should be doing to manage these symptoms. Unfortunately, back pain will only get worse as your bones spread apart to make room for baby's arrival and as you become more front-heavy. However, once your baby drops into your pelvic cavity (called lightening) you should feel relief from heartburn and be able to breathe easier and more deeply. As for exhaustion, the best way to deal with fatigue is to rest. Many women run themselves ragged these last weeks trying to get ready, only to find that after baby comes their biggest regret is that they wish they had slept more when they had the chance.

Of course, telling a near-term pregnant woman to rest is easier said than done. The discomforts of late-term pregnancy make it very difficult to get a full night's rest, so try to catch naps during the day if you can. And if you can't—take breaks with your eyes closed and your feet up.

WAYS OTHERS CAN HELP

Your partner can be a huge support to you now, so let him in on what you need. Ask for a back rub, a foot rub, a bubble bath or a break from your regular household duties. The best thing your partner can do for you right now is to take on extra responsibilities so that you may carve out some additional time to rest each day. For instance, let him do cleaning that requires use of chemicals or motions that may cause your back to ache, such as sweeping, mopping, and vacuuming. It will also be beneficial for you to share your fears and concerns with him as he is probably experiencing many of the same worries. It is also a good idea for your partner to accompany you on as many prenatal visits as possible, though once a week may be difficult for him to manage.

As for friends and family, ask a few people to come over for a cooking party where each person prepares a dish for you to freeze and have ready to prepare after baby comes home. You should also make arrangements for older children if you haven't already done so. Make sure that whomever you choose to be in charge of your older children is someone they are used to and comfortable with. Also, have a plan in place for getting your kids to the hospital to meet their new brother or sister so that family bonding can begin as soon as possible.

Notes . . . .

Week 33

Starting Weight: _________

OVERVIEW

By the end of this week your baby will take up most of the room inside your uterus. Since the amniotic fluid is at its peak level this week, your baby's size means he no longer floats in the bag of waters. Instead he is flush against the walls of your uterus. He has little room to move, and so the intensity of his kicks and punches will decrease, though now and then you will feel a big one. You should continue to do kick counts; remember that your goal is to feel at least 10 discernible movements per hour. Keep track in a notebook or a form from you doctor. It is also worth repeating that if you do not feel your baby move at least 10 times within 2 hours, call your doctor.

While you are stressing over the number of times your baby moves each hour of the day, your baby is getting ready for life on the outside. At this point, most of his vital organs are developed. His kidneys are functional, his liver is doing its job by filtering waste, and his lungs are continuing to produce enough surfactant to keep them inflated with breath. If you were to go into labor at this point your baby would have a nearly 100 percent chance of survival and would require only short-term medical care.

DAY 225: Date:___/___/___

MOM - WHAT'S HAPPENING:

Today, familiarize yourself with the terms effacement and dilate. Effacement is the thinning of your cervix. Dilation occurs as your cervix opens up to let your baby pass through. When you go into labor your cervix will dilate from 0 to 10 centimeters over the course of your labor. It can take anywhere from 2 to 20 hours for you to become completely dilated (or more, though doctors usually won't let it go on longer). Your doctor will start to check your cervix for effacement and dilation at your next appointment.

BABY - WHAT'S HAPPENING:

As fat accumulates, your baby's arms and legs will become more defined, and she may even be born with dimpled elbows and knees. Your baby is starting to fit snugly inside your uterus. As she gets longer and plumper she has less room to maneuver. She is no longer floating in the amniotic fluid, though she does continue to swallow and breathe it in.

FOR YOUR HEALTH: Sometime between now and week 35, your doctor will swab your vagina and rectum to get a culture. She is testing for Group B streptococci (GBS). Between 10 and 30 percent of women are carriers, yet most have no idea. This bacteria is often harmless for mom, but if it is passed on to baby during delivery it can cause infections such as meningitis, pneumonia, and blood infections. These can be potentially fatal for your baby. If you are a carrier, you will be given intravenous antibiotics as you labor, which should cut your baby's risk of infection.

DAILY JOURNAL

Mood:

Energy:

Cravings:

Symptoms:

Weight:

DAY 226: Date:___/___/___

MOM - WHAT'S HAPPENING:

Your uterus has grown to about 35 centimeters, making the top of your fundus about 6 inches above your belly button. This means that some part of your baby—either his head or his rump—is sitting snug inside your rib cage. For some unlucky moms this means that baby's elbow is putting pressure on her ribs, which can cause pain or an incessant ticklish feeling that cannot be relieved.

BABY - WHAT'S HAPPENING:

Your baby's kidneys are completely developed and functioning. This is an important milestone, because the kidneys are responsible for filtering out waste, toxins, and water in the form of urine. Urine travels through tubes called ureters to the bladder where it sits until baby feels the urge to urinate. Your baby has two kidneys that sit on either side of her spine, and they are partially protected by her rib cage. Interestingly, the right kidney is slightly lower than the left due to the placement of the liver.

PREGNANCY FACT: Lightening is when your baby drops into your pelvic cavity in preparation for birth. This can happen four weeks before you go into labor or just a few hours before labor begins. If it happens sooner, you will have an easier time breathing, heartburn is lessened, your appetite returns, and your organs are less crowded. However, once baby drops you will need to urinate as often as every 45 minutes. You may also experience rectal discomfort from the pressure. No matter how you feel physically, lightening is an exciting sign that your baby is almost ready to meet you.

DAILY JOURNAL

Mood:

Energy:

Cravings:

Symptoms:

Weight:

DAY 227: Date:___/___/___

MOM - WHAT'S HAPPENING:

If you frequently need to urinate today, it is likely that your baby has moved into the head-down position. He still may not have dropped low into your pelvis just yet, but the pressure of his head sitting firmly against your bladder can have you running to the bathroom up to once an hour—even during the night. You may also experience an increase in stress incontinence, which means that when you sneeze, cough, or laugh you are unable to control your bladder.

BABY - WHAT'S HAPPENING:

Your baby may be facing head down at this point, which means he is getting ready to make his grand entrance—though hopefully not before he's considered full-term, which is at 38 weeks LMP. By now, your baby has a decent amount of body fat, and when he is born, he will be comprised of about 15 percent body fat.

TIPS AND ADVICE: Consider breast-feeding. Breast milk is the perfect food for baby and there are countless benefits for children who are breastfed for even just the first six months of their life. Breast milk contains nutrients that cannot be duplicated in commercial formula. It is highly digestible, helps prevent allergies, provides baby with important antibodies, and is linked to both higher IQs and reduced rates of obesity. This is why the World Health Organization recommends that women breast-feed their children for at least one year, if possible.

DAILY JOURNAL

Mood:

Energy:

Cravings:

Symptoms:

Weight:

DAY 228: Date:___/___/___

MOM - WHAT'S HAPPENING:

As you get closer to your due date, you may notice an increase in vaginal discharge. This happens as your cervix thins out and the mucus plug starts to flush. This can be a gradual process or the plug can drop out in one piece, called bloody show. It is still early for the plug to drop out intact, so it is more likely that you will notice a thin, white or pale greenish discharge. If the consistency seems different than what you are used to or if you ever experience a rush of fluid, call your doctor. This can be an indication that your water has broken.

BABY - WHAT'S HAPPENING:

Though your baby's brain is able to regulate her body temperature and she has accumulated a nice amount of fat, if she was born today she would most likely spend a couple of weeks in an incubator. This is because she doesn't quite have enough fat just yet to keep her warm enough outside of your womb.

PREGNANCY FACT: Your doctor will estimate baby's weight at each prenatal visit. If her weight is below the 10th percentile for other babies at this fetal age, she may suffer from intrauterine growth restriction (IUGR). Sadly, babies with IUGR often have many health problems, but the severity of those problems depends on what caused IUGR, such as heart or lung disease in mom or other medical conditions. If IUGR is diagnosed, your doctor will probably want to either induce labor or perform a Cesarean section if the baby is too weak to survive vaginal delivery.

DAILY JOURNAL

Mood:

Energy:

Cravings:

Symptoms:

Weight:

DAY 229: Date:___/___/___

MOM - WHAT'S HAPPENING:

Today you might be fearing the pain of childbirth. Many women become consumed by this fear, especially if this is their first baby. If you find that you are unable to think of anything else, it is time to educate yourself. Your childbirth classes are hopefully helping with this; to enhance that experience, be sure to ask lots of questions. Many childbirth educators will give out their email addresses so that participants with more questions can get in touch. It will also help if you are able to find women to talk to who have had positive and varied birth experiences.

BABY - WHAT'S HAPPENING:

If you are having a boy it is likely that his testes have completed their descent into his scrotum by now. Some boys' testicles don't descend until sometime after birth, however. If you are having a girl, her clitoris is still prominent because her labia have not yet grown large enough to cover it.

FOR YOUR HEALTH: Each time you see your doctor she will check for your baby's presentation. This is your baby's birth position. By now in your pregnancy, she is probably head-down, the ideal position for vaginal delivery. If this is your first baby, how ever your baby sits right now is likely how she'll stay positioned. Women who have had other children will find that baby may change position up to the last week of pregnancy. If your doctor has difficulty determining your baby's presentation by external exam, she may do a vaginal exam to feel which part of baby is closest to the exit.

DAILY JOURNAL

Mood:

Energy:

Cravings:

Symptoms:

Weight:

DAY 230: Date:___/___/___

MOM - WHAT'S HAPPENING:

Today you should try the following exercise to alleviate back pain and help during labor. It is called the pelvic tilt, and it can be done in one of two ways. Get on all fours and tilt your hips and head toward each other. Make sure to keep your back flat and your movements controlled. Another way to perform this exercise is to stand against and press the small of your back into the wall and hold. This exercise stretches your lower back and eases tension while creating space between each of your vertebrae.

BABY - WHAT'S HAPPENING:

Today your baby is taking up more space in your womb, which means that the quality of his movements is changing. You may find it difficult to distinguish one movement from another. This is because your baby has such little room to move that sometimes five or six different motions feel like they blend together. As long as you feel your baby moving, don't worry too much about what he's doing.

PREGNANCY FACT: If your baby's presentation is rear end or feet first she is considered in a breech position. Vaginal delivery of a breech baby can be risky, because there is no way to tell if baby's head will fit through your pelvis. Thus, it is possible that her body will be born and that her head will become stuck. It is also common for breech babies to present a prolapsed umbilical cord, which is when the cord comes out first, slowing or cutting off blood flow to baby. Therefore, if your baby doesn't present head down before your due date, your doctor may recommend a Cesarean delivery.

DAILY JOURNAL

Mood:
Energy:
Cravings:
Symptoms:
Weight:

DAY 231: Date:___/___/___

MOM - WHAT'S HAPPENING:

You should be consuming 2,400 calories per day to provide enough energy and nutrients for your body's needs and your baby's growth. Though you should not overdo it, feel free to indulge now and then with a special delectable. After all, you only have 35 days left to go in your pregnancy, and that deserves a little celebration.

BABY - WHAT'S HAPPENING:

As your 33rd week of gestation comes to an end, your baby is at least 18 inches long and weighs about 6 pounds. His head size has increased slightly to make room for his rapidly expanding brain. Hopefully he is presenting head down and getting ready to drop into your pelvic area, which should give you a break from feeling breathless. In just a few weeks you will be able to hold him in your arms and welcome him into your world.

TIPS AND ADVICE: There are some cases in which a woman should not breast-feed. You should not breast-feed if you must take medications that will harm baby, such as sedatives, antidepressants, or lithium (check with your doctor about others). If you are HIV positive, or if you are currently abusing drugs or alcohol, you can pass harmful substances to your baby. If any of these apply to you, you are doing the right thing by abstaining from breast-feeding. You will still be able to forge an intimate bond with your baby when feeding him formula from a bottle.

DAILY JOURNAL

Mood:

Energy:

Cravings:

Symptoms:

Weight:

Week 34

Starting Weight: _________

OVERVIEW

This week, expect to experience Braxton Hicks contractions more frequently, though they should still come at irregular intervals. Though these contractions are not painful like those that accompany true labor, they will give you some idea of what to expect once labor starts. In fact, you should be ready to go to the hospital at this point, because even though you are still 4 weeks from your due date, labor can start any time. Statistically, it is more common for a first-time mother to go beyond her due date rather than to go into labor early. Still, it is always better to err on the side of caution and be prepared. Thus, if you haven't already done so, use this week to finalize your birth plan, pack a bag for the hospital, and make a list of important phone numbers to take with you to the hospital.

You are not the only one getting ready for baby's big debut! As you are preparing things on the outside, your baby is doing what she can in utero to be as strong and healthy as possible when she is born. Her main job at this point is to gain as much weight as possible at a rate of approximately an ounce each day. So, if you carry your baby until her due date, she should gain approximately 34 more ounces, though this number will vary from baby to baby.

DAY 232: Date:___/___/___

MOM - WHAT'S HAPPENING:

Your prenatal visits are becoming more exciting and informative. Your doctor will do a vaginal exam each week to determine whether you have started to dilate and if effacement has begun. These are important diagnostics for estimating when your may go into labor, though it is impossible to say for sure. Your doctor will measure the height of your fundus and baby's presentation. If baby is not presenting head down, your doctor will discuss options for trying to turn him around. She will also give you a handout with steps to take when labor starts, along with information on Cesarean delivery for you to have on hand just in case.

BABY - WHAT'S HAPPENING:

Today your baby lost a little more room in utero. Instead of feeling quick kicks or punches, you are probably feeling her push outward. If you are lucky, you can see baby's hand poking out through your belly or feel her bum somewhere above your ribs if she is presenting head-down.

FOR YOUR HEALTH: If your baby is in a breech position your doctor may suggest turning your baby around by a process called external cephalic version (ECV). ECV is done by your OB/GYN who will use manual manipulation on the outside of your abdomen in the form of massage and pressure to try to coax baby into presenting head down. This procedure has mixed results and poses some risk to baby if the umbilical cord is too short or becomes tangled. If the procedure is successful, however, it reduces the chance that you will have to deliver by Cesarean section.

DAILY JOURNAL

Mood:

Energy:

Cravings:

Symptoms:

Weight:

DAY 233: Date:___/___/___

MOM - WHAT'S HAPPENING:

Today you may feel irritable as your discomforts intensify and you become increasingly anxious for your baby to come. If you find that you are snapping at your partner, the grocer, and your best friend on a regular basis, take a step back from dealing with people and spend more time on stress management. Though most people expect pregnant women to be unpredictable, snapping often is usually a sign that mom isn't getting enough rest or downtime.

BABY - WHAT'S HAPPENING:

Though your baby's bones have been ossifying over the last few months, they remain soft enough for him to compress to fit through the birth canal. Your baby's bones will continue to harden during the first few years of his life, which is why getting enough calcium will continue to be a very important dietary concern. At this point, your baby's growth will slow down a bit. This is a good thing, because if he gets too big it can complicate your delivery.

FOR YOUR HEALTH: Your doctor will regularly monitor the level of amniotic fluid surrounding your baby. If your fluid level is too low, called oligohydramnios, you could be in for an early or complicated delivery. It depends on what is causing fluid levels to decrease, but the main concern is that the lack of protective solution will cause the umbilical cord to become compressed. Thus, your doctor may decide to induce labor, which may include pumping warm saline solution into the amniotic sac. Your doctor may also have you deliver baby by Cesarean—whichever is safest for you and your baby.

DAILY JOURNAL

Mood:

Energy:

Cravings:

Symptoms:

Weight:

DAY 234: Date:___/___/___

MOM - WHAT'S HAPPENING:

The vaginal discharge that appears today may be light yellow in color and tinged with blood. Do not be alarmed—this is how the dissolution of the mucus plug looks. It is even possible that the entire plug may become dislodged after a vaginal exam. If this is your first baby, this can be scary and cause you to fear that labor has started. Feel free to call your doctor, but remember that you can lose the mucus plug several weeks before labor starts. Once the plug drops, it is important that you not have sex or put anything inside your vagina that can cause infection. The plug is what keeps germs away from your baby and without it she becomes vulnerable to bacteria.

BABY - WHAT'S HAPPENING:

Right around now the waxy coating on your baby's skin (vernix) will start to thin out a bit. This and the lanugo she's shedding will be swallowed, digested, and added to the meconium that is building in your baby's intestines.

FOOD FOR THOUGHT: In addition to feeding baby after she is born, you and your partner will have to deal with feeding yourselves. Therefore, start collecting menus from your favorite take-out restaurants that deliver. Put them in a folder in a drawer in the kitchen. Though you will probably be stocked up on goodies from friends and family, sometimes it is easier to have a pizza delivered than to wait an hour for frozen lasagna to cook. Also, if you don't have a dishwasher, consider stocking up on recycled paper plates and napkins for those first couple of weeks after baby is born.

DAILY JOURNAL

Mood:

Energy:

Cravings:

Symptoms:

Weight:

DAY 235: Date:___/___/___

MOM - WHAT'S HAPPENING:

It is possible that you will stop gaining weight at this point. This is because your baby is absorbing and using most of the calories that you consume. Plus, if your baby hasn't dropped yet, you probably don't have much of an appetite. Still, be sure to consume at least 2,400 calories per day. If you have trouble eating enough, drink smoothies and vegetable juices with protein powder. It is possible that you may see a decrease in heartburn at this point since you are unable to eat big meals. Some women, though, have heartburn up until the minute baby is born.

BABY - WHAT'S HAPPENING:

Your baby's body is becoming an impressive little machine. Blood is circulating throughout her body just as it should be, and her immune system is gearing up to fight infections outside of your uterus. Her digestive tract will continue to mature throughout the first year of her life, which is why breast milk is ideal since it is easy on a baby's system.

PREGNANCY FACT: If your doctor is concerned with the health of your baby and needs information beyond that which the non-stress test can provide, she may ask you to come in for fetal acoustical stimulation (FAS). FAS is done by placing a device on your abdomen that produces vibrations that your baby should respond to. This test is valuable for determining if your baby is moving as much as he should be, and it will also give a more accurate read on baby's cardiac response to stimulation. FAS can also clarify other test results.

DAILY JOURNAL

Mood:

Energy:

Cravings:

Symptoms:

Weight:

DAY 236: Date:___/___/___

MOM - WHAT'S HAPPENING:

Thanks to pregnancy hormones still circulating throughout your body, your joints and ligaments will continue to loosen. This is necessary to make room for your baby's descent into your pelvic cavity but can be quite uncomfortable and cause you to walk with a bit of a waddle. The pregnancy waddle really sets in once baby presents head down and starts to work his way lower into your pelvis. This can cause pain in your hips, pelvis, and lower back as bones literally move aside to let your baby through.

BABY - WHAT'S HAPPENING:

There is an excellent chance that baby is presenting head down at this point, and may have even dropped into your pelvis. If so, your doctor will refer to this as your baby being engaged. Odds are your baby will stay in this position until he is born. He will still move from side to side, but probably will not change positions. If lightening has occurred you will know, because it will be easier to breathe.

TIPS AND ADVICE: When packing your labor bag for the hospital, be sure to include the following: at least two copies of your birth plan; a stopwatch to time your contractions; a camera and/or video camera; important phone numbers; a stress or tennis ball for squeezing; candies to keep you from getting too thirsty; warm socks; slippers; a robe; toothbrush; hairbrush; something to hold your hair back; photos of your other children or pets; a CD player with soothing music; a yoga ball to sit on; a mini DVD player and movies; and any lotions or essential oils that you find relaxing.

DAILY JOURNAL

Mood:

Energy:

Cravings:

Symptoms:

Weight:

DAY 237: Date:___/___/___

MOM - WHAT'S HAPPENING:

If you have experienced lightening by now, you should be breathing easier. This is often a huge relief because you can actually feel your lungs inflate all the way again! You will also be able to eat a little more, but try to stick to the 2,400 calorie diet since you only have a few weeks left to go. Lightening may also reduce heartburn since your upper organs are less compressed. However, depending on how low in your pelvic area your baby is, you may feel pain in your vagina, rectum, hips, and lower back.

BABY - WHAT'S HAPPENING:

Most of the lanugo has been shed except for what remains on your baby's shoulders and upper arms. He is really starting to fill out, especially his face, neck, and upper shoulder area. In fact, his skin is much less wrinkled than it was just a few weeks ago. Though no one would call him chubby, he is just a pound or two away from the size he will be at birth.

TIPS AND ADVICE: Pack a second, postpartum bag to take to the hospital. Remember to include the following in your postpartum bag: pajamas that open in the front; warm socks and slippers; a robe; nursing bras; nursing pads; a few changes of underwear; overnight maxi pads; snacks; and a homecoming outfit for both you and baby. It is also very important that you have your car seat with you. The hospital will not let you take your baby home without one.

DAILY JOURNAL

Mood:

Energy:

Cravings:

Symptoms:

Weight:

DAY 238: Date:___/___/___

MOM - WHAT'S HAPPENING:

You have gained between 25 and 30 pounds by now, though it is possible that you haven't gained anything this week. Try not to worry if that is the case. As long as you are consuming enough healthy calories your baby is just fine. The tradeoff at this point in your pregnancy is that as your upper-body discomforts are on the decline, you can expect a host of lower-body aches and pains over the next few weeks as baby nestles down into your pelvis in preparation for birth.

BABY - WHAT'S HAPPENING:

Your baby now weighs about 6 pounds and is 19 inches long. She is quickly approaching both average birth weight and height. If she was born today, not only would she survive, but she would require minimal medical assistance (assuming delivery was without complications). Baby's lungs are still maturing, though they are close to completion. If you are expecting twins, plan to go into labor any day now, since multiples are usually born between lunar weeks 34 and 36.

PREGNANCY FACT: Approximately one in 100 women will have too much amniotic fluid—a condition called hydramnios. If your uterus is measuring large for your due date and you have a host of extreme symptoms, such as severe abdominal discomfort, shortness of breath, and edema, your doctor may suspect hydramnios. If so, you will be very closely monitored for the duration of your pregnancy and have a series of non-stress tests, ultrasounds, and possibly an amniocentesis. It is likely you will deliver by Cesarean since your overfull uterus may not contract properly.

DAILY JOURNAL

Mood:

Energy:

Cravings:

Symptoms:

Weight:

Week 35

Starting Weight: _________

OVERVIEW

If this is your first pregnancy it is very likely that your baby will drop down into your pelvis this week (if she hasn't already). As mentioned earlier, this will take some pressure off your diaphragm, which should make it much easier to breathe. If this is not your first baby, then lightening may not occur until just before labor begins. Though digestion remains sluggish, once your baby drops you will experience some relief from heartburn and constipation. Be sure to continue to drink plenty of water and to eat a diet rich with fiber to keep you as regular as possible. Other side effects to expect once your baby drops are increased hip, joint, and lower back pain. You will also need to urinate often—and urgently—as baby's head presses down on your bladder. No matter how many times you feel the urge to go—or how annoying it becomes—be sure to heed the call each time so you do not end up with a late-term urinary tract infection.

At the end of this week your baby will be considered full-term. This is very exciting, because it means that all of her body systems will be operational and able to function outside of your uterus. If your pregnancy is without complications and baby is born near the end of this week, she will have an excellent of survival. She will also have an excellent chance of boarding in-room with you without requiring special medical attention.

DAY 239: Date:___/___/___

MOM - WHAT'S HAPPENING:

This is your last week for childbirth classes, and you only have three weeks until your due date. As the big day approaches you are probably oscillating back and forth between, "Get this baby out of me!" and "I don't know how to care for a newborn." You may even see these thoughts turn up in your dreams. Pregnancy dreams are vivid and thematic. In fact, many women have been dreaming for months about the sex of their baby—without finding out from the doctor. Though this is not an accurate indication of baby's gender, anecdotal evidence indicates that many women dream it right.

BABY - WHAT'S HAPPENING:

Your baby is continuing to put on weight—approximately an ounce each day. She may gain a little length, as well, before she is born, though she is close to her birth height at this point. By now her head measures 3½ inches around, and the bones in her skull have not fused together to allow for compression through the birth canal.

TIPS AND ADVICE: Stretching the perineum area by massaging it may help you avoid an episiotomy. Make sure your hands are clean and that you have a large mirror to guide you. Lubricate your thumbs and first-fingers and the perineum with water-based lubricant and sit with your legs apart. Insert your thumbs into the back of your vagina and gently push down toward your rectum and out toward the sides. Hold each stretch for a minute. Next, gently move the skin along the back side of your vagina forward and hold for 3 to 4 minutes. Make sure to be very gentle and stop if you feel any pain.

DAILY JOURNAL

Mood:

Energy:

Cravings:

Symptoms:

Weight:

DAY 240: Date:___/___/___

MOM - WHAT'S HAPPENING:

Today you might be scheduling your last three visits to your doctor. At these appointments, your doctor will check your cervix to see how much it has softened— in fact, your cervix will soften over the next three weeks and end up feeling similar to a peeled kiwi. You will also be checked for dilation—you can be 2 or 3 centimeters dilated for weeks, days, or hours before labor begins, but it is a sign that your body is getting close. Effacement will also be checked. Once your cervix is soft, 10 centimeters dilated, and 100 percent effaced, you will be ready to push.

BABY - WHAT'S HAPPENING:

Your uterus is getting stretched pretty thin, which lets more light in. Whereas a few weeks ago baby was turning away from light, now he looks toward it. His curiosity is outgrowing his environment and anything new will grab his attention—light, music, voices, and new flavors will all add excitement.

TIPS AND ADVICE: If your baby is in the posterior position when labor begins (the back of his head pressing on your spine) you will probably experience back labor. Back labor is severe back pain that accompanies contractions and does not let up between them. If this happens, don't worry too much—only 15 percent of babies are posterior at the start of labor and many will turn around before it is time to push. Getting on your hands and knees, doing pelvic tilts, and having your partner massage your lower back can help ease the pain of back labor.

DAILY JOURNAL

Mood:

Energy:

Cravings:

Symptoms:

Weight:

DAY 241: Date:___/___/___

MOM - WHAT'S HAPPENING:

Your pregnancy breast size will peak around today. Because of their size, your nipples may become flat or inverted. If so, you will likely be visited by a lactation specialist after you give birth. He or she will fit you with a nipple shield and show you how to use it along with your baby's suction to pull your nipples back out. If you plan to purchase nursing bras before you deliver, it is recommended that you buy a size larger than you currently need, because your breasts will get even bigger once your milk comes in—which will happen within a few days to a week of having your baby.

BABY - WHAT'S HAPPENING:

Your baby's hair is longer and thicker now than it will be a few months after he is born. This is because newborns shed the hair that they are born with during the first couple of months. This means that baby's hair may change color or texture within his first few months of life.

FOR YOUR HEALTH: If you delivered your older child (or children) by Cesarean, it is still possible for you to have a vaginal birth this time. The possibility of a vaginal birth after Cesarean (VBAC) depends on why you had a Cesarean delivery, the placement of your incision, your baby's health, and your doctor's willingness. There is some risk of uterine rupture during labor and delivery, and this risk is increased to 24 out of 1,000 cases when labor is induced. Before deciding, first educate yourself and weigh the pros and cons of VBAC—though, ultimately, it is up to your doctor.

DAILY JOURNAL

Mood:

Energy:

Cravings:

Symptoms:

Weight:

DAY 242: Date:___/___/___

MOM - WHAT'S HAPPENING:

Today, discharge from your vagina might be slightly thicker and have more mucus and blood in it. Be aware of its consistency so you know the difference between normal secretions and that of amniotic fluid in the event that your bag of waters ruptures or develops a slow leak. You will also leak urine at the slightest cough, sneeze, or laugh because there is so much pressure on your bladder. Wear a panty liner to absorb this excess moisture. Be sure to change them often, and never use tampons or douches while pregnant, no matter how icky you feel.

BABY - WHAT'S HAPPENING:

Your baby is sinking lower into your pelvis at this point, hopefully head down. He is still breathing and swallowing amniotic fluid, which helps him get his lungs in shape for breathing air and his digestive tract ready for breast milk (or formula). His thumb-sucking is also useful in that it strengthens the face and throat muscles he will use to nurse.

PREGNANCY FACT: If baby's body is putting too much pressure on the umbilical cord it can decrease blood flow. Cord compression can be dangerous as it decreases the amount of oxygen that gets to baby. If this occurs during labor your doctor may have you moving around like a monkey in many different positions to try to get the baby to move off the cord. Since this usually happens close to when baby is about to be born, your doctor may decide that use of forceps or a vacuum extractor is necessary. He might also skip these and do a Cesarean if your baby is still too high for them to work.

DAILY JOURNAL

Mood:

Energy:

Cravings:

Symptoms:

Weight:

DAY 243: Date:___/___/___

MOM - WHAT'S HAPPENING:

Around now, your uterus is thinning out and the amniotic fluid level is decreasing. If you have started to dilate, you may occasionally feel sharp stabbing pains deep inside your vagina. Keep in mind that before your baby can be pushed out of your uterus, your cervix must open from zero to 10 centimeters. This can happen gradually, or very quickly once labor starts.

BABY - WHAT'S HAPPENING:

Around one out of 25 babies will be breech at this point. Your baby is considered breech if she is not presenting head first. There are three basic breech positions. One is frank breech—this is when baby's bottom is in the birth canal with his legs folded up against the front of his body. Another is complete breech—when the baby's buttocks are in the birth canal and his legs are folded under him with his feet flush against his bottom. Finally, there is footling breech—when one or both of baby's feet are positioned to come out first.

TIPS AND ADVICE: Talk to your doctor about getting forms that will allow you to pre-register at the hospital. Doing so can save you a lot of time and aggravation after true labor has started. Registering in advance gives the hospital bureaucracy time to process your basic information and make sure your insurance is in order. Your information will be given to the maternity ward, and they will be expecting you. Thus, once you go into labor you can just go right to the maternity floor and bypass the emergency room.

DAILY JOURNAL

Mood:

Energy:

Cravings:

Symptoms:

Weight:

DAY 244: Date:___/___/___

MOM - WHAT'S HAPPENING:

The waiting game is truly underway at this point, since you could go into labor at any time. To avoid having a stress-related meltdown, focus on your relaxation techniques. This will help you relax and also becomes invaluable as you labor. Practice some or all of the following throughout the day to keep anxiety as low as possible: progressive muscle relaxation, deep breathing, visualization, and meditation.

BABY - WHAT'S HAPPENING:

Your baby is still putting on weight, but more slowly. All his organs are mature and ready for life outside the womb. Baby has much less room to move around, so she is limited to side-to-side maneuvers. Her low position may be putting pressure on your perineum area, which can cause your rectum to ache and make it uncomfortable for you to empty your bowels. Baby is still building his first bowel movement, meconium, which will hopefully stay put until after he is born.

TIPS AND ADVICE: Early labor is when the cervical opening goes from 0 to 3 centimeters. Contractions during early labor usually last between 30 and 60 seconds and come between 5 and 20 minutes apart. This phase of labor usually lasts the longest and is the least painful, so you may want to stay home to do your early labor for this part. You will be more comfortable and have more freedom. In fact, many hospitals will send you home and tell you to come back once contractions are coming more frequently and with more intensity.

DAILY JOURNAL

Mood:

Energy:

Cravings:

Symptoms:

Weight:

DAY 245: Date:___/___/___

MOM - WHAT'S HAPPENING:

Today might be your last day at work. Indeed, many women call it quits two weeks before their due date. This gives them two weeks of time around their house to get the nursery ready. Some begin work on a scrapbook for baby's first year of life. Just be sure that you have something to occupy your mind during the next two weeks, or you may go crazy wondering if every twitch and Braxton Hicks contraction is going to kick you into labor.

BABY - WHAT'S HAPPENING:

By now baby weighs about 7 pounds and is as long as 19½ inches. Your baby is passing time by sucking her thumb and looking around at your pelvis. She follows rays of light that are filtered into your thinning uterus, and practices her breathing. Though she is considered full-term at this point it will be beneficial for her to stay in your womb a little longer unless there is evidence of fetal distress.

PREGNANCY FACT: Once true labor starts, your body may excrete a number of bodily fluids. You may have diarrhea and feel the urge to urinate frequently. If your amniotic sac ruptures, you will feel a rush of warm fluid run down your legs. During the transition stage of labor—just before pushing—many women vomit. And as you are pushing it is not uncommon to defecate. Rest assured that you will be so consumed with what you are doing that you will care less about this at the time. And plus, the medical staff sees this every day and is prepared to clean it up before you even know what happened.

DAILY JOURNAL

Mood:

Energy:

Cravings:

Symptoms:

Weight:

Week 36

Starting Weight: ________

OVERVIEW

Congratulations! Your baby is now considered full-term. You now have no need to be concerned if you go into labor before your due date. You will definitely see your doctor this week for a checkup. At this appointment, you can expect an internal exam to determine if you are dilated and if effacement has begun. If your doctor detects problems with you or baby's health, she may schedule a Cesarean section or induction. After all, at this point all of your baby's organs are fully developed, functional, and ready for life on the outside.

Since all of baby's major development is complete you are basically just playing the waiting game until you go into labor. While you wait you can expect to alternate between feeling energetic—with the nesting instinct in full swing—to exhausted and overwhelmed. The best way to deal with these mood swings is to simply go with them. When you feel the urge to busy yourself with projects, go for it. And when you are tired and just want to veg out with your feet up—do it. You may even let yourself slip from your healthy pregnancy diet and treat yourself to take-out, as you are probably much too frazzled to cook every night. However, this is definitely not the time to indulge in any unhealthy vices, such as alcohol consumption, drug use, or smoking cigarettes. Though baby's development is complete, she is still vulnerable to whatever you consume.

DAY 246: Date:___/___/___

MOM - WHAT'S HAPPENING:

Today, take some time to monitor your swelling. It is not unusual for your ankles and wrists to swell a bit more than usual during the day, though it should subside in the evening when you are able to put your feet up and rest. If, however, you suddenly gain a few pounds or your hands and face become puffy, your vision becomes blurred, or you suffer from severe headaches, call your doctor. You may have developed preeclampsia. If such a condition develops at this point in your pregnancy your doctor will want to delivery your baby immediately either via induction or Cesarean.

BABY - WHAT'S HAPPENING:

By now, your baby's head, shoulders, and abdomen all measure the same around. What this means for you is that delivery of baby's upper body, which presents first, will be the most difficult. Once baby's shoulders make it through the birth canal, it is smooth sailing for the rest of his body.

FOR YOUR HEALTH: As the big day approaches, sit down with your partner to discuss his role as the support person when you go into labor. Hopefully, you both learned a lot in your childbirth class, but it can help to talk it out so that you feel more prepared. In general, your partner should be prepared to offer emotional support and reassure you that you are doing great; he should be your coach and remind you how and when to employ breathing techniques. He is also responsible for timing your contractions and should be familiar with how to touch you to help you relax.

DAILY JOURNAL

Mood:

Energy:

Cravings:

Symptoms:

Weight:

DAY 247: Date:___/___/___

MOM - WHAT'S HAPPENING:

If you haven't already done so, stop working. Going to work this late in your pregnancy is not advised. For one, you are probably not getting much sleep, which makes the workday drag by. Secondly, you need as many hours a day as possible to both catch up on needed rest and loose ends. In fact, it is a great idea to spend from now until delivery day work-free, because soon your life will become busier than you ever could have imagined.

BABY - WHAT'S HAPPENING:

You may find that baby's movements seem muted, but as long as you continue to feel something several times an hour, you should not worry. However, if you ever notice a decrease in fetal movement, call your doctor. He will ask you to come in and hook you up to a fetal heart monitor. He also may want to do an ultrasound. He may ask you to drink a glass of juice or eat a cookie beforehand to stimulate baby.

TIPS AND ADVICE: Your partner may not volunteer to share his fears about fatherhood because he is trying to stay calm for you. But you should ask about his feelings because, as your due date approaches, he is probably becoming progressively more nervous. He may be afraid for you and your baby's safety in labor and delivery, or concerned about finances. He is likely terrified that he will be a bad father. He may be afraid of what he will see during delivery or how you will respond to him during labor. And finally, he may be sad to see your time as "just us" come to an end.

DAILY JOURNAL

Mood:

Energy:

Cravings:

Symptoms:

Weight:

DAY 248: Date:___/___/___

MOM - WHAT'S HAPPENING:

The contractions you have been experiencing may intensify a bit today. However, they should continue to be irregular. Contractions may even become painful at this point but should be low in the abdomen and lower back. Contractions that indicate true labor start at the top of the fundus and roll downward. If you start to feel this sensation, call your doctor.

BABY - WHAT'S HAPPENING:

Your baby's brain is ready to take the job of regulating his temperature, digestion, and heartbeat outside of the womb. His brain will continue to develop throughout his childhood and into his teen years, so keeping up good nutrition will continue to be as important after he is born as it was for the nine months you housed him in your womb.

TIPS AND ADVICE: Slow, deep breathing is an effective way to become grounded and more relaxed between contractions. To practice this method, breathe in deeply through your nose while counting to 10. Hold for a few seconds, and then exhale for a 10 count. Try to expel every bit of breath from your lungs. Practice deep breathing several times daily so that you are able to easily fall into a pattern once true labor starts. You should also feel free to abandon this technique once it is no longer helpful.

DAILY JOURNAL

Mood:

Energy:

Cravings:

Symptoms:

Weight:

DAY 249: Date:___/___/___

MOM - WHAT'S HAPPENING:

Though you may be feeling incredibly unsexy, make time for intimacy with your partner today. It may be a long time after baby is born before you have the time and interest to do so. If your pregnancy is without complications and your doctor has not told you to avoid sex and orgasms—go for it. You will have to be creative in positioning but, at this point, the most comfortable positions tend to be spooning, mom on top, and mom on her hands and knees. These positions allow you to control the depth of penetration and completely avoid putting pressure on your belly.

BABY - WHAT'S HAPPENING:

If your doctor has told you it is OK to have sex, you may be concerned about how having an orgasm affects baby. When you orgasm, your baby feels something similar to the Braxton Hicks contractions she's used to by now. Also, there is little risk for orgasm kicking off labor if your pregnancy has been normal and uncomplicated.

TIPS AND ADVICE: When you are in the midst of a contraction it can be helpful to focus on what is called paced breathing. This very specific breathing technique can help you stay focused on maintaining the breathing pattern and not on your pain. To do paced breathing, practice thinking "hah" on the inhale and "hee" when you exhale. It should be shallow and fairly quickly, and go as follows: "Hah (in), hee (out); hah (in), hee (out)." Do this for as long as the contraction lasts. As with slow, deep breathing, feel free to abandon this method when it no longer benefits you.

DAILY JOURNAL

Mood:

Energy:

Cravings:

Symptoms:

Weight:

DAY 250: Date:___/___/___

MOM - WHAT'S HAPPENING:

If your baby is low in your pelvis, she is likely pressing on nerves that run from your vagina down your legs. This can feel as though there are tiny electrodes zapping up and down your legs. Unfortunately, there is little to be done for this but to deliver your baby. If you are experiencing this sensation, you may also be having some trouble with sciatica, which causes numbness in your leg or foot.

BABY - WHAT'S HAPPENING:

Most of the lanugo and vernix that covered baby has sloughed off inside the amniotic fluid. However, as mentioned earlier, both can still be seen on baby after he is born. These, plus cells that have been shed and other debris floating in the 4 to 5 cups of amniotic fluid left, are accumulating in baby's intestines as his first stool.

PREGNANCY FACT: The station is determined by figuring out the relationship between baby's presenting part—usually the head—to the spines of your pelvic bones. When doing a vaginal exam, your doctor will be able to feel two bones that stick out, called the ischial spines. If baby's head is flush with the ischial spines his station is 0, and he is ready for birth. If he is above this marker his station is negative, such as -2, and if he is below it the number is positive, such as +2, which indicates baby is close to being born. His crowning number (head visible outside of your vagina) is +5.

DAILY JOURNAL

Mood:

Energy:

Cravings:

Symptoms:

Weight:

DAY 251: Date:___/___/___

MOM - WHAT'S HAPPENING:

If your baby still has not dropped you are probably finding it increasingly difficult to breathe. Make sure to take it slow when you go up stairs, or if you have to lift groceries or an older child. Use pillows to prop you up when you sleep or consider spending the remainder of your pregnant nights sleeping upright in a recliner. This will reduce pressure on your lungs and make it easier for you to feel like you are getting a good breath. It is possible that your baby will not drop until labor starts, so just remind yourself, "Any day now!"

BABY - WHAT'S HAPPENING:

Your baby continues to practice breathing and her lungs are producing more surfactant, which allows her lungs to inflate and prevents them from sticking together when she exhales. Because her lungs have matured enough for her to breathe on her own outside of the womb if she was born today she would likely not require any medical care beyond routine cleaning and testing.

TIPS AND ADVICE: If you're home from work and resting these days, find ways to stay busy that don't involve housework or alphabetizing your bookshelves. Sign up for a service like Netflix, which delivers DVDs to your home or streams them instantly to your computer. Or, join a book swap, where you can read and exchange books with other members for a small shipping fee. Books and movies can help you put your feet up, relax, and even fall asleep. You won't have time for these extras after your baby is born, so kick back now while you can.

DAILY JOURNAL

Mood:

Energy:

Cravings:

Symptoms:

Weight:

DAY 252: Date:___/___/___

MOM - WHAT'S HAPPENING:

Around now you have hit your maximum weight gain, somewhere between 25 and 35 pounds. You probably haven't seen much of a change in your measurements lately, and you may even lose a few pounds before baby comes. Your emotions are probably all over the map, but you are definitely ready to have your baby and be done with pregnancy at this point. Many women report that they start dreaming about going into labor and wake up excited, only to find that it was just a dream.

BABY - WHAT'S HAPPENING:

Your baby may be having more frequent bouts of hiccups as he swallows increasing amounts of amniotic fluid. This will feel funny to you—as if your baby is bopping up and down at regular intervals. There is nothing to be worried about as your baby cannot be harmed by frequent hiccups. Once he is born, you and your partner will get a good laugh from seeing how surprised baby is at these bouts of hiccups.

FOR YOUR HEALTH: Bleeding in these late weeks can be completely normal and is a result of minor injury to the cervix. This type of bleeding is usually light. It is pink or red and streaked through normal discharge. It generally occurs after intercourse or a vaginal exam and is not cause for concern. However, if you have bright red spotting or heavy bleeding, there may be an issue with your placenta, which will require immediate medical intervention. And finally, any bleeding along with contractions may indicate labor has begun, and you should call your doctor.

DAILY JOURNAL

Mood:

Energy:

Cravings:

Symptoms:

Weight:

Lunar Month

Ten

PHOTO

Place a photo of you during
your tenth month here

My Monthly Update

Waist Measurement: ____________

Weight: ____________

Mood: ____________

PREGNANCY CHECKLIST

- ❑ Talk to your doctor about your options if you are overdue

MY PERSONAL CHECKLIST:

- ❑ ....
- ❑ ....
- ❑ ....
- ❑ ....
- ❑ ....
- ❑ ....
- ❑ ....
- ❑ ....

MY HOPES FOR THIS MONTH:

....

....

....

....

....

....

....

....

....

....

....

....

....

....

....

Lunar Month Ten

Third Trimester

LUNAR MONTH 10 IS DIFFERENT from the other months in that it usually only deals with the first two weeks of the month. These are an exciting two weeks, though, because so much happens, including the birth of your baby! It is important to note that only 5 percent of babies are actually born on their due dates, so there is a possibility that you will still be pregnant even after you finish reading this book. When you feel as though you cannot stand to be pregnant for another day, remind yourself that you are finally at the point where you can see the light at the end of the tunnel. That light is your sweet, little baby!

WHAT TO EXPECT THIS MONTH

This month you can expect an increase in Braxton Hicks contractions. They will happen more often, become progressively painful, and feel somewhat like menstrual cramps. They will last longer than in previous months. However, they should still be irregular and manageable. Once true labor begins, your contractions will change and be less localized. They will start at the top of your uterus and roll down through to your pelvis. These will also cause quite a bit of lower back pain and will come at regular intervals that get closer together.

You can also expect to see an increase in vaginal discharge as your cervix softens and the mucus plug is either shed in layers or is completely dislodged. You will see some brownish blood mixed in, which is not cause for concern—though you will probably look to every change as a sign that labor has started. As your general state of being escalates into this heightened awareness, you can expect to feel anxious, irritable, and impatient.

THINGS TO CONSIDER

At the start of this month you should have a birth plan in place with copies in your hospital bag handy to give to your doctor and the nursing staff. The car should be gassed up and ready to go. Your family and friends should be ready to receive "the call," because you can go into labor at any time. To pass the time, keep the house clean and make sure you have plenty of clean towels, clothes, and a well-stocked refrigerator and freezer. This will make your return from the hospital much more pleasant.

TIPS FOR COPING

The biggest favor that you can do for yourself at this point is to keep busy and rest. This many sound like conflicting advice, but it is not. Keep busy by reading, watching movies, having friends over for chats, organizing the baby's room or working on your pregnancy scrapbook. Keeping your mind off the Big Question: "When will I go into labor?" will help you maintain your sanity (and your partner's). Doing nothing but obsessing on the Big Question will not hasten labor and will only make you anxious and tense.

At the same time, you should get as much rest as possible. Nap, take baths, put your feet up, and go to bed early. You will want to be well-rested and energized for the long haul of labor and delivery.

Keep in mind that you will probably never experience anything that is so physically demanding as giving birth to your baby—so prepare by taking good care of yourself.

WHAT TO EAT

At this point, most women have very little appetite thanks to increasing nerves and anxiety. Still, you should be sure to continue to eat several small meals daily. Keep eating foods that are nutritious and high in calcium. If your stomach is unsettled, stick to bland foods, such as rice, pasta, and whole grain bread and cereal. Oatmeal is a wonderful and healthy way to consume calories and minimize the consequences of feeding an upset stomach.

HOW MUCH WEIGHT TO GAIN

You may not gain any weight at all this month and, in fact, you will probably lose a pound or two since your appetite has decreased. However, if your appetite remains intact, or you are a nervous eater, you should not gain more than 1 pound before your baby is born. If you do notice that you suddenly gain a few pounds and that your hands and face are puffy, call your doctor immediately, because this could be a sign that you have developed pregnancy-induced hypertension. In that case, your doctor may recommend that you be induced or that you have a Cesarean birth within the next day or two.

EXERCISE TIPS AND ADVICE

Unless your doctor has restricted your activity level, there is no reason that you cannot continue to swim or go for walks. Other activities are up to your common sense, but you should be careful because you are easily put off-balance and your joints are looser than ever. You should continue to do Kegel exercises, and you may want add daily squats to your routine, as they can help open up your pelvis in preparation for baby's delivery.

POTENTIAL SYMPTOMS AND HOW TO ALLEVIATE THEM

With intensified contractions, it is a good idea to practice the breathing techniques you learned in your childbirth class. To manage the general aches and pains, continue to take warm baths or ask your partner to give you a massage each night before bed. This can help relax you enough to actually get a few hours of sleep, since uninterrupted sleep has likely become a distant memory.

You can also expect to have to urinate frequently and urgently. The only way to really manage this problem is to go when nature calls. You can limit what you drink before bed, but you should not cut back your daily water intake as you need to stay hydrated. If your baby has dropped, you can expect to have an easier time breathing, which may be enough of a relief to make you care less about the other symptoms. But perhaps the most helpful thing to do these days is to remind yourself that you are almost there! Once your baby is born, the symptoms you have endured for the past 10 months will disappear.

WAYS OTHERS CAN HELP

This is your partner's month to shine. There are so many ways for him to be of assistance to you, but you must let him know what you need. Your partner can help ease your aches and pains by giving you daily massages and by taking on the majority of the housework. He should make sure the details of the household are taken care of when you are at the hospital. These include arrangements for pet care, childcare for older children, and arranging for a friend or family member to pick up your mail.

But perhaps the most important role he will play is that of your cheering section during labor and delivery. This month, your partner will get to step into the role he's been training for the past 10 months—labor coach. Once you go into labor, he will be responsible for reminding you of your breathing techniques, timing your contractions, keeping you on task, encouraging you to keep going, having labor tools handy, and running inference with visitors and medical staff.

As for friends and family, it is important that you make your wishes known to them beforehand. Many women don't mind visitors in the hospital at first but quickly become overwhelmed and need a break. Thus, it will be up to your partner to notify everyone when you are up for receiving visitors and when visiting hours are over. It is recommended that you shut off the phone and close your door to visitors for the first few days after baby is home so you can bond as a family.

Another way friends and family can help is by bringing your family food once you are home. A "food calendar" is a great way to do this. Have close family and friends sign up to bring your family one meal a day in the two weeks following the birth. With people in your community helping just one night, you can have hot, nutritious meals brought to you continuously as you settle into being a family. Not having to think about what you will eat will allow you to focus on the most important task: welcoming your new baby home!

Notes . . . .

"Having a baby is like falling in love again, both with your husband and your child."

~ Tina Brown

Week 37

Starting Weight: _________

OVERVIEW

As you get closer to your due date, less will happening with your baby physically on a daily basis. His organ development is complete at this point, except for his brain and lungs, which will continue to develop even after he is born. However, you can expect graduated changes to your cervix, such as softening, dilation, and the percentage of effacement. Some women will find they are 1-centimeter dilated with 0-percent effacement this week. But this varies and the numbers are very individualized so there is no hard and fast rule for how the cervix responds to the prostaglandins—hormones that soften the cervix and stimulate contractions—that are released by your body in preparation for labor.

As you emotionally prepare for labor, you may find that you are irritable one minute and overcome with anticipation and joy the next. This is to be expected. Also, your moods will not stabilize for some time until your body recovers from childbirth and your hormones are reset. Be sure to include your partner in your thought processes and to give him an ear as well, since he is probably facing many of the same—and some very different—fears and hopes. Something to discuss this week is what you expect from your partner during labor and delivery. You should also have several plans in place for when you go into labor based on you and your partner's location at the time it starts.

DAY 253: Date:___/___/___

MOM - WHAT'S HAPPENING:

As your baby makes room in your pelvis and your body continues to prepare for labor you can expect to feel achy all over your body. This is due to the softening of the cartilage throughout your body. Your cartilage softens in order to allow your pelvis to expand to let your baby through. The average woman's pelvis expands between 1 and 1½ centimeters. As this happens, your hips, spine, vagina, and legs will ache and feel stressed. But fortunately, you are almost there!

BABY - WHAT'S HAPPENING:

Your baby is just over 7 pounds now and may be up to 20 inches long. She has very little room in which to move. Most of her attempts will feel more like prodding than kicking. At this point, baby should be presenting head-first and sitting low in your pelvis. Do not be concerned if lightening has not yet occurred. It may not happen for you until labor begins.

FOOD FOR THOUGHT: After your baby is born, stick to a healthy diet. If you are breast-feeding, your caloric intake should be increased between 500 and 600 calories per day (from your pre-pregnancy diet), putting your total calorie intake around 2,900 to 3,000 calories per day. You can also expect to feel thirsty often, so make sure to drink at least eight glasses of water a day. Continue to take your prenatal vitamins and remember that many medications—including those sold over the counter—will still be off limits since baby will ingest them through your breast milk.

DAILY JOURNAL

Mood:

Energy:

Cravings:

Symptoms:

Weight:

DAY 254: Date:___/___/___

MOM - WHAT'S HAPPENING:

Your body is releasing prostaglandin hormones to soften your cervix. This can take a few days or weeks and makes it possible for effacement (thinning) to begin. Consider that your cervix in its normal state is 1½ to 2 inches long. Before your baby can pass through, however, it must stretch out to be as thin as a single sheet of paper—this process is effacement, and your doctor will check for this at each prenatal visit from now on. If there are no changes to your cervix, you will be 0-percent effaced. When you are ready to have your baby you will be 100-percent effaced.

BABY - WHAT'S HAPPENING:

Your baby continues to put on layers of fat and will do so until he is born. He is putting on both white and brown fat. Brown fat is deposited in the area between his shoulder blades and as a protective layer around his organs. Brown fat is heat generating and will help keep your baby warm as he adjusts to the temperature of the outside world.

PREGNANCY FACT: If you are just dying for your doctor to make an educated guess about when you will go into labor, ask him for your Bishop score. Your Bishop score is based on cervical dilation and effacement, which is given a score between 0 and 3; the station of your baby's presenting body part, which is scored from 0 to 3; and the level of softening and the position of your cervix, which is given a score from 0 to 2. If your Bishop score is 6 or higher and your cervix has thinned to 26 millimeters or less, you are likely to go into labor within the next week.

DAILY JOURNAL

Mood:

Energy:

Cravings:

Symptoms:

Weight:

DAY 255: Date:___/___/___

MOM - WHAT'S HAPPENING:

It may be hard to believe but your uterus weighs 20 times more than it did before you were pregnant. Indeed, what started out the size of a small pear is now more like the size of a large piece of sports equipment. Being aware of how much your body has stretched itself probably helps you understand better some of your symptoms, such as feeling as though your internal organs are going to drop through your body onto the floor.

BABY - WHAT'S HAPPENING:

Your baby's lungs have increased production of surfactant, which is great news, because babies who are born with insufficient pulmonary surfactant will have Infant Respiratory Distress Syndrome (IRDS). This occurs when the alveoli (branches of the lung that processes oxygen and carbon dioxide) collapse, leaving your baby unable to breathe on his own. IRDS usually affects premature babies, but can afflict full-term babies who lack adequate surfactant production.

FOR YOUR HEALTH: If your Group B strep (GBS) test came back positive, you should remind your doctor so that he or she gives you the necessary antibiotic treatment. It is extremely important to prevent transmission of GBS to your baby as she passes through the birth canal. If your baby contracts GBS at birth, she will be susceptible to sepsis, pneumonia, and meningitis. And since penicillin is the treatment used most often for GBS, make sure to let everyone who attends to you in the hospital know if you are allergic.

DAILY JOURNAL

Mood:

Energy:

Cravings:

Symptoms:

Weight:

DAY 256: Date:___/___/___

MOM - WHAT'S HAPPENING:

Though today you may be tempted to try anything to get labor started, let nature take its course. After all, your body knows best when it is time to push your baby out into the world. That said, there are many alleged natural ways to induce your own labor, such as nipple stimulation, frequent orgasms, and going for long walks. There is little evidence to support that any of these actually affect the timing of when labor starts, and the safety of doing any of these in excess is debatable. You are better off just letting your body decide on its own when it is time.

BABY - WHAT'S HAPPENING:

At this point your baby has lost her pink hue and is very light-skinned and pale. This is true for dark-skinned babies as well, who will develop dark skin pigmentation shortly after they are born. The pink color baby had up until this point has been whitened by a thick layer of fat that covers blood cells and makes her skin opaque.

FOOD FOR THOUGHT: There are several old wives tales regarding eating and drinking certain things to hasten labor. These include drinking raspberry leaf tea and castor oil. Though you are probably willing to try just about anything, you should avoid ingesting these substances. Neither will not start labor, but they can cause a host of intestinal problems, such as cramping, diarrhea, gas, and vomiting. Some women claim that eating spicy foods helps to induce labor, though you may run into many of the same problems, including heartburn and indigestion.

DAILY JOURNAL

Mood:

Energy:

Cravings:

Symptoms:

Weight:

DAY 257: Date:___/___/___

MOM - WHAT'S HAPPENING:

As your baby sinks lower and your hips spread apart, you may find that you are becoming increasingly clumsy. You are probably dropping keys, glasses, and anything else that you hold, as the pressure on the nerves in your wrists weakens your grip. It is likely that your knees and shins are bruised from repeatedly walking into the coffee table. Clumsiness is just a part of who you are for the next week or so—rest assured that you will return to your coordinated self soon after baby is born.

BABY - WHAT'S HAPPENING:

At this point, the placenta weighs in at about 1½ pounds and the umbilical cord is more than 2 feet long. Your baby is just about 20 inches long, maybe more. As you can see, your uterus is becoming a very crowded place to be. Thus, your baby does not have much room left to maneuver and is getting as ready as you are to be out in the world.

PREGNANCY FACT: If your doctor suspects a problem with your baby's health, he may bring you in for a biophysical profile (BPP) test. This combines the non-stress test with an ultrasound. It is noninvasive and safe. BPP lasts about 35 to 45 minutes and looks for evidence of baby's breathing, at least two movements, active flexing of at least one limb, increase in heartbeat in reaction to stimuli, and measures level and distribution of amniotic fluid. Your baby is given an overall score, and your doctor will decide if you should be induced or have a Cesarean delivery rather than labor naturally.

DAILY JOURNAL

Mood:

Energy:

Cravings:

Symptoms:

Weight:

DAY 258: Date:___/___/___

MOM - WHAT'S HAPPENING:

You may be feeling hungrier today than you have felt in a while. This is because as your baby drops, he puts less pressure on your organs, including your stomach. If this is the case, don't overeat or indulge in greasy foods. If you happen to go into labor after bingeing, you will very quickly become nauseous—you may also end up with diarrhea and vomiting. When you are choosing your meals at this point you may want to consider how it will feel sitting in your stomach if labor starts.

BABY - WHAT'S HAPPENING:

Approximately 30 percent of babies void their bowels before they are born. This will be evidenced in your amniotic fluid—if baby has passed meconium while in utero, the fluid will look green. This can cause pneumonia or other breathing problems for baby, so if you notice a green liquid discharge be sure to let your doctor know, as babies who move their bowels in utero are often in some kind of distress and may be delivered early.

TIPS AND ADVICE: As you wait for labor to begin, do squats several times a day. Steady yourself by either holding on to a sturdy chair or leaning your back against a wall. Keep your back straight as a board and squat down with your knees spread apart. This helps open up your pelvis, which is good practice for when you are in labor. This position can bring you some relief from the pain of labor and facilitate baby's descent into the birth canal. Soon, your baby will be ready to get pushed out of your womb and into your arms.

DAILY JOURNAL

Mood:

Energy:

Cravings:

Symptoms:

Weight:

DAY 259: Date:___/___/___

MOM - WHAT'S HAPPENING:

You have just completed the next to last week before your due date! You are probably feeling crabby and ready to have your baby out of your body and cradled in your arms. At this stage, just getting through the day can be an exercise, since your weight and loosening joints are causing you to have constant back, pelvic, and hip pain. Now is the time to treat yourself to frequent warm baths and to extended periods of rest with your feet up, which will help take the edge off your aches and pains.

BABY - WHAT'S HAPPENING:

Your baby is about 7½ pounds at this point. She may gain up to another ½ pound before she is born, depending on how much longer she remains in utero. She has shed most of the lanugo and vernix that was coating her body, and her skin is markedly less wrinkled than just four weeks ago.

TIPS AND ADVICE: There are several ways to make your Cesarean delivery more personal and feel less "surgical." Bring in your own music, ask for a mirror to be placed so that you may see when baby is delivered, or ask that the screen be let down at that moment. Request that your partner be allowed to cut the cord and insist that you want to hold your baby before she is taken to be cleaned. You may also make it known that you want to breast-feed while you are in recovery and that you want your baby with you as much as is feasible.

DAILY JOURNAL

Mood:

Energy:

Cravings:

Symptoms:

Weight:

Week 38

Starting Weight: _________

OVERVIEW

Welcome to your last week of pregnancy. This week you can expect to go into labor and have your baby! Once labor begins you will experience mild contractions that last between 25 to 45 seconds and come at 5- to 15-minute intervals. These should feel like moderate menstrual cramps accompanied by tightening in your lower abdomen. Your amniotic sac may or may not rupture, but if it does, be sure to head to the hospital and call your doctor on the way. When early labor starts, it is important to stay calm and to rest as much as possible. Although this is the longest stage—lasting between 7 and 8 hours, on average—it is the least demanding. You will want to save the majority of your energy and stamina for the later portions of labor.

While you still have a few days at home, review your birth plan and make sure you have several copies on hand. You should also have your partner gas up the car and have your hospital bag ready to go. It is also smart to make a phone tree for when the baby is born. This is a small group of people who can call the rest of the community when the baby is born, rather than you and your partner calling everyone individually. Select three or four people in your immediate circle and get them each a list of phone numbers of people you'd like alerted to the fact that you have just had a very healthy boy or girl!

DAY 260: Date:___/___/___

MOM - WHAT'S HAPPENING:

You may be concerned that your water will break while you are out at the grocery store or getting the newspaper. But the fact is only 15 percent of women experience the rupture of the amniotic sac before labor starts. So, odds are against it! However, if it will make you feel better, you can wear overnight-size sanitary pads just in case. It is much more common for women to "spring a leak" than to have a complete rupture, as it is often portrayed in the movies.

BABY - WHAT'S HAPPENING:

At this point, your baby's bones are much harder than they were just 3 weeks ago. However, her skull remains soft so that her head will be able to compress to fit through the birth canal. If you have a vaginal delivery, don't be surprised if your baby's head is somewhat cone-shaped for awhile.

FOR YOUR HEALTH: Your doctor will likely bring you in this week to do an ultrasound that will determine your amniotic fluid index (AFI). He will be looking for four pockets of fluid that cushion your baby. Each pocket will be measured for its depth and the four scores will be added up. For instance, if each pocket is 3 centimeters deep, your AFI score will be 12—which is the average. Normal scores range from 8 to 18. If you fall above or below this range, your doctor will probably discuss doing an induction or Cesarean delivery within the next couple of days.

DAILY JOURNAL

Mood:

Energy:

Cravings:

Symptoms:

Weight:

DAY 261: Date:___/___/___

MOM - WHAT'S HAPPENING:

At your prenatal appointment this week, you will likely have a non-stress test to see how baby is doing. You will be assigned an AFI score and will also be given a biophysical profile score to try to determine how close you are to labor. If there is any sign of fetal distress your doctor will discuss induction or Cesarean delivery. And if both you and baby are doing fine, he will discuss the possibility of letting you go past your due date.

BABY - WHAT'S HAPPENING:

Your baby's head size is holding steady at a diameter of 4 inches, so your cervix must dilate to 10 centimeters in order for baby to fit through the birth canal. If your baby's head grows any larger before you give birth, you are likely to have some tearing in the perinea area or will likely end up having an episiotomy. If your baby is measuring larger at this point, your doctor may try to encourage you to be induced to avoid further growth.

PREGNANCY FACT: If you are scheduled for a Cesarean section, you may be wondering what to expect during recovery. Most women are surprised how quickly the Cesarean delivery goes—usually about 1½ hours from epidural to stitching. Afterward, you can expect to feel shaky, tingly, and chilly as the drugs wear off. You will be sore around your incision, and probably slightly nauseous. You will feel exhausted and you should sleep as much as you can. You will be monitored closely for the first 24 hours and be up on your feet within eight hours of the surgery.

DAILY JOURNAL

Mood:

Energy:

Cravings:

Symptoms:

Weight:

DAY 262: Date:___/___/___

MOM - WHAT'S HAPPENING:

You might be wondering if you will actually give birth on your due date. You probably will not—only 5 percent of babies are actually born on their due dates. This means that 95 percent of births occur in the 2 weeks preceding and the 2 weeks after their projected due date. A pregnant woman is not considered overdue until she is 40 lunar weeks pregnant because of the margin of error involved in calculating due dates.

BABY - WHAT'S HAPPENING:

Your baby is nestling further into your pelvis with his legs running up the length of his body—his toes are near his forehead and his knees press against his mouth or nose. This may sound uncomfortable, but baby is used to his cramped quarters by now. His movements are limited to side to side maneuvers that may create a rolling sensation for you.

PREGNANCY FACT: Before your baby is born, his lungs are flat and his body must work extra hard to get blood to circulate through them. Once he is born, though, and the umbilical cord is cut, his body immediately craves oxygen, which causes his lungs to inflate (thanks to all that surfactant!). Baby takes his first breath out of reflex and necessity. Once his lungs are inflated, the flow in the left side of your baby's heart strengthens and his circulation increases. His lungs will continue to develop through his infancy.

DAILY JOURNAL

Mood:

Energy:

Cravings:

Symptoms:

Weight:

DAY 263: Date:___/___/___

MOM - WHAT'S HAPPENING:

Around now Braxton Hicks contractions may start to become painful. As long as true labor has not yet begun, these contractions will stay low and may radiate out to your lower back. Baby responds by either becoming perfectly still or by pushing outward during a contraction.

BABY - WHAT'S HAPPENING:

The average baby at this point weighs between 7 and 9 pounds and is between 19½ and 21 inches long. You do not want your baby to grow bigger than this, because that will make vaginal delivery very difficult. Therefore, your doctor will carefully measure baby's size this week so that you both may decide if induction is necessary. Interestingly, according to the Guiness Book of World Records, the largest baby ever born weighed 22 pounds and was 28 inches long. The baby only lived for two hours. Other large-birth babies—such as one born in Brazil in 2005, who weighed almost 17 pounds—have survived and thrived.

PREGNANCY FACT: Early labor may begin any time now. It is the longest and least-demanding phase, so be sure to rest as much as possible. You will know you are in early labor when you start having contractions every 5 to 15 minutes that last between 25 and 45 seconds. You should call your doctor to let him know, but you may not have to rush to the hospital just yet, as this stage lasts, on average, 7 or 8 hours. During this time, your cervix will open from 0 to 3 centimeters.

DAILY JOURNAL

Mood:

Energy:

Cravings:

Symptoms:

Weight:

DAY 264: Date:___/___/___

MOM - WHAT'S HAPPENING:

Today you might see an increase in vaginal discharge, and it will be slightly thicker and streaked with mucus. This is normal and means your cervix is doing its job preparing for labor by softening, which causes the protective mucus to be shed. You may lose it all in one drop in the toilet, so don't be shocked if you find your mucus plug comes out the next time you use the bathroom. Some blood streaks are normal, but bright red spotting or a constant flow should be immediately reported to your doctor.

BABY - WHAT'S HAPPENING:

The quality of your baby's movements has changed as a result of having run out of room in your uterus. As long as you feel her squirming or pushing with regularity, you should not be overly concerned. It is also worth noting that the umbilical cord is so full of blood that it should be firm enough to prevent tangling with baby's limbs, even in these very tight quarters.

PREGNANCY FACT: Once active labor begins you should be either on your way to the hospital or already there. Contractions become quite painful, are 3 to 4 minutes apart, and last between 40 and 60 seconds for 1 to 4 hours. During active labor, your cervix dilates from 4 centimeters to 7 centimeters. If you decide to have an epidural, this is the window in which to have it. Most doctors will not administer pain medication once the cervix is dilated to 7 centimeters, because of the effects pain medication can have on pushing and the delivery process.

DAILY JOURNAL

Mood:

Energy:

Cravings:

Symptoms:

Weight:

DAY 265: Date:___/___/___

MOM - WHAT'S HAPPENING:

You probably have very little appetite because you are so anxious to deliver your baby and nervous about labor. Try to eat small, nutritious meals, though, because you will need to keep your energy up for labor. Your anxiety level and loss of appetite may be kicking up stomach acids, which will increase heartburn. If you absolutely cannot stomach a full meal, be sure to at least nibble on toast or crackers to help absorb excess stomach acids.

BABY - WHAT'S HAPPENING:

Baby is ready to go! She is now engaged and her presenting part is really bearing down on your pelvis. She is putting a lot of pressure on your perineum, which can cause you to feel like she is going to fall out any minute. Some women even become afraid to take baths or use the toilet, but there are many stop-gaps in place that will prevent baby from just falling out. If pressure is followed by a tightening sensation that is accompanied by cramps, you could be in labor!

PREGNANCY FACT: The transition period of labor can last from ½ to 2½ hours and is usually the most painful part of labor. During transition, your cervix completes its dilation from 7 to 10 centimeters. At this point, you will be ready to push. Contractions during this labor phase come every 1 to 2 minutes and last for 60 to 90 seconds. Your partner is very important during transition, because you will be so focused on what is happening that you will likely forget to breathe and may want to push prematurely.

DAILY JOURNAL

Mood:

Energy:

Cravings:

Symptoms:

Weight:

DAY 266: Date:___/___/___

MOM - WHAT'S HAPPENING:

You have arrived at your official due date. Congratulations! You may not have your baby today, but soon. At this point you are just waiting for a sign that labor has begun—so be sure to pay attention to the quality of your contractions. Are they coming at regular intervals? Do they start at the top of the fundus and roll downward? Are they increasing in intensity? If you have decided to do early labor at home, be sure you have lots of magazines, movies, and light snacks on hand. And get rest—you are going to need your energy!

BABY - WHAT'S HAPPENING:

By now, your baby is engaged in the birthing position with his face toward your spine and the back of his head against your pubic bone. It is rare for babies to radically shift position at this point so however he is presenting is how he will be born. If he is in breech, you may have a Cesarean delivery. No matter how your baby comes into the world, you've done a great job and are ready to be a mother.

PREGNANCY FACT: Pushing and delivery can last between 1 and 3 hours and begins once your cervix is completely dilated and ends with the birth of your baby. Contractions will become less frequent coming at 3 to 5 minute intervals and lasting for 60 to 90 seconds. You may feel a burning sensation as baby passes through the birth canal and everything stretches. It is not unusual for mom to fall sleep for a few minutes between contractions because of how exhausting labor has been. Your partner should offer encouragement and help keep you on task.

DAILY JOURNAL

Mood:

Energy:

Cravings:

Symptoms:

Weight:

Your Birth Plan

When it comes to having your baby, the days of blindly following doctor's orders are long gone. Instead, it has become fashionable for parents-to-be to write a birth plan. Creating a birth plan establishes that you have preferences that should take priority over convenience for the medical staff that attends to your labor and delivery. Of course, the most important aspect of your delivery is that it be safe. Should safety become an issue at any point in your delivery, the parameters of your birth plan will be abandoned in favor of safer measures. Indeed, medical necessity will always supersede wishes expressed in a birth plan. Thus, when composing your plan the most important thing to bring to the table is flexibility. Remember that your birth plan is an outline of action that is applicable in the best-case scenario.

The following list of questions will help get you thinking about important issues related to your birth plan:

Where do I want to have my baby? Are you prepped for a home birth? Have you planned to deliver at a birthing center with a midwife? Or are you going to delivery in a hospital?

Where do I want to do early labor? Many women prefer to do early labor at home, since it is familiar and more comfortable. You will be able to walk around as much as you want, get in the bathtub, eat or drink, and be in control of how you spend this time.

When do I want to go to the hospital or birthing center? Some women want to get to the maternity wing the minute they feel contractions, while others prefer to wait it out. Decide at what point in your labor you want to head to the hospital and have a plan for who's taking you in what car. Make sure your bag is packed.

What is important for me to have during active labor? You may want to have some light snacks on hand, such as Jell-O or crackers. Though some hospitals will not allow you to eat or drink during active labor, eating light, bland snacks can give you the energy you need to keep going—and be sure to ask for ice chips to prevent dehydration. Some other items you may want with you include: glasses or contact lenses; labor tools, such as tennis balls or a sock stuffed with warm rice; a yoga ball; a CD player; and essential oils.

Do I want pain medication? This is a personal matter for pregnant women. Some women know at the get-go that they want to feel every pain associated with natural childbirth. Others, however, know that the experience of bringing their child into the world will be better if they do not feel pain during it. Many women change their mind about pain medication once true labor gets underway and that is perfectly fine. There is a window for when most pain medications can be given, however, so if you change your mind and decide you want it, speak up sooner rather than later.

Who do I want with me while I labor and when I deliver my baby (besides your partner)? If you want your best friend to videotape your birth so that your husband can hold your hand, write it down in your birth plan. Also, be sure to include your doula in your birth plan if you have one. She can run interference with doctors and nurses while your partner's attention is completely on you. It may also be worth listing who you do not want in the room with you, such as your brother-in-law or nosy neighbor.

How do I feel about the use of oxytocin to induce labor or to facilitate a slow labor? Keep in mind that inducting and facilitating labor are usually last-ditch efforts by your doctor to prevent a Cesarean delivery. If you would prefer to avoid the ultra-intense contractions that often accompany oxytocin injections and skip to a Cesarean section, make it known verbally and also write it down. Ultimately, though, your doctor is going to make the safest choice for you and baby.

What if I really do not want an episiotomy? This is another decision that will ultimately be up to your doctor. However, if you write it down in your birth plan, your doctor will know to avoid this option if possible.

What if I have a Cesarean delivery? Do you want a mirror set up so you can see baby as she is delivered? Be sure to state your medication preference: epidural or spinal. Also make it clear if you want baby to be placed immediately on your chest before she is cleaned up.

Does my partner want to cut the umbilical cord? This should be discussed ahead of time with your doctor, who will probably need a reminder.

Do I want to bank my baby's cord blood? If so, this should be set up before delivery day, but remind your doctor verbally and via your birth plan.

How soon after my baby is born do I want to breast-feed? Note in your birth plan if you want to try to nurse your baby before the cord is cut or the pediatric team takes her away to clean and assign her an APGAR score. If you rather your baby is cleaned and tested first, note that too. You should also decide if you will allow your baby to be bottle fed and whether it is OK to supplement with formula.

Do I want my son circumcised? This can be done while you are still in the hospital or may be done sometime within the first week.

How long are we going to stay in the hospital? If everyone is doing fine and you had an uncomplicated vaginal delivery you may go home as early as 24 hours after baby is born. If you had a Cesarean delivery you are usually able to go home within 3 to 4 days.

CREATING YOUR BIRTH PLAN

Writing a birth plan is one of the most important steps you can take to maintain control of your birth experience. Here's how to get started! Answer the following questions regarding your personal preferences pertaining to labor and delivery. Once you've completed the checklist, make a copy and discuss it with your doctor or midwife. If you decide to change your plan based on your discussion, modify your plan to create a final version. Keep in mind that childbirth doesn't always go according to plan. Aim for your ideals but keep an open mind without unreasonable expectations. What matters most is your and your baby's health and well-being.

GENERAL INFORMATION

Your first/middle/last name: ______________________

Your partner's first/last name: ______________________

Your due date: ______________________

Name of your doctor or midwife: ______________________

This birth plan is prepared for:

❒ Normal (vaginal) delivery

❒ Cesarean

❒ Induction

❒ Twins or multiple birth

❒ VBAC (vaginal birth after Cesarean)

❒ Other: ______________________

STATEMENT

Following is a statement of our birth plan and childbirth choices:

ATTENDANTS

I would like the following people to be present during labor and/or birth:

- ❒ Partner: ______
- ❒ Friend/s: ______
- ❒ Relative/s: ______
- ❒ Doula: ______
- ❒ Children: ______
- ❒ I would like my family/friends, etc. brought in to see me and meet the new baby as soon as possible after the birth.

PERSONAL REQUESTS/AMENITIES

I prefer the following personal amenities:

- ❒ Private birthing room
- ❒ Dim lights
- ❒ Peace and quiet
- ❒ My own music
- ❒ My own clothes during labor and delivery
- ❒ A private phone
- ❒ Other: ______

LABOR

I prefer the following options during labor:

- ❒ The option of returning home if I'm not in active labor
- ❒ Minimal vaginal exams
- ❒ To be free to walk around and go to the bathroom throughout labor
- ❒ To be free to move in bed only (and to use the bathroom)
- ❒ A catheter and/or regular epidural

- ❒ To have my partner to stay with me at all times
- ❒ To have only my practitioner, nurse, and guests present (i.e., no residents, medical students, or other hospital personnel)
- ❒ To wear my contact lenses, as long as I don't need a Cesarean
- ❒ To be able to eat and drink whatever I want
- ❒ To be free to drink clear fluids
- ❒ To have ice chips available to me at all times
- ❒ To have intermittent rather than continuous electronic fetal monitoring
- ❒ To be allowed to progress free of stringent time limits

During labor, I am open to try:

- ❒ A birthing stool
- ❒ A birthing chair
- ❒ A squatting bar
- ❒ A birthing pool/tub

I plan on bringing the following items:

- ❒ A birthing stool
- ❒ A beanbag chair
- ❒ A birthing pool/tub
- ❒ Other: ______________________________

Pushing and delivery preferences:

- ❒ To do so instinctively
- ❒ To be directed on when to push and the duration
- ❒ I would like to choose my positions for pushing and giving birth

I would like to try the following positions during labor:

❒ Semi-reclining

❒ Side-lying position

❒ Squatting

❒ Hands and knees

❒ Other: ______________________________

PROCEDURE

The following are my procedure preferences:

❒ I would like to avoid an enema and/or shaving of pubic hair

❒ I would like a Heparin/Saline lock (Most hospitals require this as access to a vein should an emergency occur, it can also be used in place of an IV for administration of antibiotics for complications such as MVP or Beta Strep)

❒ I would like to avoid an IV unless I become dehydrated

MONITORING

The following are my monitoring preferences:

❒ I do not wish to have continuous fetal monitoring unless it is required because of the baby's condition

In the event that I require or have chosen fetal monitoring, my preference is:

❒ Fetoscopy

❒ Doppler ultrasound

❒ External electronic monitor

❒ Internal electronic monitor

PAIN RELIEF

The following are my pain relief preferences:

- ❒ I would like not to be offered pain medication—I'll request it if I need it
- ❒ I would like pain medication administered as soon as possible
- ❒ I would like to give birth naturally without medication using the following techniques:
  - ❒ Bradley Method
  - ❒ Lamaze
  - ❒ Bath/shower
  - ❒ The Alexander Technique
  - ❒ Massage
  - ❒ Acupressure
  - ❒ Breathing techniques/distraction
  - ❒ Hot/cold therapy
  - ❒ Self-hypnosis
  - ❒ Other: ____________________

I am attempting a natural childbirth but if I ask for pain medication I would like to use:

- ❒ Stadol
- ❒ Nubain
- ❒ Demerol
- ❒ Walking epidural (low dose)
- ❒ Epidural block
- ❒ Other: ____________________

If I decide I want medicinal pain relief, I would prefer:

- ❒ Regional analgesia (an epidural and/or spinal block)
- ❒ Systemic medication

LABOR AUGMENTATION/INDUCTION

The following are my labor augmentation/ induction preferences:

- ❒ I wish to have induction/augmentation preferences included in my birth plan
- ❒ I do not wish to have the amniotic membrane ruptured artificially unless there are signs of fetal distress
- ❒ If labor is not progressing I would like to have the amniotic membrane ruptured before other methods are used to augment labor
- ❒ I would prefer to be allowed to try changing positions and other natural methods before medical methods or medications are used

If I choose to be induced or it becomes medically necessary, my preferences are:

- ❒ Pitocin
- ❒ Prostaglandin gel
- ❒ Amniotomy

VAGINAL BIRTH

During the delivery, I would prefer:

- ❒ To dim the lights for the birth
- ❒ To have the room be as quiet as possible
- ❒ To view the birth using a mirror so I can see the baby's head when it crowns
- ❒ To touch my baby's head as it crowns
- ❒ To risk a tear rather than have an episiotomy
- ❒ My partner to help "catch" our baby

After birth, I would prefer:

- ❒ To have the baby placed on my chest immediately after delivery
- ❒ To wait until the umbilical cord stops pulsating before it's clamped and cut
- ❒ My partner to cut the umbilical cord
- ❒ To breast-feed as soon as possible

PLACENTA

The following are my placenta preferences:

- ❒ I want an injection of Pitocin after the delivery to aid in expelling the placenta
- ❒ I do not want an injection of Pitocin after the delivery to aid in expelling the placenta
- ❒ I would like to see the placenta after it is delivered

EPISIOTOMY

The following are my episiotomy preferences:

- ❒ I prefer no episiotomy (massage, compresses, positioning, etc.) (Select if you would prefer no episiotomy but not to the point of tearing)
- ❒ I prefer to tear (massage, compresses, positioning, etc.) (Select if you would prefer to tear rather than have an episiotomy)
- ❒ I prefer pressure episiotomy (Done without anesthesia, although you cannot feel it due to the pressure from the baby's head)
- ❒ Local anesthesia (for repair)

CESAREAN/COMPLICATION

The following are my Cesarean/complication preferences:

- ❒ I want complications and Cesarean preferences included in my birth plan
- ❒ Unless absolutely necessary, I would like to avoid a Cesarean
- ❒ If my primary caregiver recommends a Cesarean birth, I would like a second opinion, if time warrants
- ❒ If my primary physician recommends a Cesarean, I will cooperate with the procedure at any time

If I have a Cesarean, I would like:

- ❒ My partner present at all times during the operation
- ❒ The screen lowered a bit so I can see my baby coming out
- ❒ The baby given to my partner as soon as he or she is dried off (as long as baby is in good health)
- ❒ To breast-feed my baby in the recovery room
- ❒ Spinal/epidural anesthesia
- ❒ General anesthesia
- ❒ My partner or coach present
- ❒ My partner to be able to take video/pictures
- ❒ The screen lowered to view birth
- ❒ To touch the baby as soon as possible
- ❒ My partner to cut cord
- ❒ Other: ______________________________

POST-PARTUM BABY CARE

The following are my post-partum baby care preferences:

- ❒ All newborn procedures to take place in my presence
- ❒ My partner to stay with the baby at all times if I can't be there
- ❒ To stay in a private room
- ❒ To have a cot provided for my partner

Eye-care preference:

- ❒ None
- ❒ Delayed for bonding time
- ❒ Immediate

Feeding preferences:

- ❒ I would like my baby fed on demand
- ❒ I would like my baby fed on a schedule
- ❒ Breast-feeding only
- ❒ Bottle feeding only
- ❒ Combination

The following can be offered to my baby:

- ❒ Formula
- ❒ Sugar water
- ❒ Pacifier
- ❒ Please don't offer anything to my baby at any point

Separation preferences:

- ❒ I would like 24-hour rooming-in with my baby
- ❒ I would like my baby to room-in with me only when I'm awake
- ❒ I would like my baby brought to me for feedings only
- ❒ I would like to make my decision later depending on how I'm feeling
- ❒ I would like no separation—baby/mother in same room
- ❒ Delayed (after recovery period)
- ❒ Partial rooming-in (baby with mother during day, but not night)
- ❒ Nursery (baby brought to you on your schedule)

Circumcision preferences: (Choose as many as apply)

- ❒ In the hospital
- ❒ Parents present
- ❒ Use anesthesia (depends on the practitioner)
- ❒ None (Check here if you do not intend to have the baby circumcised, or if you do not intend to have him circumcised at the birth place.)
- ❒ Do not retract the foreskin

Sick infant preferences: (Choose as many as apply)

- ❒ Breast-feeding, if possible
- ❒ Unlimited visitation for parents
- ❒ Handling the baby (holding, care of, etc.)
- ❒ If baby is transported to another facility, move us as soon as possible
- ❒ Other: ______________________________

Things You Need to Know

LABOR AND DELIVERY INFORMATION

If you are a first-time mother, you probably have many questions regarding labor and delivery. Perhaps the first question on your mind is, "How will I know when I am in labor?" Unfortunately, there is no way to accurately predict when you will go into labor or how the body decides when it is time. However, once your body is ready, it will start to produce chemicals called prostaglandins, which cause the cervix to dilate and soften. Your system will be flooded with prostaglandins as your labor progresses, which causes oxytocin receptors in your uterus to start contractions. During labor, contractions will start at the height of the fundus and roll down your uterus toward your pelvis. Contractions move this way to push baby down through your pelvic area and out through your vagina, with your help, of course. As labor continues, contractions will intensify and come closer together. It is important to remember that each woman's labor is a unique experience, which means that your labor may last anywhere from 4 to 24 hours or more.

The Pain of Labor

Your next question is probably, "How badly does labor hurt?" There is no answer to this question, as labor differs for every woman. The pain of labor depends on your threshold for pain, how intense your contractions are, and how long your labor lasts. To give you an idea of what to expect, let's review the changes your body experiences in labor. First, your baby must drop down into your pelvic area. As your baby's head settles in, bones are pushed aside and this can cause pelvic, hip, and lower-back pain. Once contractions start, your uterus will tighten and clench, which may feel like strong menstrual cramps with lots of pressure on your abdomen. This feeling will intensify as your contractions become more frequent and as you get closer to pushing. Once the contraction subsides, so too does the pain, giving you a break here and there.

Meanwhile, your cervix must be 100-percent effaced and dilated 10 centimeters before you are ready to push. To help you visualize this, consider that your cervical opening must go from being completely shut to having an opening about the size of a grapefruit. It must also thin out, or stretch, from 1½ to 2 inches thick to about the thickness of a sheet of paper. These changes can happen gradually or very quickly. This is one reason to remain flexible in the way you choose to handle the pain of labor.

Labor Tools

You have likely completed a childbirth class by now, so you know that there are many techniques that help manage your pain if you choose to avoid medication. These include breathing exercises, lower-back massage, aromatherapy, hydrotherapy, and the use of balls of varying sizes, used for sitting, bouncing, holding, and squeezing. You should have settled on a few of these tools by now. They should be packed in your hospital bag. You should also decide which breathing methods work well for you. For some women, fast, shallow breathing keeps them focused and prevents them from thinking too much about the pain. Others find that this type of breathing is distracting and ineffective. They prefer to use deep breathing and mediation. Whichever style you choose, practice it at home. If none of the natural methods appeal to you or work for you as you are laboring, you have the option of receiving childbirth pain medication.

Childbirth Medication

The most common childbirth medication is the epidural block, because it allows you to be awake, alert, and participate in pushing. If you decide to have an epidural, the anesthesiologist will administer the medication by inserting a small, flexible needle into your spine. Most often a catheter is used. This allows nurses to add doses of medication to the epidural throughout a woman's labor. You will be closely monitored as you receive an epidural because of potential side effects, such as a drop in blood pressure, partial numbness, severe "spinal" headache, and slowed labor.

THE STAGES OF LABOR

There are three stages of labor. Each has its own components and considerations. The first is early labor. The second is active labor, which is further broken down four parts: stage one, transition, pushing, and delivery. The final stage is delivery of the placenta. You should expect to experience changes to your body, pain level, mood, and energy level during each stage. Several factors influence how quickly your labor progresses. They are: the size of your baby, the location of baby's head, baby's position or presentation, the size of your pelvis, your preexisting medical issues, strength and effectiveness of your contractions, your emotional state, your energy level, and use of medications.

Early Labor

Early labor signals that true labor has begun. This is signified by contractions that come at 5- to 15-minute intervals that last between 25 and 45 seconds. They are stronger than Braxton Hicks contractions, but not unmanageable. Early labor contractions may feel like menstrual cramps with tightening and pressure. It is possible that your amniotic sac may rupture or that you will drop the mucus plug. If your water breaks, call your doctor and head to the hospital. If your water does not break, many women choose to do early labor at home where it is more comfortable.

It is common to feel excited, anxious, scared, and surprised that early labor does not hurt as much as you expected. Many women also become very talkative and want to tell those around them that labor has begun, while others want it to remain private. You may be overcome with an urge to keep moving—walking is fine, but stay close to home so you can get to the hospital in time.

Early labor is the longest phase of labor. It lasts, on average, between 7 and 8 hours. During this time your cervix will dilate to 3 centimeters. Since this can take so long, it is important to relax and rest as much as possible.

Active Labor—Stage 1

Over the course of active labor, contractions will become more intense and the peaks will last longer and be more painful. Contractions will come at 3- to 4-minute intervals and last between 40 and 60 seconds. You may start to sweat, become extremely thirsty, and feel nauseous or even vomit. It may become difficult to get a good breath because of mounting anxiety. In this case, relax and use your breathing techniques.

You will likely become irritable, quiet, and focused. It may become difficult for you to hold conversations or listen to instructions, which is why it is important that your partner be there to coach you into going with the contractions instead of fighting them. He should also encourage you to settle on a focal point and remind you to close your eyes and rest between contractions. Your partner should also do what he can to make you comfortable, which includes keeping your lips and forehead cool with a damp cloth.

Active labor will last, on average, from 1 to 4 hours. During this time, the cervix dilates from 4 to 7 centimeters. If you are receiving an epidural block, it will happen during the active phase of labor.

Transition

Transition is the most difficult phase of labor, though it is often the shortest. This period lasts from ½ to 2½ hours and completes the dilation of the cervix from 8 to 10 centimeters. Contractions will come at 1- to 2-minute intervals and last between 60 and 90 seconds. During the transitional phase you may shake, cry, vomit, experience extreme changes in body temperature, become increasingly irritable, or even fall asleep between contractions. You will likely find it impossible to follow instructions, so let your partner guide you.

During transition, your partner should remind you that you are close to having your baby and encourage you to keep going. He should remind you of your breathing techniques and help you stay focused. Your partner should also time your contractions so that he can anticipate the next one and help you prepare.

As the cervix finishes dilating, your baby is bearing down in the pelvis with his chin tucked in toward his chest. He will rotate toward your spine, which puts pressure on your perineum and bowels, thus you may feel the urge to "bear down" and push.

Pushing and Delivery

Pushing can last anywhere from just one contraction to several hours. Contractions may slow to 3- to 5-minute intervals and last between 60 and 90 seconds. If you do not have an epidural, you will feel a strong urge to push and may vomit or defecate. Do not be embarrassed about this. The medical team has seen it all before and will clean up before you realize what has happened.

Your partner's role is to encourage you to keep up the great work by helping you with good pushing posture, count as you push, keep you cool and happy with ice chips, and remind you how to breathe by breathing along with you. As baby moves through the birth canal to crowning in your vagina you may feel burning. It is possible you will feel the tearing of the perineum. Once baby is all the way out, you may cry, shake, and be very weak and exhausted. Most of all, you will be elated and relieved.

Delivery of the Placenta

Delivering the placenta can take from 5 to 15 minutes, and is followed by contractions that function to start the process of shrinking your uterus back down to about the size of a grapefruit. You may feel anxious to be alone with your family and ready to have the medical team leave you alone; they will just as soon as they are sure you and your baby are healthy and safe.

BRINGING BABY HOME

As your hospital stay draws to a close, you may feel anxious about bringing baby home where there are no experts to ask for help. This is a common fear among first-time mothers, so the top issues are addressed below. However, 99 percent of parenting is intuition and response. You will eventually be able to intuit the right response to your baby's cries. It may take some figuring out, but you will get there.

Leaving the Hospital

If you have an uncomplicated delivery you will be able to go home as soon as 24 hours after you have your baby. If you have a Cesarean, you will probably stay in the hospital for 3 or 4 days if there were no complications and your baby is doing well. Either way, when it is time to go you may feel like you have no idea how to put one foot in front of the other, let alone care for a newborn—or you may be anxious to get home and start bonding with your family in your own surroundings.

Upon leaving the hospital, you will need a weather-appropriate outfit for baby. This should include one layer more than what you are wearing yourself. Baby should also wear a newborn hat to help her to retain heat and hand covers so she doesn't scratch her face. Most important is to bring your car seat with you. The hospital will not allow you to take your child home in a vehicle (including buses, taxis, and trains) without one. It is a good idea for dad to drive and for you to sit in the backseat with baby so you can comfort her and avoid straining your weary body by constantly turning around to check on her.

The First 24 Hours at Home

The first 24 hours at home should be reserved for you, dad, baby, and any other older children. This is an important time to bond. Tell family and friends ahead of time that you do not want any visitors during this time, and feel free to turn the ringer off on your phone. You, your partner, and your baby will need some time to get used to each other and will be sleeping at odd hours. In fact, you should get into the habit of sleeping when baby sleeps. Let the chores wait, because what you need now is rest.

Crying

Your baby will let you know she is hungry by crying when she wakes up. She will let you know that her diaper is wet or soiled by crying. She will also alert you to the fact that she's had enough face time and is ready for sleep by … crying! Indeed, crying is how babies communicate—the only way they communicate. It can be stressful to get used to used hearing what sounds like serious distress, but as long as your baby is feeding regularly, producing five to six wet diapers a day (starting at 4 days old), and doesn't have a fever or other indications of illness, she is fine. If you are concerned, however, call your pediatrician. It is likely that he has you bringing baby in on day three for a checkup, so come armed with questions.

Nursing

Breast-feeding your baby can be one of the most rewarding experiences of your life. For some women it comes naturally and without complications. However, the great majority of women must conquer several issues before breast-feeding becomes routine. Some women may have inverted nipples; others may not produce much milk from one breast. Therefore, getting the hang of breast-feeding can take a few days. No matter what issues you encounter, however, you are still producing colostrum, so your baby is getting enough nourishment. Despite this, you can expect your baby to lose between 5 and 10 percent of his birth weight in the first few days after delivery. He will start to gain between 4 and 7 ounces per week once your milk supply is established and should regain his birth weight by the time he is 3 weeks old.

Doctors advise new mothers to attend a breast-feeding support group shortly after they birth their child. Some women even go on their way home from the hospital. For a one-time fee, a lactation consultant will observe you nursing your baby and give you advice on how to improve the process. You will be able to attend nursing support groups three or more times per week where you can weigh your baby before and after feedings to make sure he ate enough. This is often a good place to discuss breast-feeding challenges with other nursing moms. Indeed, breast-feeding support groups are often the start of play groups for baby and long-term friendships for mom.

Umbilical Cord Care

The umbilical cord stub will fall off sometime within the first few weeks of birth. It will change colors and end up looking like a black scab. Keep the site dry and clean. To avoid irritation, fold your baby's diapers down under the scab. If your doctor has instructed you to swab it with alcohol, wash your hands first and use a clean, sterile cotton swab. If the site oozes a green liquid, becomes red or hot, has a foul odor, or your baby has a fever, call your pediatrician right away.

Sleeping and Waking

Parents are often surprised at how much a newborn sleeps. In fact, during the first couple of weeks you may have to wake your baby up to feed him. As a rule, newborn babies should never go more than three hours during the day without feeding, and four at night. You will notice that baby often falls asleep during nursing; you will want to wake him by putting a cool cloth to his forehead. He will sleep for several hours after eating, be awake for a short time, and go back to sleep. This is normal, and as he gets older his waking periods will become longer.

Babies up to 3 months old will benefit from being swaddled for sleep. Swaddling reminds your baby of life in the womb, where she was warm, safe, and snug. It also prevents her from scratching herself in her sleep or from jerking herself awake with involuntary movements. If you are unsure how to swaddle your baby, ask your doctor for help. Many physicians keep clear how-to guides that come with pictures (these can also be found online). Always be conscious of the temperature, as making baby too hot can increase her risk for sudden infant death syndrome (SIDS). Always put your baby to sleep on her back and keep her crib empty of stuffed animals, blankets, and toys.

Pee, Poop, and Spit-up

Your baby will do these three things more times than you can believe for such a tiny person. However, it will take him a few days to build up to his reputation as a body-fluid machine. During the first 24 hours after baby is born, he will probably only produce one wet diaper since he hasn't fed enough to make more. On day two, he will likely have two wet diapers. You can expect three wet diapers on day three, and five or six beginning on day four. Also, your baby will pass meconium in the first three to four days. After the meconium has been passed, his stools will be a mustard color that is runny and appears seedy for the first month. You will notice that your baby will often poop during or just after a feeding, so it is a good idea to change him just after he has eaten.

Your baby may spit up a tablespoon of breast milk several times a day. This can be scary and have you wondering if she is keeping anything down. As long as she is gaining weight, you shouldn't worry. However, call your pediatrician if she projectile vomits or spits up more than a tablespoon of breast milk more than once, as these can signify a problem with acid reflux or an allergy to something in your diet.

Introducing Baby to Older Children and Pets

It can be overwhelming to take care of a newborn and handle other responsibilities, such as caring for older children or pets. When it comes to your other children, the very best way to get them onboard is to immediately start family bonding in the hospital.

Your older children may feel jealous, scared, or worried that they are being replaced. Though you may be exhausted, give them lots of attention and let them participate in caring for baby as much as is reasonable and safe.

As far as pets are concerned the best way to approach integrating your newest family member is to give your pet time and space. Don't force Fido to sniff or inspect the baby; if your pet decides that he or she wants to have a look, closely supervise the interaction. Don't ever leave your baby unattended with your pet and make sure to have a quiet space that your pet can retreat to when he or she is feeling stressed out by the baby's crying.

Notes . . . .

Your Labor Bag Checklist

MAKE SURE YOU ARE PREPARED FOR YOUR BIRTH. There are many things that you will want to bring with you to the hospital that you will use before, during, and after the delivery. The list includes items that you should consider packing in your labor bag.

INFORMATION AND DOCUMENTS

- ❑ Admission forms/papers
- ❑ Baby-name book
- ❑ Health insurance card/documents
- ❑ Pediatrician's name and phone number
- ❑ Pregnancy/birth reference book
- ❑ Prenatal reports
- ❑ Other: ______________________________

Your Labor Bag Checklist . . . . . .

GENERAL ITEMS

- ☐ Address book
- ☐ Books/magazines
- ☐ Birth announcement cards, envelopes/stamps/pen
- ☐ Camera and/or video
- ☐ Cash/change
- ☐ CDs/MP3 player/headphones
- ☐ Extra batteries/battery pack
- ☐ Extra pillow/s with colored pillowcases
- ☐ Gifts
- ☐ Large bag to bring home gifts and hospital supplies
- ☐ Mobile phone or prepaid phone card
- ☐ Phone number list
- ☐ Small cooler with drinks and snacks
- ☐ Thank you cards/notes
- ☐ Other: ______________________________

FOR LABOR AND DELIVERY

- ☐ Aromatherapy
- ☐ Back massager (tennis ball)
- ☐ Bathrobe
- ☐ Birth ball
- ☐ Birth plan
- ☐ Hard candy/suckers (for dry mouth)
- ☐ Hot water bottle/heating pad
- ☐ Ice pack
- ☐ Lip moisturizer
- ☐ Lotion/massage oil
- ☐ Nursing pillow
- ☐ Stopwatch/watch with second hand for timing contractions
- ☐ Personal face/wash cloth

FOR LABOR AND DELIVERY (cont)

- ❑ Personal pillow
- ❑ Ponytail holder/hairband/clips
- ❑ Relaxation materials: books, magazines, games, music, candles
- ❑ Slippers/socks
- ❑ Other: ______________________________

FOR YOUR PARTNER

- ❑ Books, magazines, and other items to stay occupied
- ❑ Change of clothes
- ❑ Hand wipes
- ❑ Snacks
- ❑ Toiletries
- ❑ Other: ______________________________

CLOTHING

- ❑ Front-opening gown or pajama top for breast-feeding
- ❑ Going-home outfit for mom
- ❑ Maternity panties
- ❑ Nursing bras
- ❑ Nursing pads
- ❑ Other: ______________________________

PERSONAL CARE

- ❑ Barrettes
- ❑ Body soap
- ❑ Brush/comb
- ❑ Contact lens case/lens supplies
- ❑ Dental floss

PERSONAL CARE (cont)

- ❑ Deodorant
- ❑ Earplugs
- ❑ Eyeshade
- ❑ Facial soap
- ❑ Glasses (if you need them)
- ❑ Handheld fan
- ❑ Lip salve/chapstick
- ❑ Makeup/cosmetics
- ❑ Mouthwash/breath mints
- ❑ Prescription medications
- ❑ Sanitary napkins
- ❑ Scented wipes or tissues
- ❑ Shampoo/conditioner
- ❑ Sponge
- ❑ Talcum powder
- ❑ Tissues
- ❑ Toothbrush/toothpaste

FOR BABY

- ❑ Approved car seat
- ❑ Baby nail clippers
- ❑ Blanket for outdoors
- ❑ Blanket for receiving
- ❑ Bunting or snowsuit for winter
- ❑ Diapers
- ❑ Going-home outfit
- ❑ Infant cap
- ❑ Pair socks/booties/mittens
- ❑ Undershirt

Conclusion

Congratulations!

AS YOUR JOURNEY THROUGH PREGNANCY comes to a close, a new adventure is about to begin—life as a mother. Caring for a newborn is unlike anything you have ever done before. It is a 24-hour job that requires a lot of work and much self-sacrifice. However, as you will discover within the first few days, weeks, and months after your baby is born, your heart never knew such love before this tiny creature came into your life. You may find yourself in tears several times a day as you watch him sleep or nurse. Of course, hormones are partially responsible for these tears, but so too is the sheer magnitude of what has just occurred. For more than nine months, you carried this baby inside you and now you are his caretaker, his provider of nourishment, and his educator. Allow yourself to relish this early time in your motherhood, because it will go by faster than you can ever imagine. Congratulations to you, your partner, and the newest addition to your family!

Notes . . . .

Essential Nutritional Facts for a Healthy Pregnancy

EATING NUTRIENT-RICH FOODS IS CRUCIAL to having a happy and healthy pregnancy. This section will be a great resource in that it provides the nutritional information for foods you may want to select for your pregnancy diet. This section provides calories per serving, as well as the content in grams for fat, protein, carbohydrates, and fiber.

Use these essential nutritional facts to help you plan meals, grocery shop wisely, and choose the best diet for you and your growing baby. A helpful exercise is to make a list of foods you like that are also healthy for you during pregnancy. Use the following chart to list those items:

COMMON ITEMS YOU LIKE TO EAT

Food/Beverages	Cal	Fat	Prtn	Carbs	Fiber

Nutritional Facts . . . .

Nutrition values for fat, protein (Prtn), carbohydrates (Cbs), and fiber (Fbr) are listed in grams per serving. Serving sizes and values are approximate.

FOOD ITEM	SERVING SIZE	CAL	FAT	PRTN	CBS	FBR
A						
Alfalfa seeds	1 tbsp	1	0	0	0	0
Allspice, ground	1 tsp	5	0	0	1	0
Almond butter, w/ salt	1 tbsp	101	10	2	3	1
Almond butter, w/o salt	1 tbsp	101	10	2	3	1
Almonds, roasted	1 oz. (12 nuts)	169	15	6	6	3
Anchovies	3 oz.	111	4	17	0	0
Apple cider, powdered	1 packet	83	0	0	21	0
Apple juice	8 fl.oz.	120	0	0	29	0
Apples, w/o skin	1 medium	61	0	0	16	2
Apples, w/ skin	1 medium	72	0	0	19	3
Applesauce	1 cup	194	1	1	51	3
Apricots	1 apricot	17	0	1	4	1
Arrowroot	1 cup, sliced	78	0	5	16	2
Arrowroot flour	1 cup	457	0	0	113	4
Artichokes	1 artichoke	76	0	5	17	9
Arugula	1 cup	4	0	1	1	0
Asparagus	1 spear	2	0	0	1	0
Avocados	1 cup, cubes	240	22	3	13	10
B						
Bacon bits, meatless	1 tbsp	33	2	2	2	1
Bacon, Canadian, cooked	1 slice	43	2	6	0	0
Bacon, meatless	1 slice	16	2	1	0	0
Bacon, pork, cooked	1 slice	42	3	3	0	0
Bagels, cinnamon-raisin	1 bagel, 4" dia	244	2	9	49	2
Bagels, egg	1 bagel, 4" dia	292	2	11	56	2
Bagels, oat-bran	1 bagel, 4" dia	227	1	10	47	3
Bagels, plain	1 bagel, 4" dia	245	1	9	47	2
Bagels, deli gourmet style	1 bagel	370	3	13	71	2
Balsam pear	1 balsam pear	21	0	1	5	4
Bamboo shoots	1 cup	41	1	4	8	3
Banana chips	1 oz.	147	10	1	17	2
Bananas	1 medium, 7"-8"	105	0	1	27	3
Barley	1 cup	651	4	23	135	32
Barley flour	1 cup	511	2	16	110	15
Barley, pearled, cooked	1 cup	193	1	4	44	6
Basil	5 leaves	1	0	0	0	0
Basil, dried	1 tsp	2	0	0	0	0
Bay leaf	1 tsp, crumbled	2	0	0	0	0
Beans, adzuki, cooked	1 cup	294	0	17	57	17
Beans, baked, canned, plain	1 cup	239	1	12	54	10
Beans, baked, canned, w/o salt	1 cup	266	1	12	52	13
Beans, baked, canned, w/ beef	1 cup	322	9	17	45	10
Beans, black, cooked	1 cup	227	1	15	40	15
Beans, cranberry, cooked	1 cup	241	1	16	43	18
Beans, fava, canned	1 cup	182	1	14	31	10
Beans, french, cooked	1 cup	228	1	12	43	17
Beans, great northern, cooked	1 cup	209	1	15	37	12
Beans, kidney, cooked	1 cup	225	1	15	40	11
Beans, lima, cooked	1 cup	216	1	15	39	13

Nutrition values for fat, protein (Prtn), carbohydrates (Cbs), and fiber (Fbr) are listed in grams per serving. Serving sizes and values are approximate.

FOOD ITEM	SERVING SIZE	CAL	FAT	PRTN	CBS	FBR
B (CONT.)						
Beans, lima, canned	1 can	190	0	12	36	11
Beans, mung, cooked	1 cup	212	1	14	39	15
Beans, mungo, cooked	1 cup	189	1	14	33	12
Beans, navy, cooked	1 cup	255	1	15	47	19
Beans, pink, cooked	1 cup	252	1	15	47	9
Beans, pinto, cooked	1 cup	245	1	15	44	15
Beans, small white, cooked	1 cup	254	1	16	46	18
Beans, snap, green, cooked	1 cup	44	0	2	10	4
Beans, snap, yellow, cooked	1 cup	44	0	2	10	4
Beans, white, cooked	1 cup	249	1	17	45	11
Beans, yellow	1 cup	255	2	16	48	18
Beechnuts, dried	1 oz.	163	14	2	10	0
Beef, choice short rib, cooked	3 oz.	400	36	18	0	0
Beef bologna	1 slice	88	8	3	1	0
Beef jerky, chopped	1 piece	81	5	7	2	0
Beef sausage, precooked	1 link	134	12	6	1	0
Beef stew, canned	1 serving	218	13	12	16	4
Beef, tri-tip roast, roasted	3 oz.	174	9	22	0	0
Beef, brisket, lean and fat, roasted	3 oz.	328	27	20	0	0
Beef, brisket, lean, roasted	3 oz.	206	11	25	0	0
Beef, chuck, arm roast, lean & fat, braised	3 oz.	283	20	23	0	
Beef, chuck, arm roast, lean, braised	3 oz.	179	7	28	0	
Beef, chuck, top blade, raw	3 oz.	138	8	17	0	0
Beef, cured breakfast strips	3 slices	276	26	9	1	0
Beef, cured, corned, canned	3 oz.	213	13	23	0	0
Beef, cured, dried	1 serving	43	1	9	1	0
Beef, cured, luncheon meat	1 slice	31	1	5	0	0
Beef, flank, raw	1 oz.	47	2	6	0	0
Beef, ground patties, frozen	3 oz.	240	20	15	0	0
Beef, ground, 70% lean, raw	1 oz.	94	9	4	0	0
Beef, ground, 80% lean, raw	1 oz.	72	6	5	0	0
Beef, ground, 95% lean, raw	1 oz.	39	1	6	0	0
Beef, rib, large end, boneless, raw	1 oz.	94	8	5	0	0
Beef, rib, shortribs, boneless, raw	1 oz.	110	10	4	0	0
Beef, rib, whole, boneless, raw	1 oz.	91	8	5	0	0
Beef, rib-eye, small end, raw	1 oz.	78	6	5	0	0
Beef, round, bottom, raw	1 oz.	56	3	6	0	0
Beef, round, eye, raw	1 oz.	49	3	6	0	0
Beef, round, full cut, raw	1 oz.	55	3	6	0	0
Beef, round, tip, raw	1 oz.	56	4	6	0	0
Beef, round, top, raw	1 oz.	48	2	6	0	0
Beef, shank crosscuts, raw	1 oz.	50	3	6	0	0
Beef, short loin, porterhouse, raw	1 oz.	73	6	5	0	0
Beef, short loin, t-bone, raw	1 oz.	66	5	5	0	0
Beef, short loin, top, raw	1 oz.	66	5	6	0	0
Beef, sirloin, tri-tip, raw	1 oz.	50	3	6	0	0
Beef, tenderloin, raw	1 oz.	70	5	6	0	0
Beef, top sirloin, raw	1 oz.	61	4	6	0	0
Beets	1 beet	35	0	2	8	4
Bratwurst, chicken	1 serving	148	9	16	0	0

Nutrition values for fat, protein (Prtn), carbohydrates (Cbs), and fiber (Fbr) are listed in grams per serving. Serving sizes and values are approximate.

FOOD ITEM	SERVING SIZE	CAL	FAT	PRTN	CBS	FBR
B (CONT.)						
Bratwurst, pork	1 serving	281	25	12	2	0
Bratwurst, veal	1 serving	286	27	12	0	0
Bread stuffing, dry mix, prepared	1/2 cup	178	9	3	22	3
Bread, banana	1 slice	196	6	3	33	1
Bread, corn	1 piece	188	6	4	29	1
Bread, cracked-wheat	1 slice	65	1	2	12	1
Bread, french	1 slice	70	1	3	15	1
Bread, garlic	1 slice	160	10	3	14	1
Bread, Irish soda	1 oz.	82	1	2	16	1
Bread, rice bran	1 oz.	69	1	3	12	1
Bread, sandwich slice	1 slice	70	1	2	13	1
Bread, sourdough	1 slice	100	1	2	20	1
Broad beans, cooked	1 cup	187	1	13	33	9
Brownies	1 brownie	220	13	1	27	1
Buckwheat	1 cup	583	6	23	122	17
Buckwheat flour	1 cup	402	4	15	85	12
Buckwheat groats, roasted, cooked	1 cup	155	1	6	34	5
Buffalo, raw	1 oz.	28	0	6	0	0
Burbot, raw	3 oz.	77	1	16	0	0
Burdock root	1 cup	85	0	2	21	4
Butter, whipped, w/ salt	1 tbsp	67	8	0	0	0
Butternuts, dried	1 oz.	174	16	7	3	1
C						
Cabbage, common	1 cup, shredded	17	1	1	4	2
Cabbage, pak choi	1 cup, shredded	9	0	1	2	1
Cabbage, pe-tsai	1 cup, shredded	12	0	1	3	1
Cake, angel food	1 slice	180	4	2	36	2
Cake, Boston cream pie	1 slice	260	9	1	32	0
Cake, carrot	1 slice	310	16	1	39	0
Cake, cheesecake	1 slice	500	30	4	50	0
Cake, chocolate	1 slice	270	13	1	36	1
Cake, chocolate mousse	1 slice	250	10	1	35	1
Cake, devil's food	1 slice	270	13	2	35	0
Cake, pineapple upside-down	1 piece	367	14	4	58	1
Cake, pound	1 slice	320	16	2	38	1
Cake, sponge w/ cream, berries	1 slice	325	8	25	38	1
Cake, yellow	1 slice	260	11	2	36	1
Candy, butterscotch	5 pieces	120	3	0	20	0
Candy, caramels	1 piece	30	1	3	6	1
Candy, carob	1 bar	470	27	7	49	3
Candy, chocolate fudge	1 oz.	125	5	0	18	0
Candy, chocolate mints	1 mint	45	1	0	9	0
Candy, milk chocolate w/ almonds	2 oz.	216	14	4	21	3
Candy, choco-coated pntbtr bites	1 piece	45	3	1	4	0
Candy, chocolate-coated peanuts	12 peanuts	160	11	20	15	7
Candy, gumdrops	4 pieces	130	0	0	31	0
Candy, hard candy	1 piece	18	0	0	5	0
Candy, jelly beans	12 beans	100	0	0	24	0
Candy, licorice	1 piece	30	0	0	7	0

Nutrition values for fat, protein (Prtn), carbohydrates (Cbs), and fiber (Fbr) are listed in grams per serving. Serving sizes and values are approximate.

FOOD ITEM	SERVING SIZE	CAL	FAT	PRTN	CBS	FBR
C (CONT.)						
Candy, lollipop	1 lollipop	20	0	0	5	0
Candy, milk chocolate bar	2 oz.	235	13	3	26	2
Candy, mints	1 mint	30	0	0	7	0
Cantaloupe	1 cup, cubed	54	0	1	13	1
Cardoon	1 cup, shredded	36	0	1	9	3
Carrots	1 medium	65	0	1	15	4
Cashew butter, w/ salt	1 tbsp	94	8	3	4	0
Cashew nuts	1 oz.	157	12	5	9	1
Cassava	1 cup	330	1	3	78	4
Celeraic	1 cup	66	1	2	14	3
Chard, swiss	1 cup	7	0	1	1	1
Cheese, American	1 slice	110	9	5	1	0
Cheese, brick	1 oz.	100	8	31	0	0
Cheese, brie	1 oz.	95	8	50	1	0
Cheese, camembert	1 oz.	90	7	49	1	0
Cheese, cheddar	1 oz.	110	9	33	1	0
Cheese, colby jack	1 oz.	110	9	31	1	0
Cheese, cottage, 2%	1 cup	203	4	31	8	0
Cheese, edam	1 oz.	100	8	7	0	0
Cheese, feta	1 oz.	100	8	21	1	0
Cheese, goat	1 oz.	128	10	9	1	0
Cheese, goat, semisoft	1 oz.	103	9	6	1	0
Cheese, goat, soft	1 oz.	76	6	5	0	0
Cheese, gouda	1 oz.	100	8	7	1	0
Cheese, monterey jack	1 oz.	110	9	32	0	0
Cheese, mozzarella	1 oz.	90	7	25	1	0
Cheese, parmesan, hard	1 oz.	110	7	10	1	0
Cheese, parmesan, shredded	1 tbsp	22	2	2	0	0
Cheese, provolone	1 oz.	100	8	34	1	0
Cheese, queso	2 tbsp	110	9	28	2	0
Cheese, ricotta	2 tbsp	50	4	28	1	0
Cheese, roquefort	1 oz.	105	9	6	1	0
Cheese, swiss	1 oz.	110	9	36	1	0
Cherries, sour	8 pieces	30	0	1	7	2
Cherries, sweet	8 pieces	30	0	2	7	2
Chewing gum	1 piece	25	0	0	5	0
Chicken, breast, w/ skin	1/2 breast	249	13	30	0	0
Chicken, breast, w/o skin	1/2 breast	130	2	27	0	0
Chicken, capons, boneless	1/2 capon	1459	74	184	0	0
Chicken, capons, giblets, cooked	1 cup	238	8	38	1	0
Chicken, cornish game hen, roast	1/2 bird	336	24	29	0	0
Chicken, cornish game hen, meat	1 bird	295	9	51	0	0
Chicken, dark meat, w/o skin	1 cup diced	287	14	38	0	0
Chicken, drumstick, w/ skin	1 drumstick	118	6	14	0	0
Chicken, drumstick, w/o skin	1 drumstick	74	2	13	0	0
Chicken, leg, w/ skin	1 leg	312	20	30	0	0
Chicken, leg, w/o skin	1 leg	156	5	26	0	0
Chicken, light meat, w/o skin	1 cup diced	214	6	38	0	0
Chicken, thigh, w/ skin	1 thigh	198	14	16	0	0
Chicken, thigh, w/o skin	1 thigh	82	3	14	0	0

Nutritional Facts . . . .

Nutrition values for fat, protein (Prtn), carbohydrates (Cbs), and fiber (Fbr) are listed in grams per serving. Serving sizes and values are approximate.

FOOD ITEM	SERVING SIZE	CAL	FAT	PRTN	CBS	FBR
C (CONT.)						
Chicken, wing, w/ skin	1 wing	109	8	9	0	0
Chicken, wing, w/o skin	1 wing	37	1	6	0	0
Chickpeas, cooked	1 cup	269	4	15	45	13
Chicory greens	1 cup, chopped	41	1	3	9	7
Chicory roots	1/2 cup	33	0	1	8	0
Chicory, witloof	1/2 cup	8	0	0	2	1
Chili con carne w/ beans	1 cup	298	13	18	28	10
Chili powder	1 tsp	8	0	0	1	1
Chili w/ beans, canned	1 cup	287	14	15	31	11
Chili w/o beans, canned	1 cup	194	7	17	18	3
Chinese chestnuts	1 oz.	64	0	1	14	0
Chives	1 tbsp, chopped	1	0	0	0	0
Chocolate chip crisped rice bar	1 bar	115	4	1	21	1
Chocolate chips	1/4 cup	210	12	3	24	1
Chocolate milkshake, ready-to-drink	8 fl.oz.	181	5	8	26	1
Chocolate, semi sweet bars, baking	1 oz.	160	8	3	20	1
Choco, unsweet baking squares	1 square	144	15	4	9	5
Chorizo, pork and beef	1 link	273	23	15	1	0
Chow mein noodles	1 cup	237	14	4	26	2
Cinnamon, ground	1 tsp	6	0	0	2	1
Cisco	3 oz.	83	2	16	0	0
Citrus fruit drink, from concentrate	8 fl.oz.	124	0	1	30	1
Clam, mixed species, raw	1 large	15	0	3	1	0
Cloves, ground	1 tsp	7	0	0	1	1
Cocktail mix, nonalcoholic	1 fl.oz.	103	0	0	26	0
Cocoa mix, powder	1 serving	113	1	2	24	1
Cocoa mix, powder, unsweetened	1 tbsp	12	1	1	3	2
Coconut meat	1 cup, shredded	283	27	3	12	7
Coconut milk	1 cup	552	57	6	13	5
Coffee, brewed, decaf	1 cup	0	0	0	0	0
Coffee, brewed, regular	1 cup	2	0	0	0	0
Coffee, café au lait	8 fl.oz.	65	3	1	6	0
Coffee, cappuccino	8 fl.oz.	70	4	1	6	0
Coffee, espresso	1 shot	4	0	0	1	0
Coffee, instant, decaf	1 tsp	0	0	0	0	0
Coffee, instant, regular	1 tsp, dry	2	0	0	0	0
Coffee, latte	8 fl.oz.	100	5	0	8	0
Coffee, mocha	8 fl.oz.	180	12	1	16	0
Coffeecake	3 oz.	230	7	4	38	4
Coleslaw	1/2 cup	41	2	1	7	1
Collards	1 cup, chopped	11	0	1	2	1
Conch, baked or broiled	1 cup, sliced	165	2	33	2	0
Cookies, animal crackers	1 cookie	22	1	0	4	0
Cookies, brownies	4 oz.	430	25	1	52	1
Cookies, butter	1 cookie	23	1	0	3	0
Cookies, choco chip, fresh baked	1 cookie	275	15	0	38	1
Cookies, choco chip, commercial	1 cookie	130	7	1	17	1
Cookies, choco chip, refrigerated	1 portion	128	6	1	18	0
Cookies, chocolate wafers	1 wafer	26	1	0	4	0
Cookies, fig bars	1 cookie	150	3	2	31	2

Nutrition values for fat, protein (Prtn), carbohydrates (Cbs), and fiber (Fbr) are listed in grams per serving. Serving sizes and values are approximate.

FOOD ITEM	SERVING SIZE	CAL	FAT	PRTN	CBS	FBR
C (CONT.)						
Cookies, fudge	1 cookie	73	1	1	16	1
Cookies, gingersnap	1 cookie	29	1	0	5	0
Cookies, graham, plain or honey	2 1/2" square	30	1	1	5	0
Cookies, marshmallow w/ choco	1 cookie	118	5	1	19	1
Cookies, molasses	1 cookie	138	4	2	24	0
Cookies, oatmeal	1 cookie	238	9	3	38	2
Cookies, oatmeal w/ raisins	1 cookie	238	9	3	38	2
Cookies, oatmeal, commercial, iced	1 cookie	123	5	1	18	1
Cookies, oatmeal, refrigerated	1 portion	68	3	1	10	0
Cookies, peanut butter sandwich	1 cookie	67	3	1	9	0
Cookies, peanut butter, refrigerated	1 portion	73	4	1	8	0
Cookies, sugar	1 cookie	66	3	1	8	0
Cookies, sugar wafers w/ cream	1 wafer	46	2	0	6	0
Cookies, sugar, refrigerated dough	1 portion	113	5	1	15	0
Cookies, vanilla wafers	1 wafer	28	1	0	4	0
Coriander leaves	9 sprigs	5	0	0	1	1
Corn flour, yellow	1 cup	416	4	11	87	0
Corn, sweet, white	1 ear	77	1	3	17	2
Corn, sweet, yellow	1 ear	77	1	3	17	2
Corn, sweet, white, cream style	1 cup	184	1	5	46	3
Corn, sweet, yellow, cream style	1 cup	184	1	5	46	3
Cornnuts	1 oz.	126	4	2	20	2
Cornstarch	1 cup	488	0	0	117	1
Couscous, cooked	1 cup	176	0	6	37	0
Cowpeas, cooked	1 cup	160	1	5	34	8
Cowpeas, catjang, cooked	1 cup	200	1	14	35	6
Cowpeas, leafy tips	1 cup, chopped	10	0	2	2	0
Crab, Alaska king, raw	1 leg	144	1	32	0	0
Crab, blue, canned	1 cup	134	2	28	0	0
Crab, dungeness, cooked	1 crab	140	2	28	1	0
Crabapples	1 cup, sliced	84	0	0	22	0
Crackers w/ cheese filling	6 crackers	191	10	4	23	1
Crackers w/ peanut butter filling	6 cracker	193	10	5	22	1
Crackers, cheese, regular	6 crackers	312	16	6	36	2
Crackers, graham	1 cracker	30	1	6	5	2
Crackers, matzo, plain	1 matzo	112	0	3	24	1
Crackers, matzo, whole-wheat	1 matzo	100	0	4	22	3
Crackers, melba toast	1 cup	129	1	4	25	2
Crackers, milk	1 cracker	50	2	1	8	0
Crackers, regular	1 cup, bite size	311	16	5	38	1
Crackers, rusk toast	1 rusk	41	1	1	7	0
Crackers, rye	1 cracker	37	0	1	9	3
Crackers, saltines	1 cracker	20	0	1	4	0
Crackers, soda	1 cracker	23	1	1	4	0
Crackers, wheat	1 cracker	9	0	0	1	0
Crackers, wheat, w/ peanut butter	1 cracker	35	2	1	4	0
Crackers, whole-wheat	1 cracker	18	1	0	3	0
Cranberries	1 cup, whole	44	0	0	12	4
Cranberry juice cocktail	1 cup	144	0	0	36	0
Cranberry-apple juice	1 cup	174	0	0	44	0

Nutrition values for fat, protein (Prtn), carbohydrates (Cbs), and fiber (Fbr) are listed in grams per serving. Serving sizes and values are approximate.

FOOD ITEM	SERVING SIZE	CAL	FAT	PRTN	CBS	FBR
C (CONT.)						
Cranberry-grape juice	1 cup	137	0	1	34	0
Crayfish, wild, raw	8 crayfish	21	0	4	0	0
Cream cheese	1 tbsp	51	5	1	0	0
Cream of tartar	1 tsp	8	0	0	2	0
Cream, half & half	1 tbsp	20	2	0	1	0
Cream, heavy whipping	1 cup, fluid	821	88	5	7	0
Crepes	1 crepe	120	6	2	14	1
Croissants, apple	1 croissant	145	5	4	21	1
Croissants, butter	1 croissant	115	6	2	13	1
Croissants, cheese	1 croissant	174	9	4	20	1
Croutons, plain	1 cup	122	2	4	22	2
Croutons, seasoned	1 cup	186	7	4	25	2
Cucumber	1 cucumber	45	0	2	11	2
Cucumber, peeled	1 cup, sliced	14	0	1	3	1
Cumin seed	1 tsp	8	1	0	1	0
Currants, black	1 cup	71	1	2	17	0
Currants, red & white	1 cup	63	0	2	16	5
Curry powder	1 tsp	7	0	0	1	1
D						
Dandelion greens	1 cup, chopped	25	0	2	5	2
Danish pastry, cheese, 4 1/4" dia	1 pastry	266	16	6	26	1
Danish pastry, cinnamon, 4 1/4" dia	1 pastry	262	15	5	29	1
Danish pastry, fruit, 4 1/4" diameter	1 pastry	263	13	4	34	1
Danish pastry, nut, 4 1/4" diameter	1 pastry	280	16	5	30	1
Danish pastry, raspberry, 4 1/4" dia	1 pastry	263	13	4	34	1
Deer, ground, raw	1 oz.	45	2	6	0	0
Deer, raw	1 oz.	34	1	7	0	0
Doughnuts, choco coated or frosted	1 doughnut	133	9	1	13	1
Doughnuts, sugared or glazed	1 doughnut	250	12	3	34	1
Doughnuts, french crullers	1 cruller	169	8	1	24	1
Doughnuts, plain	1 doughnut, stick	219	12	3	26	1
Doughnuts, wheat, sugared/glazed	1 doughnut	101	5	2	12	1
Duck liver, raw	1 liver	60	2	8	2	0
Duck, meat only, roasted	1/2 duck	444	25	52	0	0
Duck, breast w/skin, roasted	1/2 breast	242	13	29	0	0
Duck, skinless, raw	1/2 duck	400	18	55	0	0
Durian	1 cup, chopped	357	13	4	66	9
E						
Eclairs w/ chocolate glaze	1 éclair	293	18	7	27	1
Eel, mixed species, raw	3 oz.	156	10	16	0	0
Egg noodles, cooked	1 cup	213	2	8	40	2
Egg substitute, liquid	1 tbsp	13	1	2	0	0
Egg white, fried	1 large	92	7	6	0	0
Egg white, raw	1 large	17	0	4	0	0
Egg yolk, raw	1 large	53	4	3	1	0
Egg, hard-boiled	1 cup, chopped	211	14	17	2	0
Egg, omelette	1 large	93	7	7	0	0
Egg, poached	1 large	74	5	6	0	0

Nutrition values for fat, protein (Prtn), carbohydrates (Cbs), and fiber (Fbr) are listed in grams per serving. Serving sizes and values are approximate.

FOOD ITEM	SERVING SIZE	CAL	FAT	PRTN	CBS	FBR
E (CONT.)						
Egg, raw	1 large	85	5.8	7	0	0
Egg, scrambled	1 cup	365	27	24	5	0
Eggnog	8 fl.oz.	343	19	10	34	0
Eggplant	1 eggplant	110	10	5	26	16
Elderberries	1 cup	106	1	1	27	10
Elk, ground, raw	1 oz.	49	3	6	0	0
Elk, raw	1 oz.	31	0	7	0	0
Endive	1 head	87	1	6	17	16
English muffins, plain	1 muffin	134	1	4	26	2
English muffins, cinnamon-raisin	1 muffin	139	2	4	49	2
English muffins, wheat	1 muffin	127	1	5	26	3
English muffins, whole-wheat	1 muffin	134	1	6	27	4
English muffins, multigrain	1 muffin	155	1	6	31	2
European chestnuts, peeled	1 oz.	56	0	1	13	0
European chestnuts, unpeeled	1 oz.	60	1	1	13	2
F						
Farina, cooked	1 cup.	471	0	3	24	1
Fast food, biscuit w/ egg	1 biscuit	373	22	12	32	1
Fast food, biscuit w/ egg & bacon	1 biscuit	458	31	17	29	1
Fast food, biscuit w/ egg, bcn & chz	1 biscuit	477	31	16	33	0
Fast food, biscuit w/ sausage	1 biscuit	485	32	12	40	1
Fast food, caramel sundae	1 sundae	304	9	7	49	0
Fast food, chzburger, lrg, 2x patty	1 sandwich	704	44	38	40	1
Fast food, chzburger, lrg, 1 patty	1 sandwich	563	33	28	38	1
Fast food, corndog	1 corndog	460	19	17	56	1
Fast food, croissant w/ egg, cheese	1 croissant	368	25	13	24	1
Fast food, croissant w/egg, chz, bcn	1 croissant	413	28	16	24	1
Fast food, croissant w/ egg, chz, ssg	1 croissant	523	38	20	25	1
Fast food, Danish pastry, cheese	1 pastry	353	25	6	29	2
Fast food, Danish pastry, cinnamon	1 pastry	349	17	5	47	2
Fast food, Danish pastry, fruit	1 pastry	335	16	5	45	2
Fast food, fish snd w/ tartar sauce	1 sandwich	431	23	17	41	1
Fast food, french toast sticks	5 pieces	513	29	8	58	3
Fast food, fried chicken, boneless	6 pieces	285	18	15	16	1
Fast food, hamburger, lrg, 2x patty	1 sandwich	540	27	34	40	2
Fast food, hamburger, lrg, 1 patty	1 sandwich	425	21	23	37	2
Fast food, hot fudge sundae	1 sundae	284	9	6	48	0
Fast food, hot dog w/ chili	1 hot dog	296	13	14	31	1
Fast food, hot dog, plain	1 hot dog	242	15	10	18	1
FF, McDonald's Big Mac® w/ chz	1 serving	560	30	25	46	3
FF, McDonald's Big Mac® w/o chz	1 serving	495	25	23	43	3
Fast food, McDonald's chzburger	1 serving	310	12	15	35	1
FF, McDonald's Chicken McGrill®	1 serving	400	16	27	38	3
FF, McDonald's Crispy Chicken	1 serving	500	23	24	50	3
FF, McDonald's Filet-o-Fish®	1 serving	400	18	14	42	1
Fast food, McDonald's french fries	1 medium	350	11	4	47	5
Fast food, McDonald's hamburger	1 serving	260	9	13	33	1
FF McDonald's 1/4 Pounder®,chz	1 serving	510	25	29	43	3
FF, McDonald's 1/4 Pounder®	1 serving	420	18	24	40	3

Nutrition values for fat, protein (Prtn), carbohydrates (Cbs), and fiber (Fbr) are listed in grams per serving. Serving sizes and values are approximate.

FOOD ITEM	SERVING SIZE	CAL	FAT	PRTN	CBS	FBR
F (CONT.)						
Fast food, onion rings, 8-9 rings	1 portion	276	16	4	31	3
Fast food, strawberry sundae	1 sundae	268	8	6	45	0
FF, sub sandwich w/ cold cuts	1 submarine 6"	456	19	22	51	4
FF, sub sandwich w/ roast beef	1 submarine 6"	410	13	29	44	4
FF, submarine sandwich w/ tuna	1 submarine 6"	584	28	30	55	4
FF, vanilla soft-serve w/ cone	1 cone	164	6	4	24	0
Fennel bulb	1 cup, sliced	27	0	1	6	3
Fennel seed	1 tbsp	20	1	1	3	2
Fenugreek seed	1 tbsp	36	1	3	7	3
Figs	1 medium	37	0	0	10	2
Figs, dried	1 fig	21	0	0	5	1
Fireweed leaves	1 cup, chopped	24	1	1	4	2
Fish oil, cod liver	1 tbsp	123	14	0	0	0
Fish oil, herring	1 tbsp	123	14	0	0	0
Fish oil, menhaden	1 tbsp	123	14	0	0	0
Fish oil, salmon	1 tbsp	123	14	0	0	0
Fish oil, sardine	1 tbsp	123	14	0	0	0
Fish, bluefin tuna, raw	3 oz.	122	4	20	0	0
Fish, bluefish, raw	3 oz.	105	4	17	0	0
Fish, butterfish, raw	3 oz.	124	7	15	0	0
Fish, carp, raw	3 oz.	108	5	15	0	0
Fish, catfish, raw	3 oz.	81	2	14	0	0
Fish, cod, Atlantic, raw	3 oz.	70	1	15	0	0
Fish, croaker, Atlantic, raw	3 oz.	88	3	15	0	0
Fish, flatfish, raw	3 oz.	77	1	16	0	0
Fish, gefilte fish	1 piece	35	1	4	3	0
Fish, grouper, mixed species, raw	3 oz.	78	1	17	0	0
Fish, haddock, raw	3 oz.	74	1	16	0	0
Fish, halibut, raw	3 oz.	94	2	18	0	0
Fish, herring, Atlantic, raw	3 oz.	134	8	15	0	0
Fish, herring, pacific, raw	3 oz.	166	12	14	0	0
Fish, mackerel, Atlantic, raw	3 oz.	174	12	16	0	0
Fish, mackerel, king, raw	3 oz.	89	2	17	0	0
Fish, mackerel, pacific, raw	3 oz.	134	7	17	0	0
Fish, mackerel, Spanish, raw	3 oz.	118	5	16	0	0
Fish, milkfish, raw	3 oz.	126	6	18	0	0
Fish, monkfish, raw	3 oz.	65	1	12	0	0
Fish, ocean perch, Atlantic, raw	3 oz.	80	1	16	0	0
Fish, perch, mixed species, raw	3 oz.	77	1	17	0	0
Fish, pike, northern, raw	3 oz.	75	1	16	0	0
Fish, pollock, Atlantic, raw	3 oz.	78	1	17	0	0
Fish, pout, ocean, raw	3 oz.	67	1	14	0	0
Fish, rainbow smelt, raw	3 oz.	82	2	15	0	0
Fish, rockfish, pacific, raw	3 oz.	80	1	16	0	0
Fish, roe, mixed species, raw	1 tbsp	20	10	3	0	0
Fish, sablefish, raw	3 oz.	166	13	11	0	0
Fish, salmon, Atlantic, farmed, raw	3 oz.	156	9	17	0	0
Fish, salmon, Atlantic, wild, raw	3 oz.	121	5	17	0	0
Fish, salmon, chinook, raw	3 oz.	152	9	17	0	0
Fish, salmon, pink, raw	3 oz.	99	3	17	0	0

Nutrition values for fat, protein (Prtn), carbohydrates (Cbs), and fiber (Fbr) are listed in grams per serving. Serving sizes and values are approximate.

FOOD ITEM	SERVING SIZE	CAL	FAT	PRTN	CBS	FBR
F (CONT.)						
Fish, sea bass, mixed species, raw	3 oz.	82	2	16	0	0
Fish, seatrout, mixed species, raw	3 oz.	88	3	14	0	0
Fish, shad, raw	3 oz.	167	12	14	0	0
Fish, skipjack tuna, raw	3 oz.	88	1	19	0	0
Fish, snapper, mixed species, raw	3 oz.	85	1	17	0	0
Fish, striped bass, raw	3 oz.	82	2	15	0	0
Fish, striped mullet	3 oz.	99	3	16	0	0
Fish, sturgeon, mixed species, raw	3 oz.	89	3	14	0	0
Fish, swordfish, raw	3 oz.	103	3	17	0	0
Fish, trout, mixed species, raw	3 oz.	126	6	18	0	0
Fish, white sucker, raw	3 oz.	78	2	14	0	0
Fish, whitefish, raw	3 oz.	114	5	16	0	0
Fish, wolffish, Atlantic, raw	3 oz.	82	2	15	0	0
Fish, yellowfin tuna, raw	3 oz.	93	1	20	0	0
Fish, yellowtail, mixed species, raw	3 oz.	124	5	20	0	0
Flan, caramel custard	5 1/2 oz.	303	12	4	43	0
Flaxseed	1 tbsp	59	4	2	4	3
Flaxseed oil	1 tbsp	120	14	0	0	0
Frankfurter	1 serving	151	13	5	2	0
Frankfurter, beef	1 frankfurter	188	17	6	2	0
Frankfurter, beef & pork	1 frankfurter	174	16	7	1	1
Frankfurter, chicken	1 frankfurter	116	9	6	3	0
Frankfurter, meat	1 frankfurter	151	13	5	2	0
Frankfurter, meatless	1 frankfurter	163	10	14	5	3
Frankfurter, pork	1 frankfurter	204	18	10	0	0
Frankfurter, turkey	1 frankfurter	102	8	6	1	0
French fries, frozen, unprepared	18 fries	170	7	3	28	3
French toast, frozen, ready-to-heat	1 piece	126	4	4	19	1
Frosting, creamy chocolate	2 tbsp	164	7	1	26	0
Frosting, creamy vanilla	2 tbsp	160	6	0	26	0
Frozen yogurt, choco, soft-serve	1/2 cup	115	4	3	18	2
Frozen yogurt, vanilla, soft-serve	1/2 cup	117	4	3	17	0
Fruit cocktail, canned	1 cup	229	0	1	60	3
Fruit punch, from concentrate	8 fl.oz.	124	1	0	30	0
Fruit salad, canned in syrup	1 cup	186	0	1	49	3
Fruit salad, canned in water	1 cup	74	0	1	19	3
G						
Garden cress, raw	1 cup	16	0	1	3	1
Garlic	1 clove	4	0	0	1	0
Garlic powder	1 tsp	9	0	1	2	0
Gelatin dessert mix,	1/2 cup	84	0	2	19	0
Gin, 80 Proof	1 fl.oz.	73	0	0	0	0
Ginger root	1 tsp	2	0	0	0	0
Ginger, ground	1 tsp	6	0	0	1	0
Ginkgo nuts	1 oz.	52	1	1	11	0
Ginkgo nuts, dried	1 oz.	99	1	3	21	0
Goose liver, raw	1 liver	125	4	15	6	0
Goose, meat & skin, roasted	cup chopped	427	31	35	0	0
Goose, meat only, roasted	cup chopped	340	18	41	0	0

Nutrition values for fat, protein (Prtn), carbohydrates (Cbs), and fiber (Fbr) are listed in grams per serving. Serving sizes and values are approximate.

FOOD ITEM	SERVING SIZE	CAL	FAT	PRTN	CBS	FBR
G (CONT.)						
Gourd, white-flowered	1 gourd	108	0	5	26	0
Granola bars, hard, plain	1 bar	134	6	3	18	2
Granola bars, soft, plain	1 bar	126	5	2	19	1
Grape juice	8 fl.oz.	160	0	0	40	0
Grapefruit	1/2 fruit	50	0	1	12	3
Grapefruit juice, sweetened	8 fl.oz.	125	0	0	33	0
Grapefruit juice, unsweetened	8 fl.oz.	91	0	1	22	0
Grapes, canned, heavy syrup	1 cup	187	0	1	50	2
Grapes, red or green	1 cup	106	0	1	28	1
Gravy, mushroom, canned	1 can	149	8	4	16	1
Gravy, au jus, canned	1 can	48	1	4	8	0
Gravy, beef, canned	1 can	154	7	11	14	1
Gravy, chicken, canned	1 can	235	17	6	16	1
Gravy, turkey, canned	1 can	152	6	8	15	1
Guacamole dip	2 tbsp	50	4	12	4	0
Guavas	1 fruit	37	1	1	8	3
H						
Ham, chopped	1 slice	50	3	5	1	0
Ham, minced	1 slice	55	4	3	0	0
Ham, sliced	1 slice	46	2	5	1	0
Hazlenuts, dry roasted	1 oz.	183	18	4	5	3
Hazelnuts, blanched	1 oz.	178	17	4	5	3
Hominy, canned, white	1 cup	119	2	2	24	4
Hominy, canned, yellow	1 cup	115	1	2	23	4
Honey	1 tbsp	64	0	0	17	0
Honeydew melons	1 cup, diced	61	0	1	16	1
Horseradish	1 tsp	2	0	0	1	0
Hot chocolate	8 fl.oz.	200	10	9	25	3
Hummus	1 tbsp	23	1	1	2	1
Hush puppies	1 hush puppy	74	3	2	10	1
I						
Ice cream cone, rolled or sugar type	1 cone	40	0	1	8	0
Ice cream cone, wafer or cake type	1 cone	17	0	0	3	0
Ice cream, chocolate	1/2 cup	143	7	3	19	1
Ice cream, strawberry	1/2 cup	127	6	2	18	1
Ice cream, vanilla	1/2 cup	144	8	3	17	1
Iced tea, presweetened	8 fl.oz.	100	0	0	25	0
Iced tea, unsweetened	8 fl.oz.	2	0	0	0	0
Italian seasoning	1 tsp	4	0	0	1	0
J						
Jams and preserves	1 tbsp	56	0	0	14	0
Japanese chestnuts	1 oz.	44	0	1	10	0
Japanese soba noodles, cooked	1 cup	113	0	6	24	2
Japanese ramen noodles, pkg, dry	1 serving	195	7	4	28	1
Jellies	1 tbsp	55	0	0	14	0

Nutrition values for fat, protein (Prtn), carbohydrates (Cbs), and fiber (Fbr) are listed in grams per serving. Serving sizes and values are approximate.

FOOD ITEM	SERVING SIZE	CAL	FAT	PRTN	CBS	FBR
K						
Kale	1 cup, chopped	34	1	2	7	1
Kiwifruit	1 medium	45	0	2	11	5
Kumquats	1 fruit	13	0	0	3	1
L						
Lamb, cubed, raw	1 oz.	38	2	6	0	0
Lamb, foreshank, raw	1 oz.	57	4	5	0	0
Lamb, ground, raw	1 oz.	80	7	5	0	0
Lamb, leg, shank half, raw	1 oz.	52	3	5	0	0
Lamb, leg, sirloin half, raw	1 oz.	74	6	5	0	0
Lamb, leg, whole, choice, raw	1 oz.	65	5	5	0	0
Lamb, loin, choice, raw	1 oz.	79	6	5	0	0
Lamb, rib, choice, raw	1 oz.	97	9	4	0	0
Lamb, shoulder, arm, raw	1 oz.	69	5	5	0	0
Lamb, shoulder, blade, raw	1 oz.	69	5	5	0	0
Lamb, shoulder, whole, raw	1 oz.	69	5	5	0	0
Lard	1 tbsp	115	13	0	0	0
Leeks	1 leek	54	0	1	13	2
Lemon juice	1 cup	61	0	1	21	1
Lemon juice, canned or bottled	1 tbsp	3	0	0	1	0
Lemon pepper seasoning	1 tsp	7	0	0	1	0
Lemonade powder	1 scoop	102	0	0	27	0
Lemonade, pink conc, prepared	8 fl.oz.	99	0	0	26	0
Lemonade, white conc, prepared	8 fl.oz.	131	0	0	34	0
Lemons w/ peel	1 fruit	22	0	1	12	5
Lentils, cooked	1 cup	230	1	18	40	16
Lentils, sprouted, raw	1 cup	82	0	7	17	0
Lettuce, green leaf	1 cup, shredded	5	0	1	1	1
Lettuce, iceberg	1 cup, shredded	10	0	1	2	1
Lettuce, red leaf	1 cup, shredded	3	0	0	0	0
Lettuce, romaine	1 cup, shredded	8	0	1	2	1
Lime juice	1 cup	62	0	1	21	1
Limes	1 fruit	20	0	1	7	2
Liverwurst, pork	1 slice	59	5	3	0	0
Lobster, northern, raw	1 lobster	135	1	28	1	0
Luncheon meat, beef, loaved	1 oz.	87	7	4	1	0
Luncheon meat, beef, thin sliced	1 oz.	50	1	8	2	0
Luncheon meat, meatless slices	1 slice	26	2	3	1	0
Luncheon meat, pork & chicken, minced	1 oz.	56	4	4	0	
Luncheon meat, pork & ham, minced	1 oz.	88	75	4	1	
Luncheon meat, pork or beef	1 oz.	99	9	4	1	0
Luncheon meat, pork, canned	1 oz.	95	9	4	1	0
Luncheon meat, pork, ham & chicken, minced	1 oz.	87	8	4	1	
Luncheon sausage, pork & beef	1 oz.	74	6	4	0	0
M						
Macadamia nuts	1 oz. (10-12 nuts)	203	22	2	4	2
Macaroni and cheese	1 cup	259	3	11	48	2
Macaroni, cooked	1 cup	197	1	7	40	2
Malt drink mix, dry	3 heaping tsp	87	2	2	16	0

Nutritional Facts . . . .

Nutrition values for fat, protein (Prtn), carbohydrates (Cbs), and fiber (Fbr) are listed in grams per serving. Serving sizes and values are approximate.

FOOD ITEM	SERVING SIZE	CAL	FAT	PRTN	CBS	FBR
M (CONT.)						
Malt beverage	8 fl.oz.	144	0	1	32	0
Mangos	1 fruit	135	1	1	35	4
Maraschino cherries	1 cherry	8	0	0	2	0
Margarine, fat free spread	1 tbsp	6	0	0	1	0
Margarine, stick	1 tbsp	100	11	0	0	0
Margarine, stick, unsalted	1 tbsp	102	11	0	0	0
Margarine, tub	1 tbsp	102	11	0	0	0
Martini	1 fl.oz.	69	0	0	1	0
Mayonnaise	1 tbsp	100	11	0	0	0
Milk, 1% low fat	1 cup	102	2	8	12	0
Milk, 2% low fat	1 cup	138	5	10	14	0
Milk, buttermilk, reduced fat	1 cup	137	5	10	13	0
Milk, chocolate	1 cup	208	9	8	26	2
Milk, dry, nonfat, instant	1/3 cup dry	82	0	8	12	0
Milk, evaporated	1/2 cup	169	10	9	13	0
Milk, skim or nonfat	1 cup	83	0	8	12	0
Milk, sweetened condensed	1 cup	982	27	24	167	0
Milk, whole	1 cup	146	8	8	11	0
Milkshake, dry mix, vanilla	1 packet	69	1	5	11	0
Millet	1 cup	756	8	22	146	17
Miso soup	1 cup	547	17	32	73	15
Mixed nuts	1 cup	814	71	24	35	12
Molasses	1 tablespoon	58	0	0	15	0
Muffins, apple bran	1 muffin	300	3	1	61	1
Muffins, banana nut	1 muffin	480	24	3	60	2
Muffins, blueberry	1 muffin	313	7	6	54	3
Muffins, chocolate chip	1 muffin	510	24	2	69	4
Muffins, corn	1 muffin	345	10	7	58	4
Muffins, oat bran	1 muffin	305	8	8	55	5
Muffins, plain	1 muffin	242	9	4	36	2
Mushrooms	1 cup, pieces	15	0	2	2	1
Mushrooms, enoki	1 large	2	0	0	0	0
Mushrooms, oyster	1 large	55	1	6	9	4
Mushrooms, portabello	1 large	0	0	0	0	0
Mushrooms, shiitake	1 mushroom	11	0	0	3	0
Mussels, blue, raw	1 cup	129	3	18	6	0
Mustard greens	1 cup, chopped	15	0	2	3	2
Mustard seed, yellow	1 tbsp	53	3	3	4	2
Mustard spinach	1 cup, chopped	33	1	3	6	4
Mustard, prepared, yellow	1 tsp	3	0	0	0	0
N						
Natto (fermented soybeans)	1 cup	371	19	31	25	10
Nectarines	1 fruit	60	0	1	14	2
New Zealand spinach	1 cup, chopped	8	0	1	1	0
Nutmeg, ground	1 tsp	12	1	0	1	1
O						
Oat bran	1 cup	231	7	16	62	15
Oatmeal, instant, prepared w/ water	1 cup	129	2	5	22	4
Oil, canola	1 tbsp	124	14	0	0	0

Nutrition values for fat, protein (Prtn), carbohydrates (Cbs), and fiber (Fbr) are listed in grams per serving. Serving sizes and values are approximate.

FOOD ITEM	SERVING SIZE	CAL	FAT	PRTN	CBS	FBR
O (CONT.)						
Oil, canola & soybean	1 tbsp	119	14	0	0	0
Oil, coconut	1 tbsp	120	14	0	0	0
Oil, corn, peanut & olive	1 tbsp	120	14	0	0	0
Oil, olive	1 tbsp	119	14	0	0	0
Oil, peanut	1 tbsp	119	14	0	0	0
Oil, sesame	1 tbsp	120	14	0	0	0
Oil, soy	1 tbsp	120	14	0	0	0
Oil, vegetable, almond	1 tbsp	120	14	0	0	0
Oil, vegetable, cocoa butter	1 tbsp	120	14	0	0	0
Oil, vegetable, coconut	1 tbsp	117	14	0	0	0
Oil, vegetable, grapeseed	1 tbsp	120	14	0	0	0
Oil, vegetable, hazelnut	1 tbsp	120	14	0	0	0
Oil, vegetable, nutmeg butter	1 tbsp	120	14	0	0	0
Oil, vegetable, palm	1 tbsp	120	14	0	0	0
Oil, vegetable, poppyseed	1 tbsp	120	14	0	0	0
Oil, vegetable, rice bran	1 tbsp	120	14	0	0	0
Oil, vegetable, sheanut	1 tbsp	120	14	0	0	0
Oil, vegetable, tomatoseed	1 tbsp	120	14	0	0	0
Oil, vegetable, walnut	1 tbsp	120	218	0	0	0
Okra	1 cup	31	0	2	7	3
Onion powder	1 tsp	8	0	0	2	0
Onions	1 cup, chopped	67	0	2	16	2
Onions, sweet	1 onion	106	0	3	25	3
Orange juice	8 fl.oz.	109	1	2	25	1
Orange marmalade	1 tbsp	49	0	0	13	0
Oranges	1 large	86	0	2	22	4
Oregano, dried	1 tsp, ground	6	0	0	1	1
Oyster, eastern, raw	3 oz.	50	1	4	5	0
Oyster, pacific, raw	3 oz.	69	2	8	4	0
P						
Pancakes, blueberry	1 pancake	84	4	2	11	0
Pancakes, buttermilk	1 pancake	86	4	3	11	0
Pancakes, plain, dry mix	1 pancake	74	1	2	14	1
Papayas	1 cup, cubed	55	0	1	14	3
Paprika	1 tsp	6	0	0	1	1
Parsley	1 cup	22	1	2	4	2
Parsley, dried	1 tsp	1	0	0	0	0
Parsnips	1 cup, sliced	100	0	2	24	7
Passion fruit	1 fruit	17	0	0	4	2
Pasta, corn, cooked	1 cup	176	1	4	39	7
Pasta, plain, cooked	1 cup	197	1	7	40	2
Pasta, spinach, cooked	1 cup	195	1	8	38	2
Pastrami, turkey	1 oz.	40	2	5	1	0
Pate de foie gras	1 tbsp	60	6	2	1	0
Pate, chicken liver, canned	1 tbsp	26	2	2	1	0
Pate, goose liver, canned	1 tbsp	60	6	2	1	0
Peaches	1 large	61	0	1	15	2
Peaches, canned	1 cup, halved	59	0	1	15	3
Peanut butter, chunky	2 tbsp	188	16	8	7	3

Nutrition values for fat, protein (Prtn), carbohydrates (Cbs), and fiber (Fbr) are listed in grams per serving. Serving sizes and values are approximate.

FOOD ITEM	SERVING SIZE	CAL	FAT	PRTN	CBS	FBR
P (CONT.)						
Peanut butter, smooth	2 tbsp	188	16	8	6	2
Peanuts, dry roasted w/ salt	1 oz.	166	14	7	6	2
Peanuts, raw	1 oz.	161	14	7	5	2
Pears	1 pear	121	0	1	32	7
Pears, Asian	1 pear	116	1	1	29	10
Pears, canned	1 cup	71	0	1	19	4
Peas, green, fresh, cooked	1 cup	134	0	9	25	9
Peas, green, frozen, cooked	1 cup	125	0	8	23	9
Peas, split, cooked	1 cup	231	1	16	41	16
Pecans	1 oz. (20 halves)	196	20	3	40	3
Pepper, black	1 tsp	5	0	0	1	1
Pepper, red or cayenne	1 tsp	6	0	0	1	1
Pepperoni	15 slices	135	12	6	1	0
Peppers, chili, green	1 cup	29	0	1	6	2
Peppers, chili, red	1 pepper	18	0	1	4	1
Peppers, chili, sun-dried	1 pepper	2	0	0	0	0
Peppers, jalapeno	1 pepper	4	0	0	1	0
Peppers, sweet, green	1 medium	24	0	1	6	2
Peppers, sweet, red	1 medium	31	0	1	7	2
Peppers, sweet, yellow	1 medium	32	0	1	8	1
Persimmons	1 fruit	32	0	0	8	0
Pheasant, boneless, raw	1/2 pheasant	724	37	91	0	0
Pheasant, breast, sknls, bnls, raw	1/2 breast	242	6	44	0	0
Pheasant, leg, sknls, boneless, raw	1 leg	143	5	24	0	0
Pheasant, skinless, raw	/2 pheasant	468	13	83	0	0
Pickle relish, sweet	1 tbsp	20	0	0	5	0
Pickle, sour	1 large 4"	15	0	0	3	2
Pickle, sweet	1 large 4"	158	0	1	43	2
Pickles, dill	1 large 4"	24	0	1	6	2
Pie crust, graham cracker, baked	1 pie crust	1037	52	9	137	3
Pie, apple	1 piece	411	19	4	58	0
Pie, blueberry	1 piece	290	13	2	44	1
Pie, cherry	1 piece	325	14	3	50	1
Pie, lemon meringue	1 piece	303	10	2	53	1
Pie, pecan	1 piece	452	21	5	65	4
Pie, pumpkin	1 piece	229	10	4	30	3
Pine nuts	1 oz.	191	19	4	4	1
Pineapple	1 fruit	227	1	3	60	7
Pineapple, canned	1 slice	15	0	0	4	0
Pita bread, whole wheat	1 pita	170	2	6	35	5
Pistachio nuts	1 oz. (49 kernels)	161	13	6	8	3
Pizza, cheese	1 slice (3.7 oz.)	250	10	11	29	2
Pizza, pepperoni	1 slice (3.7 oz.)	288	15	12	26	2
Plantains	1 medium	218	1	2	57	4
Plums	1 fruit	30	0	1	8	1
Plums, canned	1 plum	19	0	0	5	0
Polenta	1/2 cup	220	2	2	24	1
Pomegranates	1 fruit	105	1	2	26	1
Popcorn cakes	1 cake	38	0	1	8	0
Popcorn, air-popped	1 cup	31	0	1	6	1

Nutrition values for fat, protein (Prtn), carbohydrates (Cbs), and fiber (Fbr) are listed in grams per serving. Serving sizes and values are approximate.

FOOD ITEM	SERVING SIZE	CAL	FAT	PRTN	CBS	FBR
P (CONT.)						
Popcorn, caramel-coated	1 oz.	122	4	1	22	2
Popcorn, cheese	1 cup	58	4	1	6	1
Popcorn, oil-popped	1 cup	55	3	1	6	1
Popovers, dry mix	1 oz.	105	1	3	20	1
Poppy seed	1 tsp	15	1	1	1	0
Pork, cured, strips, cooked	3 slices	156	12	10	0	0
Pork, cured, extra lean, canned	3 oz.	116	4	18	0	0
Pork, cured, ham, patties	1 patty	205	18	8	1	0
Pork, cured, extra lean, cooked	3 oz.	140	7	19	0	0
Pork, cured, salt pork, raw	1 oz.	212	23	1	0	0
Pork, fresh ground, cooked	3 oz.	252	18	22	0	0
Pork, leg, rump half, cooked	3 oz.	214	12	25	0	0
Pork, leg, shank half, cooked	3 oz.	246	17	22	0	0
Pork, leg, whole, cooked	3 oz.	232	15	23	0	0
Pork, loin, blade, cooked	3 oz.	275	21	20	0	0
Pork, loin, center loin, cooked	3 oz.	199	11	22	0	0
Pork, loin, center rib, cooked	3 oz.	214	13	23	0	0
Pork, loin, sirloin, cooked	3 oz.	176	8	24	0	0
Pork, loin, tenderloin, cooked	3 oz.	147	5	24	0	0
Pork, loin, top loin, cooked	3 oz.	192	10	24	0	0
Pork, loin, whole, cooked	3 oz.	211	12	23	0	0
Pork, shoulder, arm, cooked	3 oz.	238	18	17	0	0
Pork, shoulder, blade, cooked	3 oz.	229	16	20	0	0
Pork, shoulder, whole, cooked	3 oz.	248	18	20	0	0
Pork, spareribs, cooked	3 oz.	337	26	25	0	0
Potato chips, barbecue	1 oz.	139	9	2	15	1
Potato chips, cheese	1 oz.	141	8	2	16	2
Potato chips, salted	1 oz.	152	10	2	15	1
Potato chips, sour cream & onion	1 oz.	151	10	2	15	2
Potato chips, reduced fat	1 oz.	134	6	2	19	2
Potato chips, unsalted	1 oz.	152	10	2	15	1
Potato flour	1 cup	571	1	11	133	9
Potato salad	1 cup	358	21	7	28	3
Potatoes	1 medium	164	0	4	37	5
Potatoes, baked, w/ skin	1 medium	160	0	4	37	4
Potatoes, baked, w/o skin	1 medium	143	0	3	33	3
Potatoes, mashed	1 cup	237	9	4	35	3
Potatoes, red	1 medium	153	0	4	34	4
Potatoes, russet	1 medium	168	0	5	39	3
Potatoes, scalloped	1 cup	211	9	7	26	5
Potatoes, white	1 medium	149	0	4	34	5
Pretzels, hard, plain, salted	1 oz.	108	1	3	22	1
Prune juice	8 fl.oz.	180	0	2	43	3
Pudding, banana	1/2 cup	154	3	4	29	0
Pudding, chocolate	1/2 cup	154	3	5	28	0
Pudding, coconut cream	1/2 cup	157	3	4	28	0
Pudding, lemon	1/2 cup	157	3	4	30	0
Pudding, rice	1/2 cup	163	2	5	31	0
Pudding, tapioca	1/2 cup	154	2	4	29	0
Pudding, vanilla	1/2 cup	148	3	4	27	0

Nutrition values for fat, protein (Prtn), carbohydrates (Cbs), and fiber (Fbr) are listed in grams per serving. Serving sizes and values are approximate.

FOOD ITEM	SERVING SIZE	CAL	FAT	PRTN	CBS	FBR
P (CONT.)						
Pumpkin	1 cup	30	0	1	8	1
Pumpkin pie mix	1 cup	281	0	3	71	22
Pumpkin, canned	1 cup	83	1	3	20	7
R						
Rabbit, cooked	3 oz.	167	7	25	0	0
Radicchio	1 cup, shredded	9	0	1	2	0
Radishes	1 cup, sliced	19	0	1	4	2
Raisins	1 1/2 oz.	129	0	1	34	2
Raisins, golden	1 1/2 oz.	130	0	1	34	2
Raspberries	1 cup	64	1	2	15	8
Rhubarb	1 cup, diced	26	0	1	6	2
Rice cakes, brown rice, corn	1 cake	35	0	1	7	0
Rice cakes, brown rice, multigrain	1 cake	35	0	1	7	0
Rice cakes, brown rice, plain	1 cake	35	0	1	7	0
Rice, brown, cooked	1 cup	218	2	5	46	4
Rice, white, cooked	1 cup	242	0	4	53	1
Rice, wild	1 cup	166	1	7	35	3
Rolls, dinner	1 roll	136	3	4	23	1
Rolls, dinner, wheat	1 roll	117	3	4	20	2
Rolls, dinner, whole-wheat	1 roll	114	2	4	22	3
Rolls, french	1 roll	119	2	4	22	0
Rolls, hamburger or hotdog	1 roll	120	2	4	21	1
Rolls, hard (incl. kaiser)	1 roll	126	2	4	23	1
Rolls, pumpernickel	1 roll	119	1	5	23	2
Rosemary	1 tsp	1	0	0	0	0
Rosemary, dried	1 tsp	4	0	0	1	1
Rum, 80 proof	1 fl.oz.	64	0	0	0	0
Rutabagas	1 cup, cubed	50	0	2	11	4
Rye	1 cup	566	4	25	118	25
Rye flour, dark	1 cup	415	3	18	88	29
Rye flour, light	1 cup	374	1	9	82	15
Rye flour, medium	1 cup	361	2	10	79	15
S						
Sage, ground	1 tsp	2	0	0	0	0
Sake	1 fl.oz.	39	0	0	2	0
Salad dressing, 1000 island	1 tbsp	58	6	0	2	0
Salad dressing, bacon & tomato	1 tbsp	49	5	0	0	0
Salad dressing, blue cheese	1 tbsp	77	8	1	1	0
Salad dressing, caesar	1 tbsp	78	9	0	1	0
Salad dressing, coleslaw	1 tbsp	61	5	0	4	0
Salad dressing, french	1 tbsp	71	7	0	2	0
Salad dressing, honey dijon	1 tbsp	58	5	1	3	1
Salad dressing, Italian	1 tbsp	43	4	0	2	0
Salad dressing, mayo-based	1 tbsp	57	5	0	4	0
Salad dressing, mayonnaise	1 tbsp	103	12	0	0	0
Salad dressing, peppercorn	1 tbsp	76	8	0	1	0
Salad dressing, ranch	1 tbsp	73	8	0	1	0
Salad dressing, Russian	1 tbsp	53	4	0	5	0

Nutrition values for fat, protein (Prtn), carbohydrates (Cbs), and fiber (Fbr) are listed in grams per serving. Serving sizes and values are approximate.

FOOD ITEM	SERVING SIZE	CAL	FAT	PRTN	CBS	FBR
S (CONT.)						
Salad, chicken	6 oz.	420	33	45	11	2
Salad, egg	6 oz.	300	23	20	14	1
Salad, prima pasta	6 oz.	360	30	5	18	3
Salad, seafood w/ crab & shrimp	6 oz.	420	34	0	20	0
Salad, tuna	6 oz.	450	36	16	14	0
Salami, cooked, turkey	1 oz.	38	2	1	0	0
Salami, dry, pork or beef	3 slices	104	8	6	1	0
Salami, Italian pork	1 oz.	119	10	6	0	0
Salsa, w/ oil	2 tbsp	40	3	0	8	0
Salsa, w/o oil	2 tbsp	15	0	0	4	0
Salt	1 tbsp	0	0	0	0	0
Sauce, alfredo	1/4 cup	120	11	15	3	2
Sauce, barbecue	1 cup	188	5	5	32	3
Sauce, cheese	1 cup	479	36	25	13	0
Sauce, cranberry	1 cup	418	0	1	108	3
Sauce, hollandaise	1 cup	62	2	2	10	0
Sauce, honey mustard	1 tbsp	30	1	0	5	0
Sauce, marinara	1 cup	185	6	5	28	1
Sauce, salsa	1 cup	70	0	4	16	4
Sauce, soy	1 tbsp	10	0	0	0	0
Sauce, steak	1 tbsp	25	0	0	6	0
Sauce, teriyaki	1 tbsp	15	0	17	2	0
Sauce, tomato chili	1 cup	284	1	7	54	16
Sauce, worcestershire	1 cup	184	0	0	54	0
Sauerkraut	1/2 cup	25	0	1	5	4
Sausage, Italian pork, raw	1 link	391	35	16	1	0
Sausage, pork	1 link	85	7	4	0	0
Sausage, smoked linked, pork	1 link	265	22	15	1	0
Sausage, turkey	1 link	65	5	4	0	0
Savory, ground	1 tsp	4	0	0	1	1
Scallops	1 scallop	26	0	5	1	0
Seaweed, dried	1 oz.	50	0	0	13	0
Sesame seeds, dried	1 tbsp	52	5	2	2	1
Shallots	1 tbsp, chopped	7	0	0	2	0
Shortening	1 tbsp	113	13	0	0	0
Shrimp, mixed species, raw	1 medium piece	6	0	1	0	0
Snacks, cheese puffs or twists	1 oz.	157	10	2	15	0
Soda, club	12 fl.oz.	0	0	0	0	0
Soda, cream	12 fl.oz.	252	0	0	66	0
Soda, diet cola	12 fl.oz.	0	0	0	0	0
Soda, ginger ale	12 fl.oz.	166	0	0	43	0
Soda, lemon-lime	12 fl.oz.	196	0	0	51	0
Soda, regular, w/ caffeine	12 fl.oz.	155	0	0	40	0
Soda, regular, w/o caffeine	12 fl.oz.	207	0	0	53	0
Soda, root beer	12 fl.oz.	202	0	0	52	0
Soda, tonic water	12 fl.oz.	166	0	0	43	0
Soup, beef broth	1 cup	29	0	5	2	0
Soup, beef stroganoff	1 cup	235	11	12	22	1
Soup, beef vegetable	1 cup	82	2	3	13	1
Soup, chicken broth	1 cup	39	1	5	1	0

Nutrition values for fat, protein (Prtn), carbohydrates (Cbs), and fiber (Fbr) are listed in grams per serving. Serving sizes and values are approximate.

FOOD ITEM	SERVING SIZE	CAL	FAT	PRTN	CBS	FBR
S (CONT.)						
Soup, chicken noodle	1 cup	75	2	4	9	1
Soup, chicken vegetable	1 cup	75	3	4	9	1
Soup, chicken w/ dumplings	1 cup	96	6	6	6	1
Soup, clam chowder	1 cup	95	3	5	12	2
Soup, cream of chicken	1 cup	117	7	3	9	0
Soup, cream of mushroom	1 cup	129	9	2	9	1
Soup, cream of potato	1 cup	149	6	6	17	1
Soup, minestrone	1 cup	82	3	4	11	1
Soup, split-pea w/ham	1 cup	190	4	10	28	2
Soup, tomato	1 cup	161	6	6	22	3
Soup, vegetarian	1 cup	72	2	2	12	1
Sour cream	1 tbsp	26	2.5	0	1	0
Sour cream, fat free	1 tbsp	9	0	0	2	0
Sour cream, reduced fat	1 tbsp	22	2	1	1	0
Soy milk	1 cup	127	5	11	12	3
Soy protein isolate	1 oz.	96	1	23	2	2
Soybeans, green, cooked	1 cup	254	12	22	12	7
Soybeans, nuts, roasted	1/4 cup	194	9	17	14	3
Soyburger	1 patty	125	4	13	9	3
Spaghetti, cooked	1 cup	197	1	7	40	2
Spaghetti, spinach, cooked	1 cup	182	1	6	37	2
Spaghetti, whole-wheat, cooked	1 cup	174	1	7	37	6
Spinach	1 cup	7	0	1	1	1
Squab, boneless, raw	1 squab	585	47	37	0	0
Squab, skinless, raw	1 squab	239	13	29	0	0
Squash, summer	1 cup, sliced	18	0	1	4	1
Squash, winter	1 cup, cubed	39	0	1	10	2
Squid, mixed species, raw	1 oz.	26	0	4	1	0
Stock, beef	1 cup	31	0	5	3	0
Stock, chicken	1 cup	86	3	6	9	0
Stock, fish	1 cup	40	2	5	0	0
Strawberries	1 cup	49	1	1	12	3
Succotash	1 piece	145	1	7	31	7
Sugar, brown	1 tsp	12	0	0	3	0
Sugar, granulated	1 tsp	16	0	0	4	0
Sugar, maple	1 tsp	11	0	0	3	0
Sugar, powdered	1 tsp	10	0	0	3	0
Sunflower seeds	1 tbsp	45	10	4	2	5
Sweet potato	1 cup, cubed	114	0	2	27	4
Syrup, chocolate	1 tbsp	67	2	1	12	1
Syrup, dark corn	1 tbsp	57	0	0	16	0
Syrup, grenadine	1 tbsp	53	0	0	13	0
Syrup, light corn	1 tbsp	59	0	0	16	0
Syrup, maple	1 tbsp	52	0	0	13	0
Syrup, pancake	1 tbsp	47	0	0	12	0
T						
Taco shell, hard	1 shell	55	3	2	6	0
Tangerines	1 large	52	0	1	13	2
Tarragon, dried	1 tsp	2	0	0	0	0

Nutrition values for fat, protein (Prtn), carbohydrates (Cbs), and fiber (Fbr) are listed in grams per serving. Serving sizes and values are approximate.

FOOD ITEM	SERVING SIZE	CAL	FAT	PRTN	CBS	FBR
T (CONT.)						
Tea, instant	1 cup	2	0	0	0	0
Thyme	1 tsp	1	0	0	0	0
Thyme, dried	1 tsp	3	0	0	1	0
Tofu, firm	1/2 cup	183	11	20	5	3
Tofu, fried	1 piece	35	3	2	1	1
Tofu, soft	1/2 cup	76	5	8	2	0
Tomato juice, canned, with salt	6 fl.oz.	31	0	1	8	1
Tomato juice, canned, without salt	6 fl.oz.	30	0	1	8	1
Tomato paste, canned	1/2 cup	107	1	6	25	6
Tomato sauce, canned	1 cup	78	1	3	18	4
Tomatoes, canned, crushed	1 cup	82	1	4	19	5
Tomatoes, green	1 cup, chopped	41	0	2	9	2
Tomatoes, orange	1 cup, chopped	25	0	2	5	1
Tomatoes, red	1 cup, chopped	32	0	2	7	2
Tomatoes, sun-dried	1 cup, chopped	139	2	8	30	7
Toppings, butterscotch or caramel	2 tbsp	103	0	1	27	0
Toppings, marshmallow cream	2 tbsp	132	0	0	32	0
Toppings, nuts in syrup	2 tbsp	184	9	2	24	1
Toppings, pineapple	2 tbsp	106	0	0	28	0
Toppings, strawberry	2 tbsp	107	0	0	28	0
Tortilla chips, plain	1 oz.	142	7	2	18	2
Tortilla, corn	1 tortilla	45	1	2	9	3
Tortilla, flour	1 tortilla	160	3	18	28	3
Trail mix	1/4 cup	173	11	5	17	3
Turkey, deli sliced, white meat	1 oz.	30	1	5	1	0
Turkey, back, sknls, boneless, raw	1/2 back	180	5	31	0	0
Turkey, breast, boneless, raw	1/2 breast	541	12	103	0	0
Turkey, breast, sknls, boneless, raw	1/2 breast	433	3	96	0	0
Turkey, dark meat, boneless, raw	1/2 turkey	686	26	107	0	0
Turkey, dark meat, sknls, bnls, raw	1/2 turkey	532	13	98	0	0
Turkey, leg, boneless, raw	1 leg	412	13	70	0	0
Turkey, leg, skinless, boneless, raw	1 leg	355	8	67	0	0
Turkey, wing, boneless, raw	1 wing	204	10	27	0	0
Turkey, wing, sknls, boneless, raw	1 wing	95	1	20	0	0
Turkey, young hen, back, bnls, raw	1/2 back	650	48	52	0	0
Turkey, young hen, breast, bnls, raw	1/2 breast	1460	73	189	0	0
Turkey, young hen, dark, bnls, raw	1/2 turkey	1056	40	163	0	0
Turkey, young hen, leg, bnls, raw	1 leg	991	49	128	0	0
Turkey, young hen, wing, bnls, raw	1 wing	470	31	45	0	0
Turkey, young tom, back, bnls, raw	1/2 back	938	58	97	0	0
Turkey, young tom, breast, bnls, raw	1/2 breast	2701	113	393	0	0
Turkey, young tom, dark, bnls, raw	1/2 turkey	1884	63	307	0	0
Turkey, young tom, leg, bnls, raw	1 leg	1740	78	241	0	0
Turkey, young tom, wing, bnls, raw	1 wing	654	39	71	0	0
Turnip greens	1 cup, chopped	18	0	1	4	2
Turnips	1 cup, cubed	36	0	1	8	2
V						
Vanilla extract	1 tbsp	37	0	0	2	0
Veal, breast, raw	1 oz.	59	4	5	0	0

Nutrition values for fat, protein (Prtn), carbohydrates (Cbs), and fiber (Fbr) are listed in grams per serving. Serving sizes and values are approximate.

FOOD ITEM	SERVING SIZE	CAL	FAT	PRTN	CBS	FBR
V (CONT.)						
Veal, cubed, raw	1 oz.	31	1	6	0	0
Veal, ground, raw	1 oz.	41	2	6	0	0
Veal, leg, raw	1 oz.	33	1	6	0	0
Veal, loin, raw	1 oz.	46	3	5	0	0
Veal, rib, raw	1 oz.	46	3	5	0	0
Veal, shank, raw	1 oz.	32	1	5	0	0
Veal, shoulder, arm, raw	1 oz.	37	2	6	0	0
Veal, shoulder, blade, raw	1 oz.	37	2	6	0	0
Veal, shoulder, whole, raw	1 oz.	37	2	6	0	0
Veal, sirloin, raw	1 oz.	43	2	5	0	0
Vegetable juice	8 fl.oz.	50	0	2	12	2
Vinegar	1 tbsp	2	0	0	1	0
W						
Waffles, plain	1 waffle	218	11	6	25	0
Walnuts	1 oz. (14 halves)	185	19	4	4	2
Wasabi root	1 cup, sliced	142	1	6	31	10
Water chestnuts, Chinese	1/2 cup, sliced	60	0	1	15	2
Watercress	1 cup, chopped	4	0	1	0	0
Watermelon	1 cup, diced	46	0	1	12	1
Wheat bran	1 cup	125	3	9	37	25
Wheat flour, whole grain	1 cup	407	2	16	87	15
Wheat germ	1 cup	414	11	27	60	15
Whipped cream	1 cup	154	13	2	8	0
Wine, cooking	1 tsp	2	0	0	0	0
Wine, red	3-1/2 oz. glass	74	0	0	2	0
Wine, rose	3-1/2 oz. glass	73	0	0	1	0
Wine, white	3-1/2 oz. glass	70	0	0	1	0
Y						
Yam	1 cup, cubed	177	0	2	42	6
Yeast, active, dry	1 tsp	12	0	2	2	1
Yogurt, fruit, low fat	8 oz. container	118	0	6	24	0
Yogurt, fruit, whole milk	8 oz. container	250	6	9	38	0
Yogurt, plain, lowfat	8 oz. container	110	4	8	7	0
Yogurt, plain, whole milk	8 oz. container	138	7	12	11	0
Z						
Zucchini	1 medium	45	0	2	10	1

Notes

Notes . . . .

Notes

Notes

Notes

Notes